ORTHOPEDIC
TISSUE
ENGINEERING

ORTHOPEDIC TISSUE ENGINEERING

BASIC SCIENCE AND PRACTICE

EDITED BY

VICTOR M. GOLDBERG
ARNOLD I. CAPLAN

Case Western Reserve University
Cleveland, Ohio, U.S.A.

MARCEL DEKKER, INC.

NEW YORK · BASEL

Library of Congress Cataloging-in-Publication Data
A catalog record for this book is available from the Library of Congress.

ISBN: 0-8247-4749-6

This book is printed on acid-free paper.

Headquarters
Marcel Dekker, Inc., 270 Madison Avenue, New York, NY 10016, U.S.A.
tel: 212-696-9000; fax: 212-685-4540

Distribution and Customer Service
Marcel Dekker, Inc., Cimarron Road, Monticello, New York 12701, U.S.A.
tel: 800-228-1160; fax: 845-796-1772

Eastern Hemisphere Distribution
Marcel Dekker AG, Hutgasse 4, Postfach 812, CH-4001 Basel, Switzerland
tel: 41-61-260-6300; fax: 41-61-260-6333

World Wide Web
http://www.dekker.com

The publisher offers discounts on this book when ordered in bulk quantities. For more information, write to Special Sales/Professional Marketing at the headquarters address above.

Current printing (last digit):

10 9 8 7 6 5 4 3 2 1

PRINTED IN THE UNITED STATES OF AMERICA

Preface

During the last three decades, important advances have been made in the available treatments for the loss of skeletal tissue as a result of trauma or disease. The application of large skeletal allografts and total joint replacement have become successful and reproducible treatment options. Unfortunately there still is a significant incidence of failure because of mechanical or biological complications. A new discipline known as *tissue engineering* has developed that integrates the concepts of the life sciences, such as biology, chemistry, and engineering, with surgical techniques to develop strategies for the regeneration of musculoskeletal tissue. The basic components of any tissue-engineered treatment strategy requires viable cells, biomatrices, and bioactive factors. The cells are central to the regenerative process of any musculoskeletal tissue. They must be responsive to their environment and ultimately capable of integrating into the host tissue and synthesizing appropriate extracellular matrix. The biomatrix may have several functions, including a delivery vehicle for the cells or bioactive factors, or it may function as a scaffolding to conduct the host cells and inductive molecules. Because the musculoskeletal system demands the capability of withstanding functional loads, scaffolds must be capable of temporary supportive activities when used in highly loaded environments such as bone. The matrix also may act as an organizing guiding component for the morphogenesis of the engineered tissue. The integration of the biomatrix and cells requires a definition of the optimal number density and distribution of the cell component relative to the scaffold. Bioactive factors may function as mitogens, morphogens, or growth factors. These molecules have been shown experimentally and clinically to be important inducers of the regeneration of musculoskeletal tissue.

Orthopedic Tissue Engineering: Basic Science and Practice is a timely publication that provides a basis of both the basic science and the clinical application of this emerging discipline. The book provides a strong basis for the concepts of principles of tissue engineering and regeneration of musculoskeletal tissue and the application of these principles to specific clinical problems. The publication is directed toward a wide audience of both basic scientists and clinicians involved in the experimental and clinical applications of these new treatments. Medical students and graduate students as well as established investigators and clinicians in many disciplines of surgery will use this book in their activities.

The books is divided into sections on basic science and clinical applications. The chapters in the basic science section address the issues of principles of tissue engineering and the role of each component, namely, morphogenic proteins, cells, and biomatrices. Important areas of bioreactors and clinically applicable animal models in tissue engineering are discussed for a broad background in tissue engineering/basic science.

The clinical application section addresses each type of musculoskeletal tissue, including bone, cartilage, meniscus, intervertebral disc, and ligament/tendon. The area of gene therapy to enhance both bone and cartilage repair is discussed. The integration of the two sections will provide the reader with a broad background in tissue engineering science and clinical application. Further, it will serve as a source of material for investigators in each of the areas and provide a platform for important future developments in this emerging clinical discipline. Finally, this publication has defined the state of the science and art and, most important, the future directions and issues that must be solved for the ultimate successful application of regeneration of musculoskeletal tissue.

Victor M. Goldberg
Arnold I. Caplan

Foreword

The application of tissue engineering in orthopedics has immense possibilities yet to be realized. The discipline of tissue engineering was identified and generally defined less than 15 years ago, but the recognition of its potential to impact patient treatment has resulted in a dramatic refocusing of research activities into areas of unmet or unsatisfactory clinical needs. Already there are tissue-engineered products available in the wound care field to treat burns and chronic wounds, demonstrating the validity of this approach. This has been a dramatic success story for such a new field, and has been the catalyst for a massive focus on basic and applied research, particularly in orthopedics, where the many potential applications are clear and necessary.

The field of tissue engineering, particularly when applied to orthopedics where tissues often function in a mechanically demanding environment, requires a collaboration of excellence in cell and molecular biology, biochemistry, material sciences, bioengineering, and clinical research. For success in tissue engineering it is necessary that researchers with expertise in one area have an appreciation of the knowledge and challenges of the other areas. At the same time, the influx of researchers into tissue engineering requires a rapid learning curve of the many facets of this field to bring them into a productive mode as soon as possible. Therefore there is an obvious need for a text that brings to the researcher the critical and salient points of these areas. This book provides an up-to-date knowledge base for experts and novices alike in tissue engineering, providing a guide and resource to this rapidly expanding fields.

The topics in the book comprehensively cover the basic science (cell and molecular biology) and engineering (biomatrices, bioreactors, biomechanics) aspects that are important in tissue engineering, and considers the in vitro an in vivo growth environments. It also provides insight into the physiology and developmental biology that can help guide the researcher. Of particular importance, Chapter 9 describes the animal models that are being used in translational research, where the efficacy of tissue-engineered products will be determined. Success in an animal model is generally a prerequisite for moving into clinical trials, yet the models used often are not well understood and unfortunately the interpretation of the results are often overextrapolated. The book also describes the different tissues and the clinical applications that tissue engineering can target. These chapters therefore cover the breadth of tissue engineering in orthopedics, and can educate all of us.

Tissue engineering applications can be considered to act in one of several general ways. The most simple is for the product to assist, or facilitate, the body to repair itself. The second is to induce the body to repair itself. The third is to introduce a tissue that can remodel in vivo to become functional over time. The fourth is to provide a frank replacement that can function at the time of, or soon after, implantation. While the last type of application is the one most commonly thought of as tissue engineering, it is by far the most difficult to develop. The first two mechanisms are easier to apply, and are likely in the short to medium term to be the way that tissue engineering products will have an impact on clinical treatment. Consideration of this relatively pragmatic approach may be the way to maintain forward progress of this field, while continuing to work toward the ultimate applications.

Orthopedic applications of tissue engineering have the potential to revolutionize the field. Balancing this with reality—since the technical, regulatory, and commercial challenges may be substantial—means that the introduction of new products is likely to be slow. Hopefully researchers will use the experience already gained in tissue engineering to target applications that minimize the challenges and allow progress to be made. Aiming for the ultimate goals (for example, frank replacement of mechanically functional tissues such as articular cartilage and meniscus, etc.) is essential, but at the same time applications that are less challenging will almost certainly lead to more rapid development of products that can help patients. Replacement of tissues with a mechanically demanding function such as cartilage, meniscus, and ligament is likely to be much more difficult with subsequently long development time. Induction of a repair process, already shown to be successful in wound care tissue engineering, may lead to rapid development of products in orthopedics. Every field needs its share of success!

The use of tissue engineering in orthopedics inevitably requires that the product be commercially viable. The lengthy process times for development and regulatory approval, and the high cost of production, must be weighted. It seems likely that a strategy that encourages the development of relatively simple products with shorter time to market and lower cost of production will only serve to enhance the field. While these products may not be as technically challenging or attractive to the basic research scientists and engineers, for those who focus on translational or clinical research, these potential applications can be just as rewarding. A broad approach is, therefore, necessary.

Tissue engineering is still in its infancy, but is moving into a more rigorous, science-driven field. This is welcomed and should be encouraged, and progress will surely be made not only in the areas that are already targeted, but by new researchers not burdened by history and dogma. There is therefore a need for both the safe and incremental, as well as the high-risk entrepreneurial approaches.

The visionary leadership shown by those who introduced the field of tissue engineering, and by those who early on recognized its immense potential in orthopedics, must now be enhanced by a new group of scientists and engineers with new vision. These researchers will need to work at the forefront of their own technical discipline as well as in a multi-disciplinary environment, having an advanced appreciation of technical fields not their own. This high-level collaboration among researchers in different fields will surely result in the development of new methods and products that can address the clinical challenges in orthopedics. The future is very bright!

Anthony Ratcliffe
Gail Naughton
San Diego, California, U.S.A.

Contents

PART II   CLINICAL APPLICATION

Contributors

G. Altman   Tufts University, Medford, Massachusetts, U.S.A.

Peter Angele   University of Regensburg, Regensburg, Germany

Cynthia Boehm   The Cleveland Clinic Foundation, Cleveland, Ohio, U.S.A.

Scott P. Bruder   Case Western Reserve University, Cleveland, Ohio, and DePuy, Inc., a Johnson & Johnson Company, Raynham, Massachusetts, U.S.A.

Joseph A. Buckwalter   University of Iowa College of Medicine, Iowa City, Iowa, U.S.A.

Arnold I. Caplan   Case Western Reserve University, Cleveland, Ohio, U.S.A.

E. J. Caterson   Thomas Jefferson University, Philadelphia, Pennsylvania, U.S.A.

Robert G. Dennis   Harvard-MIT Division of Health Sciences and Technology, and MIT Artificial Intelligence Laboratory, University of Michigan, Ann Arbor, Michigan, U.S.A.

James E. Fleming, Jr.   The Cleveland Clinic Foundation, Cleveland, Ohio, U.S.A.

Freddie Fu University of Pittsburgh School of Medicine, Pittsburgh, Pennsylvania, U.S.A.

Victor M. Goldberg Case Western Reserve University, Cleveland, Ohio, U.S.A.

Farshid Guilak Duke University Medical Center, Durham, North Carolina, U.S.A.

Ernst B. Hunziker University of Bern, Bern, Switzerland

Brian Johnstone Research Institute of University Hospitals, and Case Western Reserve University, Cleveland, Ohio, U.S.A.

D. L. Kaplan Tufts University, Medford, Massachusetts, U.S.A.

Lee D. Kaplan University of Wisconsin School of Medicine, Madison, Wisconsin, U.S.A.

Safdar N. Khan Hospital for Special Surgery, New York, New York, U.S.A.

B. Kinner Brigham and Women's Hospital, Harvard Medical School, and VA Boston Healthcare System, Boston, Massachusetts, U.S.A.

Joseph M. Lane Weill Medical College of Cornell University and Hospital for Special Surgery, New York, U.S.A.

Isador H. Lieberman The Cleveland Clinic Foundation, Cleveland, Ohio, U.S.A.

Jay R. Lieberman David Geffen School of Medicine at UCLA, Los Angeles, California, U.S.A.

H. Madry Saarland University, Homburg-Saar, Germany

Robert F. McLain The Cleveland Clinic Foundation, Cleveland, Ohio, U.S.A.

Antonios G. Mikos Rice University, Houston, Texas, U.S.A.

George F. Muschler The Cleveland Clinic Foundation, Cleveland, Ohio, U.S.A.

B. Obradovic   University of Belgrade, Belgrade, Yugoslavia

A. H. Reddi   Center for Tissue Regeneration and Repair, University of California, Davis, School of Medicine, Sacramento, California, U.S.A.

M. Spector   Brigham and Women's Hospital, Harvard Medical School, and VA Boston Healthcare System, Boston, Massachusetts, U.S.A.

Emily S. Steinbis   Rice University, Houston, Texas, U.S.A.

Johnna S. Temenoff   Rice University, Houston, Texas, U.S.A.

Rocky S. Tuan   Thomas Jefferson University, Philadelphia, Pennsylvania, and National Institute of Arthritis, and Musculoskeletal and Skin Diseases, National Institutes of Health, Bethesda, Maryland, U.S.A.

G. Vunjak-Novakovic   Harvard-MIT Division of Health Sciences and Technology, Massachusetts Institute of Technology, Cambridge, Massachusetts, U.S.A.

Matthew L. Warman   Case Western Reserve University School of Medicine, Cleveland, Ohio, U.S.A.

Jung Yoo   Research Institute of University Hospitals, and Case Western Reserve University, Cleveland, Ohio, U.S.A.

ORTHOPEDIC
TISSUE
ENGINEERING

1

Principles of Tissue Engineering and Regeneration of Skeletal Tissues

Victor M. Goldberg and Arnold I. Caplan
Case Western Reserve University, Cleveland,
Ohio, U.S.A.

I. INTRODUCTION

There has been significant improvement in technologies to reconstruct musculoskeletal defects as a result of trauma or disease. During the last few decades, there has been widespread use of bone-banked, processed skeletal allografts to reconstruct large deficits of bone and cartilage (1,15,17,19,29,41) with outcomes at intermediate follow-up providing 85% satisfactory results (15,17,20,23,25). However, there still is a significant incidence of nonunions and graft failures, which usually require additional surgical intervention and result in additional morbidity. Additionally, the cost and availability of graft materials and some immunological issues still have not been completely resolved.

During the last 30 years, total joint arthroplasty has become a reproducible and a consistently successful surgical treatment with 97% satisfactory outcome at 8 years (16,28,38–40). The successful outcome has encouraged the application of the technology to younger, more active patients. As a result, an increased incidence of failure with wear of the articulating surface and loosening of the implants has been reported (39).

Although great strides have been made to improve materials and surgical techniques, the failure rate in these younger patients still approaches 10% in long-term follow-ups. The ultimate goal of any treatment that addresses musculoskeletal tissue loss is the restoration of the morphology and function of the lost tissue. The recent emergence of a new discipline, defined as tissue engineering, combines aspects of cell biology, engineering, materials science, and surgery with the outcome goal to regenerate functional skeletal tissues as opposed to replacing them (4,5,9,21,24,35,37).

Repair and regeneration of skeletal tissues are fundamentally different processes (8,10,33). In many situations, scar, which is the result of rapid repair, can function satisfactorily, such as in the early phases of bone restoration. By contrast, regeneration is a relatively slow process that ultimately results in a duplication of the tissue that has been lost. Regeneration is rarely seen in adults but is evident in very young children. Such regeneration appears to recapitulate some of the key steps that occur in embryonic development. Our approach to musculoskeletal tissue regeneration is to use principles of tissue engineering that are based upon the premise that there are important constituents that distinguish the fetal environment from that in adults and by mimicking aspects of these fetal microenvironments, we can engineer the restoration of adult tissue (8–10,27,31).

A broader understanding of and attention to basic principles of tissue engineering will result in enhanced success in regenerating specific tissues. The important constituents of embryonic development include a high proportion of undifferentiated progenitor cells with a higher cell-to-extracellular matrix ratio than in the fully formed adult tissue, and the capability to mechanically protect embryonic mesenchymal tissue from surrounding tissues, which is very difficult in adults (8,9). Further, regeneration implies the establishment of a sequence of signals to allow for the appropriate differentiation and maturation cascade to proceed. Additionally, the forming tissues are continually under the influence of inductive cytokines that provide the biological cues for molecular and cellular constituents at each stage of development. Finally, the regenerated tissue must establish an appropriate turnover dynamic with the continued capacity to grow. These considerations clearly impose certain functional constraints on the maturing tissue but this regenerating and evolving tissue should be superior to repair tissue, which does not allow growth and provides little long-term benefit. Importantly, regeneration differs significantly from repair in aspects of mechanical influences on the tissue. Musculoskeletal tissue is highly responsive to its mechanical environment, and it is only through the interaction of mechanical and biological cues that tissue differentiation proceeds to an appropriate morphological and biochemical character that successfully functions in highly loaded situations. This functional constraint imposes unusual demands on tissue engineering strategies for skeletal tissues.

II. PRINCIPLES OF TISSUE ENGINEERING

The basic component of any tissue engineering strategy is the use, either in combination or separately, of cells, biomatrices or scaffolds/delivery vehicles, and signaling molecules that provide the biological cues for the progression of cellular differentiation and its site-specific functional modulation (9,27,33,37). Significant issues remain for each component that must be addressed to develop successful and realistic tissue engineering treatment strategies. Central to our strategies is the need for cells (3,8,21,22,31,33,35,45–47). Significant issues that remain include the source of these cells, the number and density, and, most important, their age, phenotypic character, and developmental potency. We have put forth the hypothesis that mesenchymal stem or progenitor cells possess the appropriate developmental potential, are responsive to local cueing, and are capable of ultimately differentiating into the appropriate required phenotype (8,9,27). By contrast, adult differentiated cells are generally less responsive to mechanical and biological cues and may not be available in the appropriate quantities to achieve the desired tissue density.

Biomatrices, scaffolds, or delivery vehicles are important components of tissue engineering strategies. Both synthetic and natural materials have been used as delivery vehicles for cytokines or cells or both (2,21,22,26,27,32,42,43,47). It is still not clear what the ideal physical, chemical, and mechanical characteristics of the carrier should be for each specific tissue application. Ceramics, polymers of lactic and glycolic acid, collagen gels, and other natural polymers have been used to fabricate delivery vehicles and have been tested both in vivo and in vitro (2,21,32,47). The optimal properties of biomatrices for each implantation site must be defined and include their biodegradability, porosity, bonding capabilities, remodeling capacity, surface characteristics, and overall architecture (9,30). Again, for emphasis, there are critical requirements for each specific tissue implantation site. Most important, since regeneration is a multistep process with sequential cues, delivery vehicles should, in theory, possess multifunctional properties including intrinsic inductive capacities during early events, modulation capacities during the process, and, finally, the capability to contribute to the control of the integration of the newly formed tissue into that of the host (44). Ideally, delivery vehicles should be engineered to sequentially release discrete components that will accomplish these specific functions as the scaffold degrades to facilitate the seamless regeneration of specific musculoskeletal tissues.

Bioactive factors or cytokines have been used as single molecules although multiple components might be more effective (9,10,37). Since the successful engineering of a regenerative tissue depends on a cascade of events, multiple factors could be expected to enhance the process. Significant in vitro and in vivo studies indicate that powerful biological agents such as transforming growth factor-β, fibroblastic growth factors, and bone morphogenetic proteins may enhance the reparative mechanisms of otherwise inactive tissue (24,37). Although during the last decade significant advances have been made in understanding the function of these molecules, there still are unanswered issues. These include the choice of specific molecules for specific indications and the correct dose, timing, and sequence of administration. Again, for the regeneration of specific musculoskeletal tissues there are additional mechanical and biological requirements.

The musculoskeletal system is unique in that its major function is to provide weight-bearing potential, which involves a complex, multifactorial environment that places the regenerating tissue under enormous mechanical disadvantage. Therefore, an important question that remains to be answered is whether a tissue-engineered composite of cells, scaffolds, and bioactive molecules should be manufactured in an in vivo site by providing the appropriate mechanical and biological environment or whether the sequence of events should be controlled in vitro (21,44). Ultimately the use of large structural tissues to replace destroyed segments of, for example, osteoarticular structure, may well require bioreactors to manufacture materials that can withstand the detrimental loading environment in vivo. Additionally, the use of genetic engineering technology may provide an additional strategy to facilitate a complete, integrative regeneration of musculoskeletal structure.

III. RULES OF TISSUE ENGINEERING

Initially, tissue engineering approaches and concepts were empirical. It has only been recently, with focus on the scientific principles, that progress has been made toward successful replacement of lost tissue. Although we have discussed the necessity of the use of cells, biomatrices, and bioactive factors, our central hypothesis is that the management of cells is critical to any successful tissue engineering strategy since cells are responsible for tissue fabrication.

Philosophically, the increase in life expectancy requires biological solutions to orthopedic problems that were previously managed with mechanical solutions. We have developed over the years, from our research endeavors, a number of rules that we believe are critical in the refinement of successful cell-based tissue engineering treatment strategies (7).

Rule 1: Physically replace the excised tissue with biologically matched tissue. This requires that precise and discrete boundaries be established to fit the volume required by the excised or damaged tissue.

Rule 2: Regenerate the engineered tissue as opposed to repairing the excised or missing tissue.

Rule 3: Regulate or integrate the *neo* tissue with the host tissue in a seamless manner to reestablish natural function.

Rule 1 addresses the central concepts that have been developed in our laboratory, namely that key features of embryonic tissue development should be used in designing tissue engineering strategies. Embryonic development has been shown to be a continuum of genetically programmed changes that produce specific tissues with restricted functions (12). This program provides important biological cues throughout the entire life of the individual. Specifically, the tissue-engineered replacement must produce a structure that fills the entire space, since the signals or the receptors for these signals present in embryos to establish morphological boundaries are not available in adults. The *neo* tissue must be able to remodel to eventually match the morphology, biology, and mechanical function of the host tissue. If allogeneic cells are used in the tissue engineering strategy, they must either be replaced by host cells or exhibit similar developmental potential to that of the host.

The accessibility of nutrients to the *neo* tissue is critical to the long-term survivability of the construct. In the embryonic environment, because of the scale, nutrient accessibility is rarely a problem. However, since the scale of tissue engineering replacements is manyfold larger in adults, nutrient accessibility can be limiting. This usually involves the management of the initial inflammatory response that occurs with any wound. Specifically, a balance between revascularization and fibrous isolation of the *neo* tissue must be accomplished. For example, bone regeneration requires the reestablishment of functional vasculature while inhibition of vascularization will result in either chondral or fibrous tissue replacement (6,13,18,34).

Regeneration, rather than repair, is the central goal of any tissue engineering strategy. Repair is usually a rapid occurrence that is required for the survival of the individual but is not necessary for its optimal function. Repair usually results in a dense connective tissue scar that fills the space; however, it may not be responsive to the highly loaded mechanical environment required of musculoskeletal tissue. In very young animals where there are high tissue growth and turnover rates, this repair tissue may be slowly replaced by normal, morphologically specialized tissue. Regeneration is a slow process that is usually characterized by the recapitulation of aspects of embryonic development. For example, skeletal muscle regeneration exhibits distinctive transitions of molecular isoforms of glycosaminoglycans, contractile proteins, actins, and myosins, where the embryonic isoform is replaced by a neonatal form that is then replaced by the adult molecule (11). All of these isoforms are distinct gene products and appear in regenerating muscle on an accelerated timetable of weeks as compared to many months to observe these transitions in normal development (14). Regeneration also involves the transition from a relatively high progenitor-cell-to-extracellular-matrix ratio to a specialized musculoskeletal tissue with a low cell-to-extracellular-matrix ratio. The extracellular matrix is a major determinant of the skeletal tissue's chemical, physical, and mechanical properties. The *neo* tissue must be capable of matching the dynamic biological mechanisms of turnover experienced by the host tissue in the short and long term. For example, in young recipients, regenerated tissue must be capable of growth, while in older recipients the regenerated tissue must be capable of downsizing that occurs with aging of the organism. The tissue engineered construct must be either immunomatched with the host or protected from the immunological survey and responses of the host.

The integration of regenerated tissues is critical to the load-bearing function of most musculoskeletal structures. The regenerated tissue must match biologically, morphologically, and mechanically to the host tissues or it ultimately will fail. For example, the hyaline cartilage of a weight-bearing surface of a diarthrodial joint must be integrated with the *neo* cartilage of regenerated tissue. Further, the new tissue must be subject to the same regulation of its growth or metabolism as the host tissue, or a mismatch may result in disproportionate growth or functional discontinuity resulting in structural failure. Finally, the phenotypic expression of the implanted cells must match the host cells. For example, it is insufficient for the cells to merely express a cartilage program that expresses type II collagen and aggrecan, since cartilages of the articular surface of the knee are significantly different when compared to the meniscus or to the ear (36).

IV. SUMMARY

The ultimate goal of tissue engineering is the complete integrative regeneration of musculoskeletal structures providing biological solutions for clinical problems. The management of cells, either in vitro or in vivo, is the cornerstone of functional tissue engineering. The integration of these cells with biomatrices and their sensitivity to growth molecules must be accomplished to provide the necessary molecular and mechanical cues required for the functional integration of the *neo* tissue with the host. Regenerative tissue must be biochemically, morphologically, and mechanically matched with the host to perform its necessary function. Finally, the scale of the tissue being replaced by engineered constructs requires special design features to ensure the health of the constituent cells following implantation and during integration events.

REFERENCES

1. Akeson WH. Current status of cartilage grafting. West J Med 1998; 168:121–122.
2. Athanasiou KA, Agrawal CM, Barber FA, Burkhart SS. Orthopaedic applications for PLA-PGA biodegradable polymers. Arthroscopy 1998; 14:726–737.
3. Brittberg M, Lindahl A, Nilsson A, Ohlsson C, Isaksson O, Peterson L. Treatment of deep cartilage defects in the knee with autologous chondrocyte transplantation. N Engl J Med 1994; 331:889–895.
4. Buckwalter JA, Mankin HJ. Articular cartilage: degeneration and osteoarthritis, repair, regeneration, and transplantation. AAOS Instr Course Lect 1998; 47:487–504.
5. Buckwalter JA, Mankin HJ. Articular cartilage: tissue design and chondrocyte-matrix interactions. AAOS Instr Course Lect 1998; 47:477–486.
6. Caplan AI. Bone development. In: Cell and Molecular Biology of Vertebrate Hard Tissues. CIBA Foundation Symposium 136. Wiley: Chichester, England, 1988: 3–21.
7. Caplan AI. Embryonic development and the principles of tissue engineering. In: Tissue Engineering of Cartilage and Bone. Novartis Foundation. London: John Wiley & Sons Ltd., 2002. In press.
8. Caplan AI. Mesenchymal stem cells. J Orthop Res 1991; 9:641–650.
9. Caplan AI. Tissue engineering designs for the future: new logics, old molecules. Tissue Eng 2000; 6:1–8.
10. Caplan AI, Elyaderani M, Mochizuki Y, Wakitani S, Goldberg VM. Principles of cartilage repair and regeneration. Clin Orthop 1997; 342:254–269.
11. Caplan AI, Fiszman MY, Eppenberger HM. Molecular and cell isoforms during development. Science 1983; 221:921–927.
12. Caplan AI, Ordahl CP. Irreversible gene repression model for control of development. Science 1978; 201:120–130.
13. Caplan AI, Pechak DG. The cellular and molecular embryology of bone formation. In: Peck WA, ed. Bone and Mineral Research, Vol. 5. New York: Elsevier 1987; 5:117–184.
14. Carrino DA, Oron U, Pechak DG, Caplan AI. Reinitiation of chondroitin sulphate proteoglycan synthesis in regenerating skeletal muscle. Development 1988; 103:641–656.
15. Chu CR, Convery FR, Akeson WH, Meyers M, Amiel D. Articular cartilage transplantation: clinical results in the knee. Clin Orthop 1999; 360:159–168.

16. Colizza WA, Insall JN, Scuderi GR. The posterior stabilized total knee prosthesis: assessment of polyethylene damage and osteolysis after a ten-year minimum follow-up. J Bone Joint Surg 1995; 77A:1713–1720.

17. Czitrom AA, Keating S, Gross AE. The viability of articular cartilage in fresh osteochondral allografts after clinical transplantation. J Bone Joint Surg 1990; 72A:574–581.

18. Drushel RF, Caplan AI. The extravascular fluid dynamics of the embryonic chick wing bud. Dev Biol 1988; 126:7–18.

19. Eastlund DT. Bone transplantation and bone banking. In: Lonstein JE, Bradford DS, Winter RB, eds. Moe's Textbook of Scoliosis and Other Spinal Deformities. 3rd ed. Philadelphia: WB Saunders, 1995; 581–594.

20. Fitzpatrick PL, Morgan DA. Fresh osteochondral allografts: a 6–10-year review. Aust NZ J Surg 1998; 68:573–579.

21. Freed LE, Marquis JC, Nohria A, Emmanual J, Mikos AG. Neocartilage formation in vitro and in vivo using cells cultured on synthetic biodegradable polymers. J Biomed Mater Res 1993; 27:11–23.

22. Frenkel SR, Toolan B, Menche D, Pitman MI, Pachence JM. Chondrocyte transplantation using a collagen bilayer matrix for cartilage repair. J Bone Joint Surg 1997; 79B:831–836.

23. Garrett JC. Fresh osteochondral allografts for treatment of articular defects in osteochondritis dissecans of the lateral femoral condyle in adults. Clin Orthop 1994; 303:33–37.

24. Gazdag AR, Lane JM, Glaser D, Forster R. Alternatives to autogenous bone graft: efficacy and indications. J Am Acad Orthop Surg 1995; 3:1–8.

25. Ghazavi MT, Pritzker KP, Davis AM, Gross AE. Fresh osteochondral allografts for posttraumatic osteochondral defects of the knee. J Bone Joint Surg 1997; 79B:1008–1013.

26. Gilbert JE. Current treatment options for the restoration of articular cartilage. Am J Knee Surg 1998; 11:42–46.

27. Goldberg VM, Caplan AI. Biological resurfacing: an alternative to total joint arthroplasty. Orthopedics 1994; 17:819–821.

28. Goldberg VM, Ninomiya J, Kelly G, Kraay M. Hybrid total hip arthroplasty: a 7- to 11-year follow-up. Clin Orthop 1996; 333:147–154.

29. Goldberg VM, Stevenson S. The biology of bone grafts. Semin Arthroplasty 1993; 4:58–63.

30. Goldberg VM. Biological restoration of articular surfaces. AAOS Instr Course Lect 1999; 48:623–627.

31. Goldberg VM, Solchaga LA, Lundberg M, et al. Mesenchymal stem cell repair of osteochondral defects of articular cartilage. Semin Arthroplasty 1999; 10:30–36.

32. Grande DA, Halberstadt C, Naughton G, Schwartz R, Manji R. Evaluation of matrix scaffolds for tissue engineering of articular cartilage grafts. J Biomed Mater Res 1997; 34:211–220.

33. Hunziker EB. Articular cartilage repair: are the intrinsic biological constraints undermining his process insuperable? Osteoarthritis Cartilage 1999; 7:15–28.

34. Jargiello DM, Caplan AI. The establishment of vascular-derived micro-environments in the developing chick wing. Dev Biol 1983; 97:364–374.
35. Minas T. The role of cartilage repair techniques, including chondrocyte transplantation, in focal chondral knee damage. AAOS Instr Course Lect 1999; 48:629–643.
36. Naumann A, Dennis JE, Awadallah A, Carrino DA, Mansour JM, Kastenbauer E, Caplan AI. Immunochemical and mechanical characterization of cartilage subtypes in rabbit. J Histochem Cytochem 2002; 50:1049–1058.
37. Reddi AH. Regulation of cartilage and bone differentiation by bone morphogenetic proteins. Curr Opin Cell Biol 1992; 4:850–855.
38. Ritter MA, Worland R, Saliski J, Helphenstine JV, Edmondson KL, Keating EM, Faris PM, Meding JB. Flat-on-flat, nonconstrained, compression molded polyethylene total knee replacement. Clin Orthop 1995; 321:79–85.
39. Schmalzried TP, Callaghan JJ. Current concepts review: Wear in total hip and knee replacements. J Bone Joint Surg 1999; 81A:115–136.
40. Schulte KR, Callaghan JJ, Kelley SS, Johnston RC. The outcome of Charnley total hip arthroplasty with cement after a minimum twenty-year follow-up: the results of one surgeon. J Bone Joint Surg 1993; 75A:961–975.
41. Shelton WR, Treacy SH, Dukes AD, Bomboy AL. Use of allografts in knee reconstruction: II. Surgical considerations. J Am Acad Orthop Surg 1998; 6:169–175.
42. Solchaga LA, Gao J, Dennis JE, Awadallah A, Lundberg M, Caplan AI, Goldberg, VM. Treatment of osteochondral defects with autologous bone marrow in a hyaluronan-based delivery vehicle. Tissue Eng 2002; 8:333–347.
43. Solchaga LA, Yoo JU, Lundberg M, Dennis JE, Huibregtse BA, Goldberg VM, Caplan AI. Hyaluronan-based polymers in the treatment of osteochondral defects. J Orthop Res 2000; 18:773–780.
44. Solchaga L, Goldberg VM, Caplan AI. Cartilage repair with bone marrow in a hyaluronan-based scaffold. In: Phillips GO, Kennedy JF eds. Hyaluronan 2000. Abington, Cambridge, England: Woodhead Publishing Ltd. 2000.
45. Specchia N, Gigante A, Falciglia F, Greco F. Fetal chondral homografts in the repair of articular cartilage defects. Bull Hosp Joint Dis 1996; 54:230–235.
46. Wakitani S, Goto T, Pineda SJ, Young RG, Mansour JM, Caplan AI, Goldberg VM. Mesenchymal cell-based repair of large, full-thickness defects of articular cartilage. J Bone Joint Surg 1994; 76A:579–592.
47. Wakitani S, Goto T, Young RG, Mansour JM, Goldberg VM, Caplan AI. Repair of large full-thickness articular cartilage defects with allograft articular chondrocytes embedded in a collagen gel. Tissue Eng 1998; 4:429–444.

2

Tissue Engineering and Morphogenesis: Role of Morphogenetic Proteins

A. H. Reddi
University of California, Davis,
School of Medicine, Sacramento, California, U.S.A.

I. INTRODUCTION

Morphogenesis is the sequential cascade of pattern formation, establishment of body plan including mirror-image bilateral symmetry of musculoskeletal structures, and culmination in the adult form. The form of the skeleton is intimately linked to function in locomotion. Locomotion of the organisms is intertwined with evolution in terms of maintenance and propagation of species and foraging for food for the energetics of metabolism. Tissue engineering is the emerging scientific endeavor of the design and fabrication of spare parts for the skeleton for functional restoration based on principles of morphogenesis and embryonic growth and differentiation (1,2). Since regeneration is a recapitulation of embryonic development it is likely morphogenes can be redeployed during regeneration of orthopedic tissue including bone and cartilage. The purpose of this chapter is to present recent progress in morphogenetic proteins with special reference to tissue engineering.

II. TISSUE ENGINEERING TRIAD

Tissue engineering is based on inductive morphogenetic signals, responding stem cells, and the biomimetic entracellular matrix functioning as a scaffold (1). This triad of cues, cells, and context constitutes the holy trinity for tissue engineering (2), and also governs morphogenesis and development. The principles and molecular basis of tissue engineering of musculoskeletal tissues are based on the realization that among all the tissue in the human body, bone has the highest potential for regeneration and is a prototype model. On the other hand, cartilage has a limited ability for repair and regeneration. Despite the fact that articular cartilage and subchondral bone are adjacent tissues, they exhibit marked differences in their regenerative potential. This is in part due to the relatively avascular nature of articular cartilage. What are the signals initiating new bone morphogenesis in the developing limb bud? Implantation of demineralized bone matrix resulted in new bone morphogenesis locally at the site of implantation (3–5). This experimental model mimics bone morphogenesis in the limb bud and permitted the identification isolation and cloning of the first bone morphogenetic proteins (BMPs).

III. BONE MORPHOGENETIC PROTEINS

Bone grafts have been used by orthopaedic surgeons to aid in the recalcitrant bone repair for many years. Decalcified bone implants have been used to treat patients with osteomyelitis (3). Lacroix hypothesized that bone contains a substance, osteogenin, that initiates bone growth (4). Urist made the key discovery that demineralized, lyophilized segments of rabbit bone when implanted intramuscularly induced new bone formation (5). Bone induction is a sequential multistep cascade (6–8). The key steps in this cascade are chemotaxis, mitosis, and differentiation. Chemotaxis is the directed migration of cells in response to a chemical gradient of signals released from the insoluble demineralized bone matrix. The demineralized bone matrix is predominantly composed of type I insoluble collagen and it binds plasma fibronectin (9). Fibronectin has domains for binding to collagen, fibrin, and heparin. The responding mesenchymal cells attached to the collagenous matrix and proliferated as indicated by [3H]-thymidine autoradiography and incorporation into acid-precipitable DNA (10) on day 3. Chondroblast differentiation was evident on day 5, chondrocytes on days 7–8, and cartilage hypertrophy on day 9. There was concomitant vascular invasion on day 9 with osteoblast differentiation. On days 10–12 alkaline phosphatase was maximal. Osteocalcin, bone carboxyglutamic acid containing gla protein (BGP), increased on day 28. Hematopoietic marrow differentiated in the ossicle and was maximal by day 21. This entire sequential bone development cascade is reminiscent of cartilage and bone morphogenesis in the limb bud. Hence, it has immense implications for isolation of inductive signals initiating cartilage and bone morphogenesis. A prerequisite for any quest for novel morphogens is the establishment of a battery of bioassays for bone formation. A panel of in vitro assays was established for chemotaxis, mitogenesis, and chondrogenesis, and an in vivo assay for osteogenesis. Although the in vitro assays are expedient, we utilized a labor-intensive in vivo bioassay as it is the only bona fide bone induction assay.

A major stumbling block in the approach was that the demineralized bone matrix is insoluble. In view of this, dissociative extractants such as 4 M guanidine HCl or 8 M urea as 1% sodium dodecyl sulfate (SDS) at pH 7.4 was used (11). Approximately 3% of the proteins were solubilized from demineralized bone matrix, and the remaining residue was mainly insoluble type I bone collagen. The soluble extract alone or the insoluble residue alone was incapable of new bone induction. However, addition of the extract to the residue (insoluble collagen) and then implantation in a subcutaneous site resulted in bone induction. Thus, there was a collaboration between soluble extract and the insoluble collagenous substratum (11) for optimal osteogenesis. This bioassay was a key advance in the final purification of BMPs and led to determination of limited tryptic peptide sequences leading to the eventual cloning of BMPs (12–14).

Demineralized bovine and human bone was not osteoinductive in rats. However, when the guanidine extracts of demineralized bovine bone were fractionated on a S-200 molecular sieve column, fractions less than 50 kDa were consistently osteogenic when bioassayed after reconstitution with allogeneic insoluble collagen (15,16). Thus, fractions inducing bone were not species-specific and are homologous among mammals. It is likely that larger molecular mass fractions and/or the insoluble xenogeneic (bovine and human) collagens were inhibitory or immunogenic. The amino acid sequences revealed homology to TGF-β1 (16). The incisive work of Wozney and colleagues cloned BMP-2, BMP-2B (now called BMP-4) and BMP-3 (also called osteogenin). Osteogenic protein-1 and 2 (OP-1 and OP-2) were cloned by Ozkaynak and colleagues (13). There are nearly 15 members of the BMP family. The other members of the extended TGF-β/BMP superfamily include inhibins and activins Mullerian duct inhibitory substance (MIS), growth/differentiation factors (GDFs), and nodal factors.

BMPs are dimeric molecules and the conformation is critical for biological actions. Reduction of the single intermolecular disulfide bond resulted in the loss of biological activity. The mature monomer of BMPs consists of about 120 amino acids, with seven canonical cysteine residues. There are three intrachain disulfides and one interchain disulfide bond. The cysteine knot is the critical central core of the BMP molecule. The crystal structure of BMP-7 has been determined (17). The BMP-7 monomer has β-pleated sheets in the form of two pointed fingers. In the dimer the pointed fingers are oriented in opposite directions. Such information will speed up the approaches to design and synthesize peptidomimetic BMPs by combinatorial library techniques using robotic, high-throughput assays. Other innovative approaches include screening for small molecules in natural products based on promoter-reporter constructs and receptor activation.

IV. GROWTH AND DIFFERENTIATION FACTORS FOR CHONDROGENESIS

Morphogenesis of the cartilage is the key rate-limiting step in the dynamics of bone development. Cartilage is the initial blueprint for the architecture of bones. Bone can form either directly from mesenchyme, as in intramembranous bone formation observed in limited craniofacial bones, or with an intervening cartilage stage, as in endochondral bone development (7). All BMPs induce, first, the cascade of chondrogenesis, and therefore in this sense are cartilage morphogenetic proteins. The hypertrophic chondrocyte matrix in the epiphyseal growth plate mineralizes and serves as a template for appositional bone morphogenesis. Cartilage morphogenesis is critical for both bone and joint morphogenesis. The two lineages of cartilage are clear-cut. The first, at the ends of bone, forms articulating articular cartilage. The second is the growth plate chondrocytes, which proliferate, mature, and hypertrophy, synthesize cartilage matrix destined to calcify acts as a nidus for replacement by bone, and are the "organizer" centers of longitudinal and circumferental growth of cartilage and endochondral bone formation. The phenotypic stability of the articular (permanent) cartilage is at the crux of the osteoarthritis problem. The "maintenance" factors for articular chondrocytes include TGF-β isoforms and the BMP isoforms.

An in vivo chondrogenic bioassay with soluble purified proteins and insoluble collagen identified a chondrogenic fraction in articular cartilage. A concurrent RT-PCR approach with degenerate oligonucleotide primers was undertaken. Two novel genes for cartilage-derived morphogenetic proteins (CDMPs) 1 and 2 were identified and cloned (18). CDMPs 1 and 2 are also called growth and differentiation factors 5 and 6 (19) and may play a critical role in initiation and maintenance of articular cartilage and joint morphogenesis.

V. BMP RECEPTOR KINASES

Recombinant human BMP-4 binds to type I BMP receptors, BMPR-IA and BMPR-IB, called ALK-3 and ALK-6, respectively. BMP-2, BMP-7, and CDMP-1 (GDF-5) bind to both BMPR-IA and -IB. The type I and II BMP receptors are membrane-bound serine/threonine kinases (2). The type II receptors phosphorylate type I receptor. The BMP type I receptor kinases phosphorylate the Smads. Smads are related to *Drosophila* Mad (mothers against dpp) and three related nematode genes, Sma 2, 3, and 4. The terms "Sma" and "Mad" have been fused as Smad to unify the nomenclature for the signaling Smads. There are nine members of the Smad family. Phosphorylated Smads 1, 5, and 8 are functional mediators of BMP family signaling in partnership with common partner Smad 4. Smads 2 and 3 are signal transducers for actions of TGF-β and activins. Smad 6 and Smad 7 function as inhibitory Smads to inhibit TGF-β/BMP superfamily signaling. The phosphorylated Smad 1 enters as a heteromeric complex with Smad 4 into the nucleus and activates transcription of early BMP response genes. The BMP receptors also appear to signal via the MAP kinase (mitogen-activated protein kinase). It is likely that BMPs regulate cell cycle progression and thus govern differentiation of mesenchymal stem cells.

VI. MORPHOGENS AND BIOMIMETIC BIOMATERIALS

The natural biomaterials in the composite tissue of bones and joints are collagens, proteoglycans, and glycoproteins of cell adhesion such as fibronectin and the mineral phase. The mineral phase in bone is predominantly hydroxyapatite. In native state the associated citrate, fluoride, carbonate, and trace elements constitute the physiological hydroxyapatite. The high protein-binding capacity makes hydroxyapatite a natural delivery system. Comparison of insoluble collagen, hydroxyapatite, tricalcium phosphate, glass beads, and polymethylmethacrylate as carriers revealed collagen to be an optimal delivery system for BMPs (20). It is well known that collagen is an ideal delivery system for growth factors in soft- and hard-tissue wound repair (21).

It is well known that extracellular matrix components play a critical role in morphogenesis. The structural macromolecules and their supramolecular assembly in the extracellular matrix do not explain their role in epithelial-mesenchymal interaction and morphogenesis. This riddle can now be explained by the binding of BMPs to heparan sulfate, heparin, and type IV collagen (22) of the basement membranes. In fact, this might explain in part the necessity for angiogenesis and vascular invasion into cartilage prior to osteogenesis during development. The actions of activin in development, in terms of dorsal mesoderm induction, is modified to neuralization by binding and termination of activin action by follistatin (23). Similarly, Chordin and Noggin from the Spemann organizer induce neuralization by binding and inactivation of BMP-4 (24,25). Thus neural induction is likely to be a default pathway when BMP-4 is rendered non-functional (24,25). Thus, this is an emerging principle in development and morphogenesis that BMP binding proteins can terminate a dominant morphogen's action and initiate a default developmental pathway. Further, the binding of a soluble morphogen to extracellular matrix (ECM) converts it into an insoluble matrix-bound morphogen to act locally in the solid state (22) and may protect it from proteolysis and prolong its half-life. In this sense, extracellular matrix is both structural and functional as a delivery system for morphogens.

During the course of systematic work on hydroxyapatite of two pore sizes (200 or 500 μm) in two geometrical forms (beads or discs) an unexpected observation was made. The geometry of the delivery system is critical for optimal bone induction. The discs were consistently osteoinductive with BMPs in rats, but the beads were inactive (26). The chemical compositions of the two hydroxyapatite configurations were identical. In certain species the hydroxyapatite alone appears to be "osteoinductive" (27). In subhuman primates the hydroxyapatite induces bone, albeit at a much slower rate. One interpretation is that osteoinductive endogenous BMPs in circulation progressively bind to implanted disc of hydroxyapatite. When an optimal threshold concentration of native BMPs is achieved, the hydroxyapatite becomes osteoinductive. Strictly speaking, most hydroxyapatite substrata are ideal osteoconductive materials. This example in certain species also serves to illustrate how an osteoconductive biomimetic biomaterial may progressively function as an osteoinductive substance by binding to endogenous BMPs.

VII. PROSPECTS

The symbiosis of biotechnology and biomaterials has set the stage for systematic advances in tissue engineering (28,29). Biomechanics is a critical component of the context for orthopedic tissue engineering. The recent advances in the enabling platform technology include molecular imprinting (30) of specific recognition and catalytic sites on a surface. The applications range from biosensors, catalytic applications to antibody, and receptor recognition sites. For example, the cell-binding RGD site in fibronectin or YIGSR domain in laminin of basement membranes can be imprinted on a synthetic biomaterial (2).

Finally, one can fabricate a mold by computer-aided design and manufacture (CAD and CAM). Such a mold reproduces the structural features of a bone such as femur and may be imprinted with morphogens, inductive signals, and cell adhesion sites. This assembly can be loaded with stem cells and BMPs with a nutrient medium to form new bone in the shape of femoral head. In fact, such a biological approach to tissue engineering with vascularized muscle flap and BMPs yielded new bone with a defined shape (31) and is proof of principle and concept for further refinement and validation. We indeed are in a brave new world of prefabricated biological spare parts for the human body based on tissue engineering and sound architectural rules of inductive signals for morphogenesis, responding stem cells, and a template of biomimetic biomaterial based on extracellular matrix. It is indeed very satisfying to note the contributions of bone and BMPs to the more wide-ranging concepts of tissue engineering in orthopedic surgery and regenerative medicine (32).

ACKNOWLEDGMENTS

This work is supported by the Lawrence Ellison Chair in Musculoskeletal Molecular Biology and grants from the Department of Defense and the Shriners Hospital for Children. I thank Rita Rowlands for her outstanding bibliographic assistance and enthusiastic help.

REFERENCES

1. Reddi AH. Symbiosis of biotechnology and biomaterials: applications in tissue engineering of bone and cartilage. J Cell Biochem 1994; 56:192–195.
2. Reddi AH. Role of morphogenetic proteins in skeletal tissue engineering and regeneration. Nature Biotechnol 1998; 16:247–252.
3. Senn N. On the healing of aseptic bone cavities by implantation of antiseptic decalcified bone. Am J Med Sci 1889; 98:219–240.
4. Lacroix P. Recent investigations on the growth of bone. Nature 1945; 156:576.
5. Urist MR. Bone: formation by autoinduction. Science 1965; 150:893–899.
6. Reddi AH, Huggins C. Biochemical sequences in the transformation of normal fibroblasts in adolescent rats. Proc Natl Acad Sci USA 1972; 69:1601–1605.
7. Reddi AH. Cell biology and biochemistry of endochondral bone development. Coll Relat Res 1981; 1:209–226.
8. Reddi AH. Extracellular matrix and development. In: Piez KA, Reddi AH, eds. Extracellular Matrix Biochemistry. New York: Elsevier, 1984:247–291.
9. Weiss RE, Reddi AH. Synthesis and localization of fibronectin during collagenous matrix- mesenchymal cell interaction and differentiation of cartilage and bone in vivo. Proc Natl Acad Sci USA 1980; 77:2074–2078.

10. Reddi AH, Anderson WA. Collagenous bone matrix-induced endochondral ossification hemopoiesis. J Cell Biol 1976; 69:557–572.
11. Sampath TK, Reddi AH. Dissociative extraction and reconstitution of extracellular matrix components involved in local bone differentiation. Proc Natl Acad Sci USA 1981; 78:7599–7603.
12. Wozney JM, Rosen V, Celeste AJ, et al. Novel regulators of bone formation: molecular clones and activities. Science 1988; 242:1528–1534.
13. Ozkaynak E, Rueger DC, Drier EA, et al. OP-1 cDNA encodes an osteogenic protein in the TGF-beta family. EMBO J 1990; 9:2085–2093.
14. Luyten FP, Cunningham NS, Ma S, et al. Purification and partial amino acid sequence of osteogenin, a protein initiating bone differentiation. J Biol Chem 1989; 264:13377–13380.
15. Sampath TK, Reddi AH. Homology of bone-inductive proteins from human, monkey, bovine, and rat extracellular matrix. Proc Natl Acad Sci USA 1983; 80:6591–6595.
16. Reddi AH. Bone and cartilage differentiation. Curr Opin Genet Dev 1994; 4:737–744.
17. Griffith DL, Keck PC, Sampath TK, Rueger DC, Carlson WD. Three-dimensional structure of recombinant human osteogenic protein 1: structural paradigm for the transforming growth factor beta superfamily. Proc Natl Acad Sci USA 1996; 93:878–883.
18. Chang SC, Hoang B, Thomas JT, et al. Cartilage-derived morphogenetic proteins; new members of the transforming growth factor-beta superfamily predominantly expressed in long bones during human embryonic development. J Biol Chem 1994; 269:28227–28234.
19. Storm EE, Huynh TV, Copeland NG, Jenkins NA, Kingsley DM, Lee SJ. Limb alterations in brachypodism mice due to mutations in a new member of the Tgf-beta-superfamily. Nature 1994; 368:639–643.
20. Ma S, Chen G, Reddi AH. Collaboration between collagenous matrix and osteogenin is required for bone induction. Ann NY Acad Sci 1990; 580: 524–525.
21. McPherson JM. The utility of collagen-based vehicles in delivery of growth factors for hard and soft tissue wound repair. Clin Mater 1992; 9:225–234.
22. Paralkar VM, Nandedkar AK, Pointer RH, Kleinman HK, Reddi AH. Interaction of osteogenin, a heparin binding bone morphogenetic protein, with type IV collagen. J Biol Chem 1990; 265:17281–17284.
23. Hemmati-Brivanlou A, Kelly OG, Melton DA. Follistatin, an antagonist of activin, is expressed in the Spemann organizer and displays direct neuralizing activity. Cell 1994; 77:283–295.
24. Piccolo S, Sasai Y, Lu B, De Robertis EM. Dorsoventral patterning in *Xenopus*: inhibition of ventral signals by direct binding of chordin to BMP-4. Cell 1996; 86:589–598.
25. Zimmerman LB, De Jesús-Escobar JM, Harland RM. The Spemann organizer signal noggin binds and inactivates bone morphogenetic protein 4. Cell 1996; 86:599–606.

26. Ripamonti U, Ma S, Reddi AH. The critical role of geometry of porous hydroxyapatite delivery system in induction of bone by osteogenin, a bone morphogenetic protein. Matrix 1992; 12:202–212.
27. Ripamonti U. Osteoinduction in porous hydroxyapatite implanted in heterotopic sites of different animal models. Biomaterials 1996; 17:31–35.
28. Langer R, Vacanti JP. Tissue engineering. Science 1993; 260:920–926.
29. Hubbell JA. Biomaterials in tissue engineering. Bio-Technology 1995; 13: 565–576.
30. Mosbach K, Ramstrom O. The emerging technique of molecular imprinting and its future impact on biotechnology. Bio-Technology 1996; 14:163–170.
31. Khouri RK, Koudsi B, Reddi H. Tissue transformation into bone invivo—a potential practical application. JAMA 1991; 266:1953–1955.
32. Reddi AH. Bone Morphognetic proteins: from basic science to clinical application. J Bone Joint Surg 2001; S1:1–6.

3

Cell-Based Approaches to Orthopedic Tissue Engineering

E. J. Caterson
Thomas Jefferson University, Philadelphia, Pennsylvania, U.S.A.

Rocky S. Tuan
Thomas Jefferson University, Philadelphia, Pennsylvania, U.S.A. and National Institutes of Arthritis, and Musculoskeletal and Skin Diseases, National Institutes of Health, Bethesda, Maryland, U.S.A.

Scott P. Bruder
Case Western Reserve University, Cleveland, Ohio, U.S.A. and DePuy, Inc., a Johnson & Johnson Company, Raynham, Massachusetts, U.S.A.

I. INTRODUCTION

The cornerstone of tissue engineering is the dynamic interplay between three basic components: bioactive factors, extracellular matrix, and responding cells. From a functional perspective, the bioactive factors provide the instructional cues that direct the behavior of the cellular components. The extracellular matrix molecules provide a substrate for bio-active factor presentation and/or cellular attachment, proliferation, and differentiation. Finally, the responding cells provide the biosynthetic machinery responsible for creating the new structural tissues. Within that context, the aims of this chapter are threefold: first, to define the role of specialized cells in the musculoskeletal system; second, to describe functional relationships of precursors, mature cells, and cellular turnover in the hierarchy of tissue formation and maintenance; and third, to use this understanding to establish a logic and rationale for selecting one cell source over another for each tissue-specific tissue-engineered product.

Tissue engineering is the intersection of clinical medicine, biological sciences, and materials and mechanical engineering. The challenge is that these individual disciplines must cross-fertilize and propagate their ideas within this burgeoning discipline, and build upon current knowledge to give respite to injury and disability caused by trauma and/or disease. The broad concepts explored in this chapter, namely, cells and their relationships to signals and the extracellular matrix scaffolding, are but a few of the areas in which advances are needed. To develop innovative therapeutic strategies, tissue engineers need to have a thorough understanding of the basic science of tissue morphogenesis as a foundation for innovation. Intrinsic to this is a fundamental grasp of embryonic development that can guide our effort to mimic the mechanisms and events of tissue construction in the repair and regeneration of musculoskeletal tissue.

II. FUNDAMENTALS OF MORPHOGENESIS

The musculoskeletal system develops from one of the three primary germ layers, the mesoderm, and neural crest cells. In development, lateral to the notochord and neural tube, a coalescence of tissue called the paraxial mesoderm serves as the foundation for the musculoskeletal system. Toward the third week of development in the human embryo, blocks of segmented tissue called somites are formed from the paraxial mesoderm on the dorsolateral surface. Each somite differentiates into two parts: (1) the sclerotome, which forms the vertebrae and the ribs; and (2) the dermatomyotome, the raw material for the dermis and the musculature of the developing embryo. The mesodermal cells from these areas give rise to mesenchyme, a loosely organized connective tissue filled with the cells that serve as progenitors for musculoskeletal tissues. Regardless of their source, these mesenchymal cells have the ability to differentiate in a number of ways, including into osteoblasts, adipoblasts, myoblasts, chondroblasts, and fibroblasts (Fig. 1). It is the differentiation of these specialized cells, which often maintain, secrete, and modulate their associated extracellular matrices, that

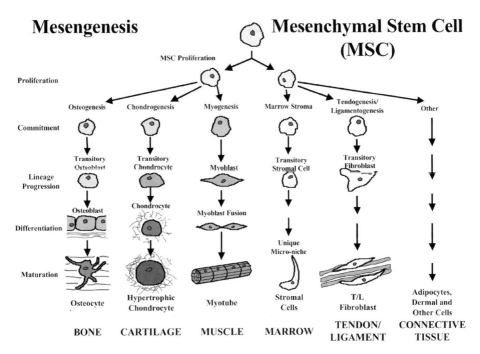

FIGURE 1 The mesengenic process. MSCs have the potential to differentiate into a variety of mesenchymal tissues, such as bone, cartilage, tendon, muscle, marrow, dermis, and fat. Proliferating MSCs enter a lineage, following their commitment to that particular pathway. The commitment event involves the action of specific growth factors and/or cytokines, as does the next phase, in which the lineage-committed cells progress through a number of transitory stages in the lineage progression process. Terminal differentiation involves the cessation of proliferation and the massive biosynthesis of tissue-specific products. Finally, these differentiated cells go through a maturation stage in which they acquire an ability to function in aspects of tissue homeostasis as opposed to high levels of synthetic activity. All of these end-stage-differentiated cells have fixed half-lives and can be expected to expire; these cells are replaced by newly differentiated cells arising from the continuous transition down the lineage pathway. The lineages are arranged from left to right based on the relative information known about definitive lineage stages. (From Ref. 46. Reprinted with permission from Elsevier Science Ltd.)

heralds the dawn of organized tissue formation. These specialized tissues, with their associated resident cells, are defined as bone, fat, muscle, cartilage, tendon, and ligament.

As in other organs, there is a hierarchical process in the formation of the musculoskeletal system. It begins with the development and differentiation of specialized cells. These events lead to the great diversity of form and function that makes orthopedic tissue engineering challenging. The musculoskeletal system has additional complexity because of its composite tissues such as bone-ligament-bone unions, osteochondral interfaces, myotendinous junctions, muscle motor units, and vertebral endplates coupled with intervertebral discs. In orthopedic tissue engineering we must not only regenerate or restore the function of an ailing portion of the musculoskeletal system, but also recreate the interaction of that portion with its natural partner. To achieve this goal, one must have a thorough understanding of the biology of the cells that serve as the functional components in extracellular matrix secretion and remodeling.

In defining the role of the specialized cells in the musculoskeletal system one must understand how the cells progress during development along a maturational continuum. That is, how do cells navigate through their beginnings as stem cells to a more restricted progenitor cell population, to a precursor of a differentiated phenotype, and finally, to a mature cell secreting and maintaining a functional matrix (1)? Though studied widely of late, the regulation of these transitions is a central feature of developmental biology that is not well understood. Occasionally, this progression continues past a mature cell phenotype to quiescence or even apoptosis. Bone formation is one example of the many musculoskeletal tissues in which this developmental progression from progenitor to differentiated cell-producing functional matrix is preserved.

Both intramembranous and endochondral bone formation occur through the regulation of precursor or transitional cells to a more differentiated phenotype. Intramembranous bone formation, as is found in the cranial and parietal bones, is the direct conversion of mesenchymal cells into osteoblasts. Intramembranous ossification occurs when the mesenchyme condenses and is subsequently invaded by vasculature directly. As a consequence, cells begin to secrete a matrix, which is later mineralized, in response to a variety of biological cues such as the bone morphogenetic proteins (BMPs). Endochondral ossification at the growth plate is responsible for the longitudinal growth of the long bones, and occurs through a cartilaginous intermediate. It occurs principally in long bones that bear weight. In these bones, the condensed embryonic mesenchyme transforms into cartilage, which reflects in position and form the eventual bone to be formed at that site (Fig. 2). In the central part of such a developing bone, intramembranous ossification is responsible for the initial diaphyseal shaft, while elongation of the proximal and distal ends results from the endochondral process.

Endochondral ossification encompasses a linear, interstitial proliferation of columns of chondrocytes, their progressive hypertrophy,

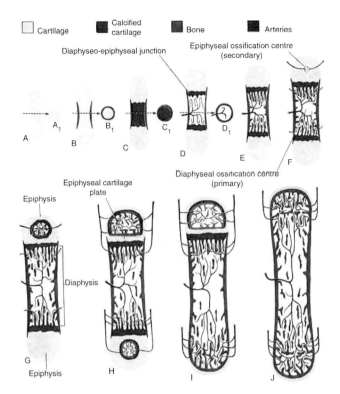

FIGURE 2 Schematic diagrams illustrating intracartilaginous or endochondral ossification and the development of a typical long bone. Panels A–J are longitudinal sections, and A_1–D_1 are cross-sections at the levels indicated. (A) Cartilage model of the bone. (B) A subperiosteal ring of bone appears. (C) cartilage begins to calcify. (D) Vascular mesenchyme enters the calcified cartilage. (E) At each diaphyseal-epiphyseal junction there is a zone of ossification. (F) Blood vessels and mesenchyme enter the superior epiphyseal cartilage. (G) The epiphyseal ossification center grows. (H) A similar center develops in the inferior epiphyseal cartilage plate. (I) The inferior epiphyseal cartilage plate is ossified. (J) The superior epiphyseal cartilage plate ossifies, forming a continuous bone marrow cavity. When the epiphyseal plates ossify, the bone can no longer grow in length. (From Moore, Persaud. The Developing Human Clinically Oriented Embryology. 5th ed. Philadelphia: WB Saunders Company, 1993. Reprinted with permission from WB Saunders Company.)

mineralization of the intercolumnar cartilage matrix in the long axis of the bone, and the persistence of the mineralized matrix after disappearance of its cells as a scaffold for the deposition of subchondral metaphyseal bone (2). Together, this structure is referred to as the growth plate. The peripheral osteoblasts in the periosteum arrive with a blood supply to penetrate the central hypertrophied, mineralized cartilage core and carry skeletal cell progenitors to the interior of the anlagen for the formation and turnover of bone. It seems that a subset of cells within the medullary cavity and the periosteum serve as an adult reservoir for cells that, as a part of normal physiology and in the case of injury, can participate in the perpetuation of the periosteum and other processes of bone growth and fracture repair.

Other components of the musculoskeletal system such as tendons and ligaments, like the cartilage found in the menisci, have their origins in the lateral plate mesenchyme. The tendon and ligament cells take a position on both sides of the mesenchymal lamina, dorsal and ventral to developing digital cartilage (3). Unlike these tissues, the intervertebral disc arises from developmentally distinct regions. The annulus and cartilage endplates are derived from the mesenchyme and the nucleus, with its mucoid matrix differentiates from the notochord. The common thread between bone formation and all of these other processes is that each specialized cell involved in musculoskeletal tissue morphogenesis has undergone a progression from an undifferentiated progenitor to a functionally mature cell, which can produce and modulate matrix. Finally, once these cells have finished their developmental program, they remain to serve as integral components in the maintenance of the tissues in which they are housed.

III. MUSCULOSKELETAL CELLS

The cellular diversity of the musculoskeletal system results from a number of tightly regulated and coordinated dynamic events. A detailed analysis of these molecular events is discussed elsewhere in this book; however, it is useful to understand the major phenotypic properties that make each of these musculoskeletal cells unique (Table 1). With appreciation for the molecular diversity of each cell type, one can apply this knowledge to better assess the success of tissue-engineered constructs designed to restore both form and function.

IV. OSTEOBLASTS

Osteoblast differentiation occurs by a linear progression from an immature progenitor cell to a preosteoblast and through the osteoblastic lineage into an osteocyte. This lineage description is based, in part, on the cellular features, the biochemical and molecular gene expression profiles, and the contribution and expression of transcription factors toward differentiation. Developmental control and modifications of transcription

TABLE 1 The Major Phenotypic Properties of Cells Comprising the
Musculoskeletal System

Cell type	Phenotypic features
Osteoblast	Cuboidal morphology, eccentric nucleus Expresses alkaline phosphatase, osteopontin, bone sialoprotein, osteocalcin, collagen type I Prostaglandin E2 and parathyroid hormone responsiveness Reacts with antibodies SB-2, SB-3, SB-5, SB-20, and others Osteocytes, or terminally differentiated osteoblasts, possess a unique stellate morphology and little biosynthetic activity
Osteoclast	Large, multinucleated morphology with a ruffled border Ability to carry out lacunar bone resorption Derived from the monocyte-macrophage lineage Expresses CD 45, CD 51, vitronectin alpha chain, tartrate-resistant acid phosphatase (TRAP), receptor activator of nuclear kappa B (RANK)
Chondrocyte	Round morphology, central nucleus Expresses collagen types II, VI, IX, XI, aggrecan, cartilage proteoglycan link protein, hyaluronic acid Survives in avascular environment (low oxygen tension) Hypertrophic chondrocytes express collagen type X Nucleus pulposus cells secrete a collagen type IV pericellular matrix
Ligament- and tendon-forming fibroblast	Fibroblastic, spindle-shaped morphology; high matrix-to-cell ratio Longitudinally aligned extracellular matrix fibrils Expresses collagen types I, III, and XII, tenascin, fibronectin, elastin
Myoblast	Multinucleated cells in striated muscle; precursors are myoblasts Reacts with antibody L4, and polyclonal antibodies against tensin Expresses muscle-specific intermediate filament protein (desmin), slow and fast contractile protein isoforms of actin and myosin, transcription factors MyoD, Myf5, myogenin, Mrf4

(Continued)

TABLE 1 Continued

Cell type	Phenotypic features
Mesenchymal stem cell	Fibroblastic, spindle-shaped morphology; rare to find in situ Expresses collagen types I, IV, fibronection, laminin Reacts with antibodies SB-10, SH-2, SH-3, SH-4, STRO-1

These are the major cell types that comprise orthopedic tissues. Both phenotypic and molecular characterization is often necessary to illustrate the specific cell type and its state of differentiation. Many of the relevant cells are characterized through biological markers that are components of the matrix they produce.

to regulate cell and tissue function are modulated by a complex series of physiological regulatory signals. On a morphological basis it is difficult to distinguish the preosteoblast from the osteoblast; therefore, it has been necessary to implement biochemical characterization of isolated cells such as the expression patterns of alkaline phosphatase and the responsiveness to factors such as parathyroid hormone (PTH), prostaglandin (PGE2), and epidermal growth factor (EGF). Although responsiveness to these factors is not unique to the osteoblastic lineage, it can serve to identify cells as more or less mature (4). Preosteoblasts in the proliferative stages are associated with histones and proto-oncogenes such as c-fos and c-myc (5), as well as low levels of parathyroid hormone/parathyroid hormone–related protein (PTH)/(PTHrP) receptor, fibroblast growth factor receptor-1 (FGFR-1), and platelet-derived growth factor (PDGF) receptor alpha (6). Members of the early-response gene family that regulates growth and development of the osteoblastic phenotype, such as c-fos, c-jun, and c-myc, have also been shown to increase when osteoblasts are exposed to PTH and various serum cytokines (7–9). Cell surface alkaline phosphatase increases initially and then decreases after mineralization has reached homeostasis; osteopontin appears before other certain matrix proteins including bone sialoprotein (BSP) and osteocalcin in differentiated osteoblasts forming bone. Osteocalcin synthesis is most closely associated with osteoblasts that are undergoing active mineralization (10,11). Collagen type I expression can be found throughout the lineage stages, but appears to peak at the late maturational stage of the osteoblast (12). Monoclonal antibodies directed against stage-specific cell surface epitopes can also characterize the developmental progression. Preosteoblasts or stromal progenitors are labeled by the antibodies, SB-10, SH-2, SH-3, SH-4 as well as STRO-1, but do not label osteoblasts or osteocytes (13–15). The osteocyte-specific antibody SB-5, in combination with other monoclonal antibodies such as SB-1, SB-2, and SB-3, helps to discriminate stages from the osteoblast to an osteocytic osteoblast to a terminally differentiated osteocyte (16). Osteocytes are stellate-shaped cells encased in mature matrix with slender cytoplasmic processes that radiate into the lacunar network of bone. This unique morphology, in part, supports the function of osteocytes as mechanosensors. One of the best markers of the osteocyte is its typical morphology; however, osteocytes strongly express the cell surface antigen known as CD44. This is in contrast to osteoblasts and other bone lining cells, which are negative for CD44 (17,18). Osteocytes are postproliferative cells considered to be relatively inactive metabolically, evidenced by the loss of many of their cytoplasmic organelles necessary for matrix production and secretion, thereby making them smaller than the osteoblast and preosteoblast. Nevertheless, like other cells of the osteoblastic lineage, osteocytes have been associated with both protein and mRNA expression of osteocalcin, osteonectin, osteopontin, fibronectin, and collagen type I (19–21).

V. OSTEOCLASTS

The osteoblast and its lineage partners are in a state of delicate balance with the multinucleated osteoclast that forms through the fusion of mononuclear precursors of hematopoietic origin. Proliferation of the osteoclast has never been documented. The osteoclast is derived from the monocyte-macrophage lineage distinct from the connective tissue cells of bone arising from the marrow stroma. The process of osteoclast differentiation involves a number of steps associated with the proliferation and commitment of mononuclear precursor cells into mature functional osteoclasts. Expression of cell surface antigens reveals that mature osteoclasts maintain a number of antigenic markers associated with macrophages, such as CD45 and CD51, and the α chain of vitronectin. Mononuclear osteoclast precursors can be found in areas that are being prepared for bone resorption. Osteotropic hormones and cytokines interact to regulate the progression of osteoclast precursor cells to mature osteoclasts through three independent signal transduction pathways: $1\alpha,25 \, (OH)_2$ vitamin D_3, cAMP, and gp130-mediated signals (22–24) (Fig. 3). Osteoblastic cells serve as the target cells for the osteotropic hormones and cytokines, and they in turn secrete soluble factors such as M-CSF and complement C3, which regulate osteoclast development (25). Tartrate-resistant acid phosphatase has been used as a cell-specific marker for osteoclasts and macrophages as well as the expression of RANK (receptor activator of nuclear kappa B). Osteoprotegerin interacts with RANK to activate bone resorptive functions in mature

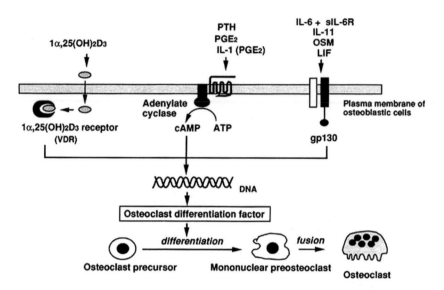

FIGURE 3 A hypothesis on the signal transduction pathways induced by osteotropic hormones and cytokines in osteoclast differentiation. Three signal transduction pathways [cAMP, gp130, and 1α, 25(OH)$_2$D$_3$ receptor-mediated pathways] are involved in the process of differentiation of postmitotic osteoclast precursors into functional osteoclasts. Signals mediated by cAMP are transduced by bone-resorbing factors such as PTH, PGE$_2$, and IL-1. Effect of IL-1 on osteoclast formation is mediated by a mechanism involving PGE$_2$. Cytokines such as IL-1, oncostatin M (OSM), and leukemia inhibitory factor (LIF), and a complex of a soluble IL-6 receptor (sIL-6R) and IL-6, stimulate osteoclast formation through a gp130-mediated signal-transducing pathway. Osteoclast formation induced by 1α, 25(OH)$_2$D$_3$ is independent of the mechanisms involving cAMP and gp130. The target cells for these osteotropic hormones and cytokines appear to be osteoblastic stromal cells. Signals induced by cAMP, gp130, and 1α, 25(OH)$_2$D$_3$ activate the same or an overlapping gene to induce an osteoclast differentiation factor(s), which is expressed in stromal cells to support osteoclast differentiation through a cell-to-cell interaction. (From Ref. 25. Reprinted with permission from Academic Press.)

osteoclasts as well as to induce osteoclastic differentiation in progenitor cells. However, the true measure of a mature osteoclast is its ability to carry out lacunar bone resorption in response to a host of signals, including the ones mentioned above, using V-type ATPases that pump protons to create the acid environment necessary for resorption of the lacuna (26). The osteoclast then employs matrix metalloproteinases (MMPs) and cysteine proteases to complement the matrix degradation and resorption process. These osteoclastic activities occur in a coordinated fashion with the osteoblastic activities to maintain the balance of bone resorption and degradation in the case of normal homeostasis. In tissue-engineered bone constructs, these same interactions will be responsible for construct maturation and longevity.

VI. CARTILAGE CELLS

Cartilage, like other tissues of the musculoskeletal system, possesses cells that progress from an undifferentiated phenotype (mesenchymal stem cell) to a mature matrix-producing phenotype (chondrocyte). Chondrocytes, similar to other differentiated cell types, have their own program of gene expression, which is understood to be under the control of transcription factors capable of inducing cartilage-specific genes. This allows the chondrocyte to exhibit unique properties, or markers, specific to its lineage, but at the same time also express markers that accompany other cells derived from mesenchyme. The expression of cartilage-specific genes leads to the assembly of a matrix with a high osmotic pressure, which in turn imparts key functional properties to foster smooth movement and shock-absorbing ability in joints. The chondrocytes produce this matrix in great abundance, yielding a tissue with a high matrix-to-cell ratio. This extracellular matrix is the platform for the physical interactions of water, and anionic proteoglycans within a retaining meshwork of collagens, which all work in concert to endow the tissue with its characteristic load-bearing properties (Fig. 4).

The primary collagen serving to scaffold the anionic molecules is type II, giving the extracellular matrix tensile strength and compressive stiffness. Aggrecan interacts with a strand of hyaluronan (HA) and the cartilage proteoglycan link protein to form large supramolecular aggregates embedded and trapped in the collagenous meshwork (27). The resulting fixed-negative-charge density, balanced by mobile counterions, gives rise to high osmotic pressures that are offset by the cross-linked collagen fibrils (28). Thus, water gives a swelling pressure to the tissue, which allows for compliance upon loading through the redistribution of water. In addition to the components already mentioned, mature chondrocytes also produce additional molecules that contribute to the cohesiveness of the matrix and the regulation of chondrocyte function, such as collagen types IX and XI, that cross-link and stabilize the fibrillar network. Additionally, collagen type VI is produced as a capsular matrix around the cell, which helps to modulate the osmotic and mechanical stresses induced by joint loading (29).

Since cartilage is an avascular tissue, the chondrocytes housed within cell-matrix units, termed chondrons, must receive nutrition via diffusion.

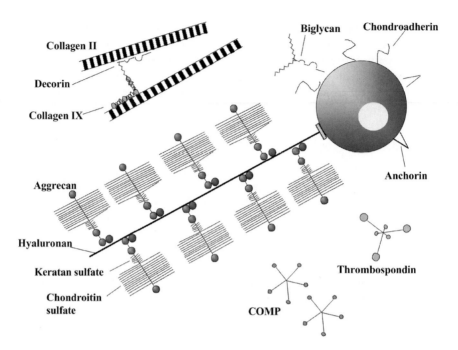

FIGURE 4 Schematic representation of the constituents of cartilage matrix. The predominant collagen, collagen type II, is decorated by the Decorin and further cross-linked by minor collagens, such as collagen type IX. In the cartilage matrix a fixed-negative-charge density, balanced by mobile counterions, gives rise to high osmotic pressures that are counteracted by the cross-linked collagen fibrils. Aggrecan interacts with a strand of hyaluronan and the cartilage proteoglycan Link protein to form supramolecular aggregates of large size embedded and trapped in the collagen meshwork. This ion trapping, coupled with the resulting hydrostatic pressure, conveys the exceptional ability of cartilage matrix to withstand compressive force. (Courtesy of Dr. Frank Barry.)

The oxygen tension in normal cartilage may be as low as 1-3% compared with the 20% found in the atmosphere (30). As a result, the chondrocyte survives in a relatively acidic environment and at a higher osmolarity than any other type of cell (31). Since they must respond to dynamic changes in hydrostatic pressure, their metabolic activities appear to be modulated through integrin and other adhesion mediators whereby oscillating loads stimulate matrix production, and static loads reduce the synthesis of aggrecan and link protein (32). To this end, joint immobilization causes a marked decrease in tissue proteoglycan content, resulting from both a decline in synthesis and an increase in catabolism of the matrix by the chondrocytes

(33). Therefore, the chondrocyte secretes a large amount of matrix with properties that allow for smooth articulation of the opposing bone ends against each other and this matrix is constantly monitored and regulated by the mature chondrocyte. However, even though the matrix is closely monitored, the postmitotic chondrocytes have a limited capacity for endogenous repair. Therefore, the major biological hurdle in constructing tissue-engineered cartilage revolves around the limited proliferation of chondrocytes themselves, and the requirement to provide all necessary nutrients in the absence of angiogenesis (i.e., by diffusion only).

VII. INTERVERTEBRAL DISC CELLS

The intervertebral disc is an important target for tissue engineering because the prevalence of disc pathology is an enormous problem facing orthopedics and neurosurgery. The annular cells or the periphery share some properties of tendon- and ligament-forming fibroblastic cells, and at the same time they share some characteristics of chondrocytes. The cells of the annulus produce type I collagen as the main fibril-forming collagen of the matrix, and the highest concentration of this collagen is localized within the outer lamellae. Type III collagen is also associated with the pericellular environment of the annular cells, as well as the nucleus pulposus cells (34). The annular cells serve an important structural role by secreting a matrix that provides significant tensile strength, thus serving to encapsulate the nucleus pulposus. The cells of the nucleus pulposus, like other chondrocytes, have a pericellular environment rich in collagen type IV, with collagen type II as the main fibril-forming collagen associated with its matrix (34). The large aggregating proteoglycan, aggrecan, is the major proteoglycan species in both the annulus and the nucleus pulposus; however, the small proteoglycans, biglycan and decorin, predominate in the annulus (34). While the precise characterization of intervertebral disc proteoglycans is still an active area of study, it is clear that there is considerable heterogeneity in proteoglycan type, molecular size, and topographic distribution within the disc. This variability is even further dispersed by disease and aging (35,36). As our understanding of these constituents improves, so will our ability to create functional tissue equivalents through bioengineering.

VIII. LIGAMENT- AND TENDON-FORMING FIBROBLASTS

Ligaments and tendons are characterized by closely packed fibers composed chiefly of collagen fibrils longitudinally aligned in the axis of tension, with flattened fibroblasts scattered between them. In adult life, the fibroblasts become relatively dormant and since the intercellular substance requires only nominal nutrition, blood supply is minimal. This reduced cell activity and turnover accounts for the inadequate natural response to injury, especially in the case of ligaments. Further complicating the healing response is the fact that the repair matrix secreted has to recreate the original organization and integrate with the old tissue for function to be restored. Important to the developing tissue is the application of mechanical forces, which help guide and mature the matrix secreted by the fibroblasts. The fibroblastic phenotype does not have a cadre of specific markers, and this appears to be one possible default differentiation pathway for mesenchymal cells. Such fibroblasts often secrete a disorganized matrix of collagen type I; however, the tendon- and ligament-forming fibroblasts are highly organized, spindle-shaped cells that produce collagen types I and III. These cells express varying compositions of fibronectin, tenascin, and elastin as they differentiate into mature tendons and ligaments.

Furthermore, tendons and ligaments contain primarily types I and XII collagen, which serve to coat and cross-link the type I collagen fibrils, thereby increasing the tensile strength of the tissue (37). The fibers are oriented parallel to the long axis in both tendons and ligaments, although compared to tendons, ligaments contain less total collagen and more proteoglycans and have a higher basal metabolic rate, a greater cellular density, a larger amount of reducible cross-links, and more collagen type III (38).

IX. MUSCLE CELLS

Skeletal muscle fibers arise from the fusion of precursor cells called myoblasts. Early progenitors of skeletal myoblasts migrate out from the somites, proliferate, and differentiate into mature, multinucleated striated muscle. The myoblasts differentiate from a multipotential cell in the mesoderm to eventually form myotubes. With further differentiation occurring under the control of the innervating nerve, there is the appearance of mature myofibers. The myoblast is a dividing cell, which can be identified as a member of the myogenic lineage by its expression of cell surface antigens that react with monoclonal antibodies such as L4 and the polyclonal antitensin antibody (39,40). Additionally, the myoblast can be identified by the expression of the muscle-specific intermediate filament protein known as desmin (41). The commitment to terminal differentiation by myogenic cells is dependent on the anchoring of integrin receptors on the myoblast (41). The basic helix-loop-helix transcription factors (bHLH), which include MyoD, Myf5, myogenin, and Mrf4, belong to the MyoD family and have been shown to induce a muscle-specific program of gene expression (42). With terminal differentiation and other stages of muscle development, diverse types of fast- and slow-twitch fibers are formed as a result of modulation of contractile protein isoforms, including actin and myosin. Each muscle fiber is, in fact, a thin and markedly elongated, multinucleated cell that varies tremendously in length depending upon the muscle in which it is situated. Interspersed within these structures are a small number of cells known as satellite cells, which act as progenitor cells, often in response to injury (43). The muscle fibers act as part of an interconnected network of fibers and neurons, which work in concert to orchestrate coordinated muscle contraction and locomotion.

X. MESENCHYMAL PROGENITOR CELLS

In many musculoskeletal tissues reside cells that are competent to respond to injury. These cells are often referred to as mesenchymal stem cells, although some local cells may only possess a limited genetic repertoire compared to the stem cell in bone marrow. The cells have no distinct morphology, other than that they are fibroblastic in appearance. Their molecular phenotype is characterized by a constellation of cell surface markers that are used in an experimental setting to identify their presence (44). Experimentally, the cells have been shown to possess extensive replicative capacity and to undergo differentiation under appropriate conditions into an ever-expanding list of mesenchymal cell types, including osteoblasts, chondrocytes, adipocytes, myoblasts, fibroblasts, tenocytes, and marrow stroma (Fig. 5). Mesenchymal stem cells are exceedingly difficult to identify in situ, in part because they represent roughly 0.001% of nucleated cells in bone marrow (1,14,15,44), and an even smaller proportion elsewhere. As a means of better understanding this interesting cell type, numerous laboratories have focused their efforts on isolating and cultivating these cells from bone marrow and other sources. Through these efforts, these cultured progenitor cells are now known to secrete an extracellular matrix rich in collagen types I and IV, fibronectin, and laminin, and can be identified in most cases by the SB-10, SH-2, SH-3, SH-4 and STRO-1 monoclonal antibodies (13–15,45). As the stem cell moves toward a more differentiated phenotype, it is the intrinsic genomic potential and the extrinsic local signaling cues that intersect at each lineage step to propel the immature cell through specific developmental pathways for each distinct tissue (46).

XI. FOUNDATIONS OF CELL-BASED TISSUE ENGINEERING STRATEGIES

Our collective objective is to create living tissue equivalents that serve to restore both organ function and form. This chapter reviews the paradigms

Controls   Differentiated

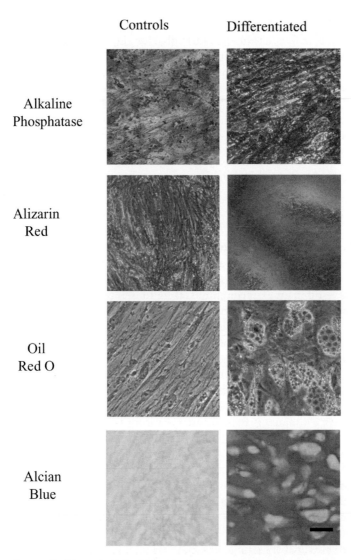

Alkaline
Phosphatase

Alizarin
Red

Oil
Red O

Alcian
Blue

FIGURE 5 Histochemical demonstration of the multiple-lineage potential of MSCs isolated by density gradient fractionation. Differentiated cells from the same population of mesenchymal stem cells were grown under appropriate conditions to differentiate the cell populations along the osteogenic, adipogenic, and chondrogenic lineages. Alkaline phosphatase and Alizarin red are selective for osteoblastic differentiation, while oil red O and Alcian blue are selective histochemical stains for adipogenesis and chondrogenesis, respectively. Bar = 10 μm.

needed to achieve these goals through the implantation of living cells from a variety of sources. This basic strategy is founded on the fact that cells are the synthetic machinery of tissues; they interact with, and produce, extracellular matrix through association with bioactive factors, other cells, and matrix molecules. In cell-based therapies, the goal is to replace the cellular machinery that has been lost to disease and/or trauma. Through these cell-based approaches one can expect to accelerate matrix deposition and overcome the possible limitations in endogenous cell activity, or number, associated with diseased or injured tissue. Therefore, success in cell-based therapy depends on two key elements: (1) an adequate number of responding cells with sufficient potential to respond to various stimuli, and (2) the appropriately coordinated spatial and temporal expression of these stimuli, including growth factors, nutrients, blood supply, and mechanical stresses or strains.

There is considerable flexibility in the selection of cell sources for repair of musculoskeletal dysfunction; however, the common thread is maintained by providing cells with sufficient machinery to repair or enhance biological function. Cells can be derived from the local environment, from the marrow, or from the invading blood supply when the appropriate cues are provided. Recruitment of cells, as in bone repair, can be enhanced by using growth factors with chemotactic properties such as recombinant human osteogenic protein-1 (rhOP-1) (47) or recombinant human bone morphogenetic protein-2 (BMP-2) (48,49). Cells may also be delivered in their precursor state. The bone marrow contains mesenchymal progenitor cells, often termed mesenchymal stem cells (MSCs), which can be readily harvested and cultured in an undifferentiated state and then induced to differentiate along several discreet mesodermal lineages (1,44). These MSCs can be delivered and directed to regenerate skeletal tissues through loading onto specific carriers (50,51), by providing exogenous growth factors in addition to the scaffold (52), or by transfecting specific genes into the cells to aid in differentiation (52,53). These insights came from earlier success in the use of marrow-containing progenitor cells, without ex vivo purification of the MSCs from the marrow. Unfractionated bone marrow contains MSCs, and as a result, delivery of whole bone marrow has been shown to offer clinical benefit in fracture repair and the treatment of nonunions (54,55).

XII. AUTOLOGOUS CELL SOURCES

The Carticel procedure (Genzyme Tissue Repair, Cambridge, MA) uses autologous chondrocytes for repair of articular cartilage defects (Fig. 6). This direct tissue source overcomes the problems associated with

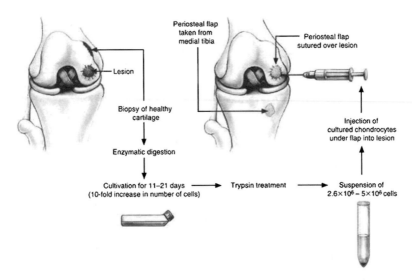

FIGURE 6 Carticel (Genzyme BioSurgery, Cambridge, MA) is the first FDA-approved cellular implant for the regeneration of musculoskeletal tissue. Shown are the steps involved in autologous chondrocyte transplantation. (From Ref. 56. Reprinted with permission from Massachusetts Medical Society.)

immunorejection of allograft materials. In this technique, chondrocytes are taken from a normal region of cartilage via biopsy, sent to a central processing facility for ex vivo replication, and then returned to the surgeon several weeks later for implantation into a cartilage defect during a second surgery (56). One key challenge of this mitotic expansion process is retention of the chondrocyte phenotype. That is, since chondrocytes from mature cartilage are not mitotically active, once they are stimulated to divide in vitro, they tend to lose their chondrocyte-specific function. A more detailed exposition of this technology is provided elsewhere in this book.

The Carticel approach is not the only strategy in musculoskeletal tissue repair that employs autologous cells. It does, however, serve as an example by which the patients' own cells can be integrated into the repair and regeneration of tissue. Variations in repair strategies include using cells that are manipulated intraoperatively and returned to the patient in the course of a single operation, as well as clinical attempts in which the cells are genetically engineered to express growth factors or other specific proteins to aid in the remediation of disease overall (57,58). Additionally, cells may be delivered as part of a cell-seeded product that is created in the laboratory prior to implantation, as was the case when an avulsed phalanx was replaced with tissue-engineered bone (59). The latter two strategies may incorporate autologous cells, but are not dependent upon them as the only source of reparative machinery. Alternatives to autologous therapy need to be further explored owing to several technical and logistical problems. The lengthy time and cumbersome procedures required to harvest the cells, culture the cells, and create an implant to suit the individual needs of each patient make it difficult for the economical development of readily available tissue products. The high cost and variability of each custom device has limited the clinical applicability of such products. For this reason, in part, alternatives such as allogeneic cell sources are being investigated aggressively, even though several autologous cell products are in clinical use today.

XIII. ALLOGENEIC CELL SOURCES

The major hurdle to overcome in allogeneic cell implantation, and to a greater extent in xenotransplantation, is graft rejection. Immunological rejection of allo- or xenograft tissue is T-cell-mediated destruction of the donor cells. Often in organ transplantation, passenger leukocytes accelerate the immune-mediated destruction by stimulating the expansion of donor-reactive T helper cells, which induce the cytotoxic T-cell response (60). In transfusions, leukocytes are filtered from donor blood to reduce the chance of an adverse reaction. Certain cell types of cells are strongly allostimulatory; for example, leukocytes and endothelial cells are two that are often found in organ transplantation to be immunogenic (61). These cell types constitutively express major histocompatibility complex (MHC) class I, II, and costimulatory molecules capable of stimulating naïve T cells, resulting in a cytotoxic-mediated immune reaction.

It is obvious that orthopedic tissue engineering will have little value if the therapy initiates the cascade of immune rejection. However, there are clinically applicable products in use that have overcome the obstacles presented by the immune system. Apligraf (Novartis Pharmaceuticals, East Hanover, NJ), an allogeneic skin replacement construct consisting of keratinocytes and fibroblasts, is one example of such a product. Cartilage repair may be achieved through autologous chondrocyte transplantation currently; however, emerging evidence in the field of mesenchymal stem cell biology indicates that allogeneic cells do not elicit a host immune response in experimental animal models. This may be the foundation for an allogeneic tissue regeneration therapy, with MSCs serving as a multipotential cell source, thus eliminating the need to harvest the patient's own cells and culture-expand them for several weeks prior to reimplantation.

The demand for an off-the-shelf therapy, as well as the high cost of producing a culture-expanded autologous product, will further drive the effort to make allogeneic cell sourcing a safe and efficacious tissue engineering strategy. However, in orthopedic tissue engineering, patient acceptance of an allogeneic product may be a barrier to implementation. In other, more life-threatening conditions, where disease progression leaves few therapeutic alternatives, the patient population may be more accepting of an allogeneic therapy. Once the medical community becomes more comfortable with this approach, allogeneic cell transplants may be used more broadly after screening for infectious agents, abnormal karyotype, tumorigenicity, phenotypic changes, and retention of tissue-forming ability. These measures could yield a product that is safer and more rigorously tested than what is traditionally used for blood and organ transplantation. In addition, sufficient quality controls could assure surgeons that the transplanted cells possess the regenerative potential necessary to recreate functional tissue. If these efforts can demonstrate a track record of both safety and efficacy, then the public will accept these therapeutic interventions.

XIV. IMMORTALIZED CELLS

Cells derived from immortalized cell lines, or from xenogeneic sources, are even less likely than allogeneic cells to have widespread clinical use and patient acceptance. Immortalized cells can replicate indefinitely, are often genetically pliable, and as such are good sources for gene transfer. On the other hand, they often have lost some measure of function and differentiation insofar as the normal regulatory controls on the cell cycle have been lifted. This loss of normal function is counterbalanced by the benefits of transferring one or more specific gene sequences to the immortalized cells. In this way, cells can be engineered directly to synthesize structural proteins, soluble bioactive factors that participate in a larger signal transduction cascade, or even intracellular regulatory proteins. In practice, cell lines serve as valuable in vitro models to study the function of specific genes and the effects of these gene products in vitro and in vivo. A principal concern in implanting cell lines is their propensity to exhibit characteristics of neoplastic cells, such as uncontrolled growth and tumor formation. Tissue engineering strategies must take into consideration appropriate precautions to protect against such potential risk. One solution is the cotransfer of genetic material that can be called upon to cause suicide in the host cell once expression of the inserted gene product is no longer required (62). Specific examples of tissue engineering strategies that

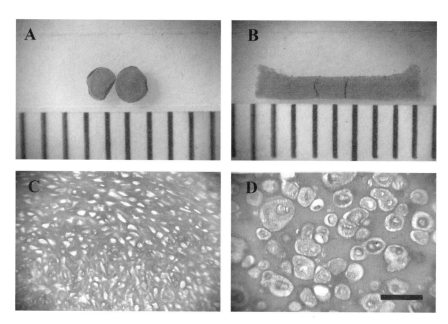

FIGURE 7 Histology demonstrating Alcian blue staining of the bone-marrow-derived cells induced to produce cartilage matrix in two different three-dimensional culture systems, in a cell pellet culture system (A), and in an alginate culture system (B), with (C) and (D) being higher-power views of the cartilage matrix. Growing the cells in a three-dimensional culture format fosters cartilage differentiation. Similar experiments in monolayer cultures do not support the cartilage phenotype or the production of cartilage-specific matrix. This illustrates the need in the case of cartilage tissue engineering for strategies to manipulate cells to enhance differentiation and prevent dedifferentiation. Both the alginate culture system and the cartilage pellet culture system facilitate the production of cartilage specific matrix; however, the histology in the alginate system (B, D) more closely resembles that of hyaline cartilage. In (A) and (B) the distance between each line is 1 mm, in (D) the bar = 50 μm.

employ such cells have been investigated in almost every musculoskeletal tissue, and are detailed in the subsequent chapters of this book.

XV. CELL MANIPULATION

Regardless of the cell source for tissue engineering, it is apparent that techniques must be optimized to enhance the number and/or function of implanted cells. These manipulations can take many forms, and may be as dramatic as genetic modification. They can also be more subtle, and

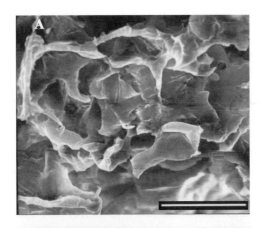

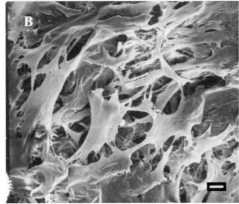

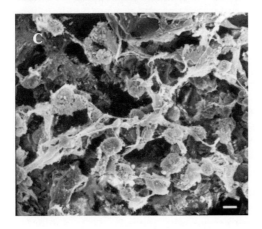

thus it may be potentially more difficult to quantify or predict their downstream effects, as is the case with extensive ex vivo cell proliferation prior to implantation in vivo. Culture expansion for a limited number of cycles for some cells, like mesenchymal stem cells, does not seem to lead to a loss of biosynthetic function or inherent potential to fully differentiate counterparts (44,63). However, chondrocytes are notorious for dedifferentiating in monolayer cell culture, thus acquiring a fibroblastic phenotype and altering their collagen expression patterns from type II to type I (64,65). Different strategies have evolved to grow chondrocytes in three-dimensional culture formats, which can prevent this dedifferentiation (Fig. 7). Still, in many instances, the chondrocyte phenotype cannot be maintained in cells whose number is rapidly expanded (66–69) (Fig. 8). Furthermore, following a period dedifferentiation, the cells are not as responsive to chondrogenic stimuli and do not produce as much cartilage-specific matrix as native chondroprogenitor cells (64,70,71).

Manipulations of cells can be chemically mediated, as is the case with growth factors, or they can be physical in nature. Combining cells with specific scaffolds, as will be discussed in other chapters of this book, confers both mechanical and geometrical stimuli, as well as chemical cues, that modulate cell function (Fig. 8). The application of "macro"-mechanical stress, strain, compression, and shear forces exert effects on the cell, regionally, as a whole or even on the entire cell population contained in a construct. Alternatively, "micro"-mechanical properties exert their effects on the cell cytoskeleton and can serve as inductive signals for further dynamic changes leading to matrix remodeling. Finally, the chemical foundation of these scaffolds can play a major role not only in the transduction of the gross physical signals, but through the delicate cell surface–scaffold

---

FIGURE 8 Scanning electron micrograph views of cells combined with two biodegradable scaffolds demonstrating that the matrix can manipulate the cells and be engineered to confer unique properties to the cells that are seeded into them. PLA scaffold alone (A), PLA seeded with bone-marrow-derived cells (B), and a PLA/alginate amalgam construct seeded with bone-marrow-derived cells (C) after 7 days in culture in defined medium that induces chondrogenic differentiation. Bone-marrow-derived cells in the PLA/alginate amalgam construct (C) exhibited a round cell shape and produced extracellular matrix. Bone-marrow-derived cells on plain PLA (B) appeared more spindle shaped and fibroblastic. In (A) bar = 100 μm; in (B, C) bar = 10 μm. (From Caterson EJ, Nesti LJ, Albert T, Vacarro A, Danielson K, Tuan RS. Three-dimensional cartilage formation by bone marrow-derived cells seeded in polylactide/alginate amalgam. J. Biomed Mater Res 2001; 57:394–403. Reprinted with permission from John Wiley and Sons.)

binding characteristics. These properties can be deliberately engineered to enhance tissue repair, as it is well known that mechanical stimuli of biological tissues can produce ultrastructural and histological variations. Tendon and ligament remodeling, like bone, depends upon the mechanical stress to which it is subjected in vivo (38,72). Therefore, it is possible to modulate tissue organization by dynamic or static mechanical stimuli in vitro for the production of specific bioengineered tissues (73,74).

XVI. CONCLUSION

In summary, there exists a wonderous diversity of cell types required for musculoskeletal morphogenesis, maintenance, and remodeling. Consequently, the cell-based strategies of tissue engineering are equally diverse. Cell biology studies aid in the design and optimization of tissue-engineered constructs. Since cells are the molecular machinery responsible for matrix production, deposition, maturation, and degradation, an appreciation of their control is a key ingredient in the recipe for creating therapeutic success. For example, regulation of appropriate matrix deposition, and the prevention of inappropriate degradation, are key control points in tissue repair. Exquisitely balanced matrix remodeling is of paramount importance in orthopedic tissue engineering because the rationale for cell-based therapy is to implant cells with the goal of rapidly creating a functional matrix that is properly integrated within the tissue as a whole.

Orthopedics is a discipline in which there exist obvious failures of the extracellular matrix. Indeed, the matrix originates from and is maintained by the cells normally housed in it; however, pathological matrix is the hallmark of disease. Methodologies and clear goals must be defined for each type of tissue restoration to replace the biomechanical functions of complex, and often composite, tissues in the musculoskeletal system. It is with further study of the cell biology and potential of various cell sources that rational cell-based interventions can become part of the practice of clinical orthopedics. This chapter has introduced the role of specialized cells and their functional relationships in the musculoskeletal system, and provided a general framework for the selection of cell sources used in repair.

A new breed of physicians will be practicing orthopedics in the future. These orthopedists will bring a knowledge of cell and molecular biology to their patient care efforts. They will understand the molecular mechanisms underlying orthopedic pathology, deformities, and diseases, and will know how to use biotechnology as an effective treatment modality (75). It seems likely that the basis for molecular orthopedics will be built partly by orthopedic scientists and partly by extension from the efforts of basic scientists in other areas of medicine and engineering. Given the extraordinary rate of new molecular, genetic, and cell biology discoveries, it seems reasonable to believe that the implants of tomorrow will resemble normal anatomical structures more than the plastic and metal of today. The foundation of this accomplishment will be therapeutic tissue engineering interventions that harness basic science to regenerate tissue that has been destroyed by disease and/or trauma.

REFERENCES

1. Caplan AI, Bruder, SP. Mesenchymal stem cells: building blocks for molecular medicine in the 21st century. Trends Mol Med 2001; 7:259–264.
2. Hunziker, EB. Mechanism of longitudinal bone growth and its regulation by growth plate chondrocytes. Microsc Res Tech 1994; 28:505–519.
3. Hurle JM, Ros MA, Ganan Y, Macias D, Critchlow M, Hinchliffe JR. Experimental analysis of the role of ECM in the patterning of the distal tendons of the developing limb bud. Cell Differ Dev 1990; 30:97–108.
4. Aubin JE, Liu F, Malaval L, Gupta AK. Osteoblast and chondroblast differentiation. Bone 1995; 17(suppl 2):S77–S83.
5. McCabe LR, Kockx M, Lian J, Stein J, Stein, G. Selective expression of fos- and jun-related genes during osteoblast proliferation and differentiation. Exp Cell Res 1995; 218:255–262.
6. Liu F, Aubin JE. Identification and characterization of preosteoblasts in the osteoblast differentiation sequence. J Bone Miner Res 1994; 9(suppl 1):S125.
7. Kano J, Sugimoto T, Kanatani M, Kuroki Y, Tsukamoto T, Fukase M, Chihara K. Second messenger signaling of c-fos gene induction by parathyroid hormone (PTH) and PTH-related peptide in osteoblastic osteosarcoma cells: its role in osteoblast proliferation and osteoclast-like cell formation. J Cell Physiol 1994; 161:358–366.
8. Lee K, Deeds JD, Chiba S, Un-No M, Bond AT, Segre GV. Parathyroid hormone induces sequential c-fos expression in bone cells in vivo: in situ localization of its receptor and c-fos messenger ribonucleic acids. Endocrinology 1994; 134:441–450.
9. Okazaki R, Ikeda K, Sakamoto A, Nakano T, Morimoto K, Kikuchi T, Urakawa K, Ogata E, Matsumoto T. Transcriptional activation of c-fos and c-jun protooncogenes by serum growth factors in osteoblast-like MC3T3-E1 cells. J Bone Miner Res 1992; 7:1149–1155.
10. Liu F, Malaval L, Gupta AK, Aubin JE. Simultaneous detection of multiple bone-related mRNAs and protein expression during osteoblast differentiation: polymerase chain reaction and immunocytochemical studies at the single cell level. Dev Biol 1994; 166:220–234.
11. Owen TA, Aronow MS, Barone LM, Bettencourt B, Stein GS, Lian JB. Pleiotropic effects of vitamin D on osteoblast gene expression are related to the proliferative and differentiated state of the bone cell phenotype: dependency upon basal levels of gene expression, duration of exposure, and bone matrix compe-

tency in normal rat osteoblast cultures. Endocrinology 1991; 128: 1496–1504.

12. Malaval L, Modrowski D, Gupta AK, Aubin JE. Cellular expression of bone-related proteins during in vitro osteogenesis in rat bone marrow stromal cell cultures. J Cell Physiol 1994; 158:555–572.

13. Bruder SP, Ricalton NS, Boynton RE, Connolly TJ, Jaiswal N, Zaia J, Barry FP. Mesenchymal stem cell surface antigen SB-10 corresponds to activated leukocyte cell adhesion molecule and is involved in osteogenic differentiation. J Bone Miner Res 1998; 13:655–663.

14. Gronthos S, Graves SE, Ohta S, Simmons PJ. The STRO-1+ fraction of adult human bone marrow contains the osteogenic precursors. Blood 1994; 84: 4164–4173.

15. Haynesworth SE, Baber MA, Caplan AI. Cell surface antigens on human marrow-derived mesenchymal cells are detected by monoclonal antibodies. Bone 1992; 13:69–80.

16. Bruder SP, Caplan AI. Osteogenic cell lineage analysis is facilitated by organ cultures of embryonic chick periosteum. Dev Biol 1990; 141:319–329.

17. Hughes DE, Salter DM, Simpson R. CD44 expression in human bone: a novel marker of osteocytic differentiation. J Bone Miner Res 1994; 9:39–44.

18. Nakamura H, Kenmotsu S, Sakai H, Ozawa H. Localization of CD44, the hyaluronate receptor, on the plasma membrane of osteocytes and osteoclasts in rat tibiae. Cell Tissue Res 1995; 280:225–233.

19. Aarden EM, Burger EH, Nijweide PJ. Function of osteocytes in bone. J Cell Biochem 1994; 55:287–299.

20. Aarden EM, Wassenaar AM, Nijweide PJ. Extracellular matrix protein synthesis by osteocytes. J Bone Miner Res 1994; 9(suppl 1):S168.

21. Hirota S, Takaoka K, Hashimoto J, Nakase T, Takemura T, Morii E, Fukuyama A, Morihana K, Kitamura Y, Nomura S. Expression of mRNA of murine bone-related proteins in ectopic bone induced by murine bone morphogenetic protein-4. Cell Tissue Res 1994; 277:27–32.

22. Udagawa N, Takahashi N, Akatsu T, Tanaka H, Sasaki T, Nishihara T, Koga T, Martin TJ, Suda T. Origin of osteoclasts: mature monocytes and macrophages are capable of differentiating into osteoclasts under a suitable microenvironment prepared by bone marrow-derived stromal cells. Proc Natl Acad Sci USA 1990; 87:7260–7264.

23. Roodman GD, Kurihara N, Ohsaki Y, Kukita A, Hosking D, Demulder A, Smith JF, Singer FR. Interleukin 6: a potential autocrine/paracrine factor in Paget's disease of bone. J Clin Invest 1992; 89:46–52.

24. Akatsu T, Takahashi N, Debari K, Morita I, Murota S, Nagata N, Takatani O, Suda T. Prostaglandins promote osteoclastlike cell formation by a mechanism involving cyclic adenosine 3′,5′-monophosphate in mouse bone marrow cell cultures. J Bone Miner Res 1989; 4:29–35.

25. Suda T, Udawaga N, Takahashi, N. Cells of bone: osteoclast generation. In: Bilezikian JP, Raisz LG, Rodan GA, eds. Principles of Bone Biology. New York: Academic Press, 1996:87–102.

26. Bekker PJ, Gay CV. Biochemical characterization of an electrogenic vacuolar proton pump in purified chicken osteoclast plasma membrane vesicles. J Bone Miner Res 1990; 5:569–579.

27. Hardingham TE, Fosang A, Dudhia J. Aggrecan the chondroitin sulfate/keratan sulfate proteoglycan from cartilage. In: Knuettner KE, Schleyerbach JG, Peyron G, Hascall VC, eds. Articular Cartilage and Osteoarthritis. New York: Raven Press 1992:5–20.

28. Mow VC, Holmes MH, Lai WM. Fluid transport and mechanical properties of articular cartilage: a review. J Biomech 1984; 17:377–394.

29. Poole CA. The chondron and its pericellular environment. In: Knuettner KE, Schleyerbach JG, Peyron G, Hascall VC, eds. Articular Cartilage and Osteoarthritis. New York: Raven Press 1992:201–220.

30. Brighton CT, Heppenstall RB. Oxygen tension in zones of the epiphyseal plate, the metaphysis and diaphysis: an in vitro and in vivo study in rats and rabbits. J Bone Joint Surg Am 1971; 53:719–728.

31. Urban JP, Hall AC, Gehl KA. Regulation of matrix synthesis rates by the ionic and osmotic environment of articular chondrocytes. J Cell Physiol 1993; 154:262–270.

32. Kim YJ, Sah RL, Grodzinsky AJ, Plaas AH, Sandy JD. Mechanical regulation of cartilage biosynthetic behavior: physical stimuli. Arch Biochem Biophys 1994; 311:1–12.

33. Palmoski M, Perricone E, Brandt KD. Development and reversal of a proteoglycan aggregation defect in normal canine knee cartilage after immobilization. Arthritis Rheum 1979; 22:508–517.

34. Urban JP, Roberts S. Development and degeneration of the intervertebral discs. Mol Med Today 1995; 1:329–335.

35. Johnstone B, Bayliss MT. The large proteoglycans of the human intervertebral disc: changes in their biosynthesis and structure with age, topography, and pathology. Spine 1995; 20:674–684.

36. Oegema TR Jr. Biochemistry of the intervertebral disc. Clin Sports Med 1993; 12:419–439.

37. Davison PF. The contribution of labile crosslinks to the tensile behavior of tendons. Connect Tissue Res 1989; 18:293–305.

38. Amiel D, Frank C, Harwood F, Fronek J, Akeson W. Tendons and ligaments: a morphological and biochemical comparison. J Orthop Res 1984; 1:257–265.

39. Bockholt SM, Otey CA, Glenney JR Jr., Burridge K. Localization of a 215-kDa tyrosine-phosphorylated protein that cross-reacts with tensin antibodies. Exp Cell Res 1992; 203:39–46.

40. George-Weinstein M, Decker C, Horwitz A. Combinations of monoclonal antibodies distinguish mesenchymal, myogenic, and chondrogenic precursors of the developing chick embryo. Dev Biol 1988; 125:34–50.

41. Boettiger D, George-Weinstein M, Menko SA. Triggering terminal myogenic differentiation. Disord Voluntary Muscle 1989:57–66.

42. Rudnicki MA, Jaenisch R. The MyoD family of transcription factors and skeletal myogenesis. Bioessays 1995; 17:203–209.

43. Schultz E, McCormick KM. Skeletal muscle satellite cells. Rev Physiol Biochem Pharmacol 1994; 123:213–257.
44. Pittenger MF, Mackay AM, Beck SC, Jaiswal RK, Douglas R, Mosca JD, Moorman MA, Simonetti DW, Craig S, Marshak DR. Multilineage potential of adult human mesenchymal stem cells. Science 1999; 284:143–147.
45. Friedenstein AJ, Chailakhyan RK, Gerasimov UV. Bone marrow osteogenic stem cells: in vitro cultivation and transplantation in diffusion chambers. Cell Tissue Kinet 1987; 20:263–272.
46. Caplan AI. Mesenchymal stem cells. J Orthop Res 1991; 9:641–650.
47. Cook SD, Dalton JE, Tan EII, Whitecloud TS, Rueger DC. In vivo evaluation of recombinant human osteogenic protein (rhOP-1) implants as a bone graft substitute for spinal fusions. Spine 1994; 19:1655–1663.
48. Reddi AH, Anderson WA. Collagenous bone matrix-induced endochondral ossification hemopoiesis. J Cell Biol 1976; 69:557–572.
49. Zegzula HD, Buck DC, Brekke J, Wozney JM, Hollinger JO. Bone formation with use of rhBMP-2 (recombinant human bone morphogenetic protein-2). J Bone Joint Surg Am 1997; 79:1778–1790.
50. Ohgushi H, Caplan AI. Stem cell technology and bioceramics: from cell to gene engineering. J Biomed Mater Res 1999; 48:913–927.
51. Bruder SP, Kurth AA, Shea M, Hayes WC, Jaiswal N, Kadiyala, S. Bone regeneration by implantation of purified, culture-expanded human mesenchymal stem cells. J Orthop Res 1998; 16:155–162.
52. Lieberman JR, Le LQ, Wu L, Finerman GA, Berk A, Witte ON, Stevenson S. Regional gene therapy with a BMP-2-producing murine stromal cell line induces heterotopic and orthotopic bone formation in rodents. J Orthop Res 1998; 16:330–339.
53. Noshi T, Yoshikawa T, Ikeuchi M, Dohi Y, Ohgushi H, Horiuchi K, Sugimura M, Ichijima K, Yonemasu K. Enhancement of the in vivo osteogenic potential of marrow/hydroxyapatite composites by bovine bone morphogenetic protein. J Biomed Mater Res 2000; 52:621–630.
54. Connolly JF, Guse R, Tiedeman J, Dehne R. Autologous marrow injection as a substitute for operative grafting of tibial nonunions. Clin Orthop 1991:259–270.
55. Cummine J, Armstrong L, Nade S. Osteogenesis after bone and bone marrow transplantation: studies of cellular behaviour using combined myeloosseous grafts in the subscorbutic guinea pig. Acta Orthop Scand 1983; 54:235–241.
56. Brittberg M, Lindahl A, Nilsson A, Ohlsson C, Isaksson O, Peterson L. Treatment of deep cartilage defects in the knee with autologous chondrocyte transplantation. N Engl J Med 1994; 331:889–895.
57. Oakes DA, Lieberman JR. Osteoinductive applications of regional gene therapy: ex vivo gene transfer. Clin Orthop Rel Res 2000; 379(Suppl):S101–112.
58. Oligino T, Ghivizzani S, Wolfe D, Lechman E, Krisky D, Mi Z, Evans C, Robbins P, Glorioso J. Intra-articular delivery of a herpes simplex virus IL-1Ra gene vector reduces inflammation in a rabbit model of arthritis. Gene Ther 1999; 6:1713–1720.

59. Vacanti CA, Bonassar LJ, Vacanti MP, Shufflebarger J. Replacement of an avulsed phalanx with tissue-engineered bone. N Engl J Med 2001; 344:1511–1514.

60. Adams PW, Lee HS, Ferguson RM, Orosz CG. Alloantigenicity of human endothelial cells. II. Analysis of interleukin 2 production and proliferation by T cells after contact with allogeneic endothelia. Transplantation 1994; 57:115–122.

61. Pober JS, Collins T, Gimbrone MA Jr., Libby, P, Reiss CS. Inducible expression of class II major histocompatibility complex antigens and the immunogenicity of vascular endothelium. Transplantation 1986; 41:141–146.

62. Kobayashi N, Noguchi H, Totsugawa T, Watanabe T, Matsumura T, Fujiwara T, Miyazaki M, Fukaya K, Namba M, Tanaka N. Insertion of a suicide gene into an immortalized human hepatocyte cell line. Cell Transplant 2001; 10:373–376.

63. Bruder SP, Jaiswal N, Haynesworth SE. Growth kinetics, self-renewal, and the osteogenic potential of purified human mesenchymal stem cells during extensive subcultivation and following cryopreservation. J Cell Biochem 1997; 64:278–294.

64. Benya PD, Shaffer JD. Dedifferentiated chondrocytes reexpress the differentiated collagen phenotype when cultured in agarose gels. Cell 1982; 30:215–224.

65. Bonaventure J, Kadhom N, Cohen-Solal L, Ng KH, Bourguignon J, Lasselin C, Freisinger P. Reexpression of cartilage-specific genes by dedifferentiated human articular chondrocytes cultured in alginate beads. Exp Cell Res 1994; 212:97–104.

66. Paige KT, Cima LG, Yaremchuk MJ, Schloo BL, Vacanti JP, Vacanti CA. De novo cartilage generation using calcium alginate-chondrocyte constructs. Plast Reconstr Surg 1996; 97:168–178; discussion 179–180.

67. Marijnissen WJ, van Osch GJ, Aigner J, Verwoerd-Verhoef HL, Verhaar JA. Tissue-engineered cartilage using serially passaged articular chondrocytes. Chondrocytes in alginate, combined in vivo with a synthetic (E210) or biologic biodegradable carrier (DBM). Biomaterials 2000; 21:571–580.

68. Gruber HE, Fisher EC Jr., Desai B, Stasky AA, Hoelscher G, Hanley EN Jr. Human intervertebral disc cells from the annulus: three-dimensional culture in agarose or alginate and responsiveness to TGF-beta1. Exp Cell Res 1997; 235:13–21.

69. Diduch DR, Jordan LC, Mierisch CM, Balian G. Marrow stromal cells embedded in alginate for repair of osteochondral defects. Arthroscopy 2000; 16:571–577.

70. Gagne TA, Chappell-Afonso K, Johnson JL, McPherson JM, Oldham CA, Tubo RA, Vaccaro C, Vasios GW. Enhanced proliferation and differentiation of human articular chondrocytes when seeded at low cell densities in alginate in vitro. J Orthop Res 2000; 18:882–890.

71. Marijnissen WJ, van Osch GJ, Aigner J, Verwoerd-Verhoef HL, Verhaar JA. Tissue-engineered cartilage using serially passaged articular chondrocytes.

Chondrocytes in alginate, combined in vivo with a synthetic (E210) or biologic biodegradable carrier (DBM). Biomaterials 2000; 21:571–580.

72.   Young RG, Butler DL, Weber W, Caplan AI, Gordon SL, Fink DJ. Use of mesenchymal stem cells in a collagen matrix for Achilles tendon repair. J Orthop Res 1998; 16:406–413.

73.   Huang D, Chang TR, Aggarwal A, Lee RC, Ehrlich HP. Mechanisms and dynamics of mechanical strengthening in ligament- equivalent fibroblast-populated collagen matrices. Ann Biomed Eng 1993; 21:289–305.

74.   Langelier E, Rancourt D, Bouchard S, Lord C, Stevens PP, Germain L, Auger FA. Cyclic traction machine for long-term culture of fibroblast-populated collagen gels. Ann Biomed Eng 1999; 27:67–72.

75.   Gartland JJ. A challenge for orthopedic surgeons. J Bone Joint Surg Am 1982; 64:159–160.

4

Intraoperative Harvest and Concentration of Human Bone Marrow Osteoprogenitors for Enhancement of Spinal Fusion

James E. Fleming, Jr., George F. Muschler, Cynthia Boehm, Isador H. Lieberman, and Robert F. McLain

The Cleveland Clinic Foundation,
Cleveland, Ohio, U.S.A.

I. INTRODUCTION

Bone marrow harvested by aspiration contains connective tissue progenitor cells (CTPs) that contribute to the efficacy of bone grafts. Bone marrow can be aspirated from the iliac crest with minimal morbidity, in contrast to traditional harvest of autogenous graft. Many investigators are studying additional methods to increase the number and procurement sources of CTPs for a variety of orthopedic tissue engineering uses. Spinal fusion rates using allograft alone do not approach that of autograft, in part owing to a deficiency of local CTPs. Methods that increase the concentration and prevalence of these osteogenic cells have been shown to further enhance bone formation in spinal fusion.

Recent studies have shown that bone-marrow-derived cells and CTPs can be rapidly concentrated using the surface of a porous implantable matrix as an affinity column. Composite cellular grafts prepared in this fashion deliver an increased concentration of CTPs to the graft site, compared with fresh marrow alone, and improve bone formation and bone union. An additional approach under investigation utilizes the vertebral body at the time of preparation for pedicle screw insertion. Bone marrow aspirated from this site can serve as a supplemental source of osteoblastic progenitors when marrow available from the pelvis is compromised by prior surgery or irradiation, and may reduce the magnitude and morbidity of surgical intervention.

In this chapter we will review the cell biological principles of intraoperative enhancement of CTPs, and will report a current clinical application in a human pilot study in which allograft bone is augmented with autogenous bone marrow aspirate for lumbar interbody fusion. Furthermore, we will review the technique of vertebral marrow aspiration during pedicle screw preparation. These methods underscore how tissue engineering is rapidly becoming a clinical reality in orthopedic spine surgery. Methods under current evaluation may obviate the need for traditional autogenous iliac crest graft.

Classic bone grafting techniques are used in over 1 million procedures each year in the United States, and approximately one half of these applications involve spinal fusion (1). Autogenous bone harvested from iliac crest continues to be the gold standard in lumbar fusion with up to 95% fusion rates (2–5). However, the procurement of autogenous bone comes at a significant cost. Complications and morbidity related to harvest of the autogenous bone graft from the iliac crest donor site can approach 30%, and include chronic pain, blood loss, wound problems, infection, and pelvic fractures (6,7). As a result of these problems arising from the use of autogenous grafts, clinicians and scientists have had a significant interest in developing alternatives to autogenous bone.

Allograft bone has historically been a widely used alternative to autograft. Allograft bone can be procured in essentially unlimited quantities and provides both osteoconductive and some osteoinductive properties while avoiding the morbidity of autograft harvest. However, the clinical effectiveness is generally inferior to autograft, manifest by an increased risk of nonunion, refracture, infection, and graft resorption. In addition, allograft processing is expensive, and there is a small but genuine risk of immune reaction and disease transmission associated with allografts (8). Finally, spinal fusion rates with allograft alone do not approach that of autograft, in posterolateral or lumbar interbody fusion (4,9,10). The compromised biological efficacy of allograft may in part be related to a deficiency in the local population of osteoprogenitors. Methods that amplify the number or concentration of osteoprogenitors within the graft site may enhance spinal fusion in a variety of clinical settings.

II. FACTORS AFFECTING SPINAL FUSION

Several well-established biological principles are germane to the success of bone grafting during spinal fusion, and the manipulation and augmentation of these variables are the focus of many tissue engineering approaches. The factors critical to the success of spinal fusion include the presence of osteogenic cells, an osteoconductive environment, appropriate osteo-inductive signals, an appropriate mechanical environment, and vascularity and host-related factors. Since clinical bone grafting strategies for spinal fusion involve the manipulation or augmentation of one or several of these core concepts, each of these entities is briefly reviewed below.

A. Osteogenic Cells

Bone tissue formation requires a sufficient number of *osteogenic cells* at the wound-healing site to promote the osseous repair. These cells can be either stem cells, progenitor cells, or osteoblastic cells that are capable of forming new bone. In young individuals, or in some tissue beds, such as healthy can-cellous bone or periosteum, these cells may be relatively abundant. In these cases, simply providing an effective osteoconductive matrix may be suffi-cient to initiate an effective bone healing response. Unfortunately, there are many clinical settings in which there are likely to be a locally deficient number and concentration of osteoblastic progenitors (11). Examples include large-bone defects, sites containing extensive scar tissue from pre-vious surgery or trauma, sites of previous infection or radiation, sites of nonunion, regions of osteonecrosis or other osseous disease states, loca-tions of compromised vascularity, and patients compromised by systemic illness, nutritional or immune system compromise, or pharmacological toxicity. In addition, recent data have shown that human aging is associated with a significant diminution in the number or prevalence of osteoprogeni-tors (12). Optimizing the chances of success in these situations may require augmentation of the local population of stem cells and progenitors.

B. Osteoconductive Environment

Osteoconduction can be defined as a scaffold function of a graft material or matrix that facilitates the attachment, migration, and proliferation of osteogenic cells, and therefore the distribution of the bone healing response through the desired volume. Allograft bone matrix also has osteoconductive properties, whether used as a structural graft or as minera-lized or demineralized chips, fibers, granules, or powder. Many synthetic graft matrices also have osteoconductive properties, including hydroxyapa-tite and tricalcium phosphate ceramics, and porous surfaces of titanium, tantalum, and cobalt chrome alloy. Osteoconductive properties are often mediated through specific interactions between cells and the chemical sur-face of the material. For example, allograft matrix contains many molecules that serve as adhesion ligands for extracellular matrix proteins such as integrin receptors that are present on cells. Examples of osteoconductive matrices in use for bone grafting or spinal fusion applications include ceramic matrices, allografts such as demineralized bone matrix or cortical cancellous chips, hydroxyapatite, corals, synthetic collagen, calcium sulfate salts, ceramic cements, degradable polymers, hyaluronic acid, and customized composites.

C. Osteoinductive Environment

Osteoinduction is a term that has evolved in recent years to refer to properties of various biological stimuli that induce proliferation, migration, or differ-entiation of osteoblastic cells. The classic osteoinductive stimuli are mem-bers of the family of bone morphogenetic proteins (BMPs), particularly BMP-2, BMP-4, BMP-6, and BMP-7 (a.k.a osteogenic protein-1, or OP-1) (13). Additional growth factors and cytokines that are known to influence the activation, proliferation, migration, and differentiation of osteogenic cells may become useful clinically as local agents, including epidermal growth factor (EGF), platelet-derived growth factors (PDGFs), basic fibroblast growth factor (FGF), transforming growth factor beta (TGF-β), IGFs, and parathyroid hormone (PTH) (14). Most of these factors are present in and/or released during remodeling of bone matrix or frac-ture hematoma. They can also be delivered on the surface of synthetic matrices or through the degradation of synthetic matrices, with appropri-ate chemical properties (15). For example, BMP-2 in a fibrillar collagen delivery system has been used in spinal fusion and is currently being eval-uated in a human clinical trial (16).

D. Mechanical Environment

The *mechanical environment* in a wound site or site of bone tissue engineering has a profound effect on the success or failure of the local bone healing response. Bone formation is promoted in a mechanically stable environ-ment, e.g., less than 2–3% strain (17). Greater amounts of micromotion and undesirable tissue strain may promote the formation of a fibrocartilaginous repair tissue, leading to pseudoarthrosis (11). The advent of rigid internal fixation for fractures and the improvement in spinal fusion rates associated with more rigid pedicle screw fixation reaffirm the validity of this principle.

E. Vascularity and Host Factors

Meticulous preparation of the graft site tissue bed, including the maintenance of a satisfactory blood supply, is mandatory in spinal fusion even in the face of maximized osteogenic, osteoconductive, and osteoinductive properties. The process of angiogenesis and revascularization promotes transport of oxygen and nutrients to the repair site, delivers inflammatory cells and stimulatory factors for bone healing, and acts as a conductive pathway for endothelial cells and osteoblastic progenitors. This response can be augmented by several growth factors, including basic fibroblast growth factor (FGF-2) and vascular endothelial growth factor (VEGF), as well as through effects mediated by fibrin split products formed by the breakdown of local fibrin clot.

Optimization of host factors is also germane to the success of bone grafting applications. Health and nutritional status should be optimized preoperatively, including the avoidance of harmful pharmacological agents and the cessation of smoking (18).

An understanding of the factors that affect spine fusion has led to a variety of tissue engineering strategies to manipulate cells, cytokines, or specific matrices alone or in combination to provide alternatives to autogenous grafts. Examples in use or under investigation include bone marrow aspiration, allograft, customized ceramic matrices, collagen, degradable polymers, the delivery of local osteoinductive factors such as BMPs, culture expansion of selected cells, and various gene therapy approaches. Although it is clear that there has been an expanding number and diversity of available materials and products for the surgeon to consider to enhance or stimulate the site of spinal fusion, it is useful to remind ourselves that fundamental biological principles must remain constant. One of the most basic and fundamental of these principles is that, when it comes to the formation or regeneration of any tissue, including bone, *cells* do all the work. No unique prosthetic surface, no matrix, no growth factor, no medication is capable of forming new bone. None of these tools or agents has any influence on bone formation, except through the specific effects that it has on the biological behavior of cells. Of particular importance is the small subset of stem cells and progenitor cells that are capable of generating new bone tissue. A sufficient and competent population of osteogenic progenitor cells in the graft site is mandatory, since the implantation of an osteoconductive material or delivery of a bioactive osteoinductive stimulus alone would be entirely ineffective in the absence of local cells capable of bone formation. Recognizing this fact, the authors have evaluated an intraoperative spinal fusion strategy that aims to amplify and concentrate the number of osteoprogenitor cells at the fusion site to enhance local bone formation and potentially eliminate the need for autogenous graft harvest. In addition, alternative repositories to enhance the number of osteoprogenitor cells to a graft site, such as bone marrow obtained during preparation for transpedicular screw fixation, are under study.

III. CONNECTIVE TISSUE PROGENITORS

Pleuripotential progenitor cells from bone marrow have been referred to by a variety of names, including mechanocytes, bone marrow stromal cells, mesenchymal stem cells, and colony-forming units fibroblastic. We use the term connective tissue progenitors (CTPs) to define the population of cells that can be harvested from bone marrow or other tissues and are capable of proliferating and differentiating into one or more connective tissue phenotypes (19,20). These cells are required for applications in orthopedic tissue engineering since only cells with this biological potential can form the desired connective tissue in a graft site. A variety of cell culture systems for isolation and characterization of these cells and their osteogenic progeny exist, including several molecular markers for distinct stages of the osteogenic pathway (21–24). Furthermore, assays for CTPs that proliferate and subsequently differentiate into the osteogenic phenotype can be readily accomplished using colony-forming unit assays in vitro (25). These assays have been used as a practical means of studying the clinical variables associated with the significant differences in concentration and prevalence of osteoblastic CTPs between individuals (e.g., age, gender, disease, pharmacological agents) (26). They have also been effective in the clinical evaluation of methods for selection of CTPs for bone and tissue grafting (27,28).

To provide a low-risk biological adjuvant and to supplement the osteogenic capacity of bone graft, some surgeons have procured bone marrow aspirated from the iliac crest (29). The value of bone marrow as a graft has been supported by many studies (30–32). Connolly et al. reported successful treatment of 18 of 20 tibial nonunions treated closed or with intramedullary nails plus percutaneous injection of nonheparinized bone marrow (31). In a separate experiment using a rabbit diffusion chamber model, Connolly et al. reported that concentration of the progenitor population by gradient centrifugation could increase the amount of bone formed after transplantation (30). Information that has guided surgeons on the technical considerations to optimize the use of bone-marrow-derived osteoprogenitors has yet to reveal any significant morbidity or complications, and has shown that a 2-mL aspiration volume minimizes the undesirable effect of dilution by peripheral blood seen in larger aspirate volumes (26). Further improvements in harvest and delivery of connective tissue progenitors are likely to significantly increase the efficacy of bone-marrow-derived grafts. This improvement may in part be achieved by the development of carrier matrices that improve the concentration of these progenitors (28).

Muschler et al. have observed that connective tissue progenitors and other bone-marrow-derived cells can be rapidly concentrated from bone marrow aspirates using selected materials that have surface properties to which osteoblastic progenitors will rapidly attach (28). Allograft bone matrix is a material found to demonstrate this property. Recent studies have shown that bone-marrow-derived cells and CTPs can be rapidly concentrated using the surface of the porous implantable allograft matrix as an affinity column. Composite cellular grafts prepared in this fashion deliver an increased concentration of CTPs to the graft site, compared with fresh marrow alone, and improve bone formation and bone union. Using a canine posterior spinal fusion model, Muschler et al. have reported an improved frequency and quality of union when the concentration of bone-marrow-derived connective-tissue progenitors was increased (27,28).

Improvements may also be achieved through alternative methods for harvesting osteoprogenitor cells with little morbidity or alteration in surgical technique. The vertebral body represents a potential reservoir of CTPs, which cannot typically be tapped during spinal surgery or instrumentation. The mechanical harvesting of autogenous bone graft requires the removal of structurally important bone from the harvest site. If the iliac crest is harvested, there is usually no impact on skeletal integrity, as the site is non-weight-bearing and remote from the area requiring reconstruction. If, however, structural bone were removed from the vertebral body, the stability of the site being surgically treated would be further compromised, even as the surgeon was trying to mechanically reinforce it.

However, the potential for harvesting CTPs through a marrow aspiration, as opposed to a trabecular bone harvest, allows us to reconsider the vertebral body as a source of CTPs for use in spinal fusion augmenting elements. The vertebral body is a reservoir of hematopoietic marrow. There is, therefore, reason to expect that pleuripotential stem cells and CTPs will be found in abundance comparable to that seen within the iliac crest. Initial studies have suggested that this is true, and that aspiration of marrow elements can be carried out effectively without altering the technique for pedicle screw placement.

In summary, even in settings where the osteoconductive and osteoinductive properties of the graft site are optimized, bone formation at the site is entirely dependent on having a sufficient number of connective-tissue progenitor cells. There are a variety of clinical settings in which the number of osteoblastic progenitor cells is suboptimal, a concept that is strongly supported by extensive animal and clinical data that indicate the addition of bone-marrow-derived cells to osteoconductive or osteoinductive materials results in a significant improvement in efficacy. Evidence of the importance of optimizing the number of osteoprogenitors is also seen in the large differences in lumbar fusion rates using autogenous bone graft compared to allograft (10,33). Although autologous bone currently remains the most effective bone graft for use in spine fusion, significant morbidity is associated with the harvest procedure (34,35).

IV. ONGOING INVESTIGATIONS

We believe that optimizing the efficacy of bone grafting procedures in most common clinical settings will require some means of enhancing the number of local CTPs. Since it is clear that amplifying the concentration of CTPs on selected matrices improves the quality of spinal fusion in animal models, one method under investigation evaluates whether CTPs in bone marrow harvested from the iliac crest by aspiration can be concentrated intraoperatively using selected allograft matrices and used to achieve a high rate of clinical success. This question is being assessed in a human clinical pilot study of lumbar interbody fusion procedures. Identification and characterization of additional potential sources of osteoblastic progenitor cells is also necessary. Therefore, an additional investigation involves the harvest of CTPs from bone marrow from the vertebral body at the time of preparation for pedicle screw fixation. Transpedicular bone marrow aspiration may reduce the magnitude of surgical intervention, reduce surgical time and blood loss, and provide cells for graft procedures of equal or greater biological capabilities than conventional iliac crest bone marrow for enhancement of spinal fusion. The vertebral body bone marrow may also serve as an alternative source of osteoblastic progenitors for patients when marrow that may be available from the pelvis is compromised by prior surgery or irradiation. These combined efforts may result in reduced surgical morbidity and may obviate the need for autogenous iliac crest graft harvest procedures entirely.

A. Aspiration of the Vertebral Body
During Pedicle Preparation

Segmental pedicle screw fixation has become a mainstay of surgical fixation of the spinal column and has been indicated for reconstruction of spinal tumors, stabilization following osteotomies, posttraumatic spinal injuries or spondylarthropathy, isthmic and degenerative spondylisthesis, acquired hypermobility above or below a previously fused segment, or for repair and stabilization of lumbar pseudoarthrosis (36). The methods of anatomical preparation and technical placement of the pedicle screw have been previously published (36,37). Briefly, after breaching of the laminar cortex with a standard starter awl, the Tuhey needle and trochar are driven coaxially down the center of the pedicle until the tip is 3.5 cm deep to the lamina. The central trochar is removed and 2.0 mL of marrow is aspirated. The trochar is then reinserted and the needle driven 1.0 cm deeper for the second aspirate. The needle is then withdrawn and a standard pedicle probe passed down the pilot hole to prepare for screw placement. Screws and instrumentation constructs are then placed in the usual fashion.

Osteoblastic Progenitor Assay

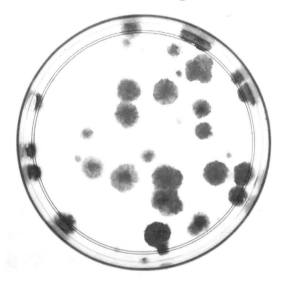

Stained for alkaline phosphatase

FIGURE 1 Osteoblastic progenitor assay. Human bone marrow aspirates are placed into culture and a subpopulation of fibroblastic cells attaches, and rapidly proliferates to form colonies. These initial colonies, called colony-forming units-fibroblastic, are stained with the osteoblastic marker alkaline phosphatase and quantitated to allow an estimate of connective-tissue progenitors.

The described methodology allows for aspiration of a total of 8 mL of vertebral body bone marrow and CTPs assuming tandem pedicle screw placement for each vertebral level. The present study involves direct comparison of the prevalence of CTPs in vertebral body marrow by harvesting control aspirates from the iliac crest in the standard fashion (26). The number of nucleated cells and CTPs is determined through published techniques using a colony-forming unit assay on labtech chamber slides (Fig. 1) (26). Preliminary data reveal that an equivalent or greater number of CTPs and bone marrow cells per unit volume can be obtained from vertebral marrow during preparation for transpedicular pedicle screw placement compared to standard aspirations from the iliac crest. If the preliminary data continue to be supported through additional investigations, an additional and commonly available reservoir to supplement the osteogenic capacity for spinal fusion applications may become a reality.

B. Intraoperative Concentration of Human Bone Marrow Progenitors

The technique of bone marrow aspiration from the iliac crest has been previously described including the recommendation of separate 2 mL volume aspirates to optimize the concentration of osteoprogenitor cells and avoid the undesirable hemodilution seen with larger aspirate volumes (34). Intraoperative concentration of human bone marrow progenitors has not been previously published. In our initial pilot study, 15 of 20 patients scheduled for anterior or posterior lumbar interbody fusion were recruited to evaluate the use of allograft matrix enriched by intraoperative concentrations of CTPs. Briefly, a matrix composed of demineralized human allograft cancellous bone chips (10 mL, ~2.7 g dry weight) and demineralized cortical bone fibers (~1.8 g dry weight) was hydrated and placed in a 60-mL syringe with a retaining filter. One 2-mm incision was made over each iliac crest and 24 2-mL-volume bone marrow aspirations were pooled to provide 48 mL of fresh marrow. Forty milliliters of the marrow was heparinized to maintain cells in suspension and 8 mL was allowed to clot in a 10-mL syringe. The heparinized marrow was then passed through the allograft matrix bed in a 60-mL syringe to deliver an effluent containing nonattached cells. The number of nucleated cells and CTPs in the initial sample and the effluent was determined using published techniques (25,26). The enriched graft was then mixed with the marrow clot portion (Fig. 2).

Results of the study revealed nine men and six women were recruited (mean age 46, range 20–66). An average of 745 million (±460 million) cells were harvested from each patient. A mean of 257 ± 238 million cells

Selective Attachment Method

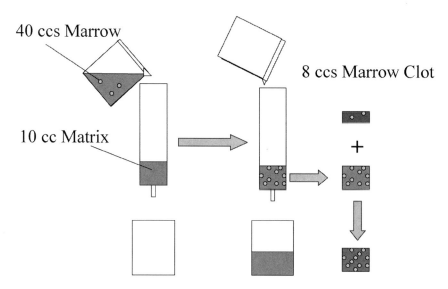

FIGURE 2 Selective attachment method. Human bone marrow aspirates are pooled and passed through a selective allograft matrix that acts as an affinity column to selectively attach connective-tissue progenitors. The enriched graft is then combined with the marrow clot to provide platelets, fibrin clot, and additional growth factors, which further improves graft efficacy.

were retained in the enriched graft. After addition of the marrow clot a total of 435 million ($\pm$326 million) cells were implanted. This represented retention of $34 \pm 14\%$ of the cells exposed to the matrix and a 2.5 ± 0.8-fold increase in number of marrow derived cells over that of the marrow clot alone. The pooled heparinized marrow aspirate was also found to contain 17,500 CTPs ($\pm$19,800). A mean of $75 \pm 22 \%$ of the CTPs were retained in the graft implant. After combination with the fresh marrow graft, $18,700 \pm 23,400$ CTPs were delivered in the graft site. This represents a 4.2 ± 1.1-fold increase in total CTPs compared to the marrow clot alone. No immediate or late morbidity was associated with marrow harvest.

The method described provides a rapid and minimally invasive means of providing composite cellular graft that is enriched in the number of CTPs delivered to the graft site (Fig. 3). The clinical and radiographic efficacy of this approach will be documented in long-term follow-up of

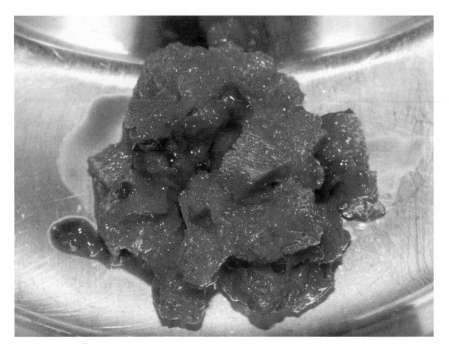

FIGURE 3 Composite cellular graft. A matrix composed of demineralized human allograft cancellous bone chips and demineralized cortical bone fibers enriched with concentrated connective-tissue progenitors is shown for use in spinal fusion applications.

these patients, though there have been no suspected failures and clinical improvement in 10 patients with at least 1-year follow-up as assayed by standard outcome measurements SF36 and Oswestry Scale.

Efforts to further optimize this strategy have been shown that the attachment and selection of CTPs from bone marrow is influenced by many factors, particularly the surface area and pore size of the matrix bed through which cells are passed, the surface chemistry of the matrix, and the method of preparation, as well as the flow rate of cells through the matrix, the thickness of the matrix bed, and the number of times that cells are passed through the matrix. Control of these variables will be necessary to optimize the concentration and delivery of CTPs using this strategy. The authors are currently collaborating with Depuy Acromed in the design of a kit and appropriate matrix materials that will allow surgeons to use these methods efficiently and reproducibly to improve bone grafting for clinical spine fusion procedures.

V. CONCLUSIONS

The cell biological principles and the necessary components for optimization of a graft in spinal fusion have been illustrated. Core concepts of bone tissue engineering have supported the rationale that no tissue engineering effort in the musculoskeletal arena can be expected to provide an optimal result if the initial population of CTPs is suboptimal. These tenants have fostered investigations in spinal fusion that aim to enhance the local number and concentration of bone-forming connective-tissue progenitors. Our human pilot study in lumbar interbody fusion in which allograft bone is enriched with autogenous bone marrow aspirate via manipulation of cellular and matrix interactions has shown a substantial increase in CTPs and good clinical outcome. A significant increase in the concentration of CTPs delivered to the graft site can be obtained using the methodology. Furthermore, the technique of aspiration of vertebral marrow during pedicle screw preparation is under investigation, as an alternative source of osteogenic cells to supplement spinal fusion. These methods underscore how tissue engineering is rapidly becoming a clinical reality in orthopedic spine surgery. The rationale suggested may eventually obviate the need for traditional autogenous iliac crest graft.

ACKNOWLEDGMENTS

The authors thank Mary Kay Reinhardt, R. N., for her invaluable contribution to the Spine Osteoprogenitor Cell Program at the Cleveland Clinic Foundation.

REFERENCES

1. Chaput C, Selmani A, Rivard CH. Artificial scaffolding materials for tissue extracellular matrix repair. Curr Opin Orthop 1996; 7:62–68.
2. An HS, Lynch K, Toth J. Prospective comparison of autograft vs. allograft for adult posterolateral lumbar spine fusion; differences among freeze dried, frozen, and mixed grafts. J Spinal Disord 1995; 8(2):131–135.
3. An HS, Simpson JM, Glover JM, Stephany J. Comparison between allograft plus demineralized bone matrix versus autograft in anterior cervical fusion: a prospective multicenter study. Spine 1995; 20:2211–2216.
4. Jorgenson SS, Lowe TG, France J, Sabin J. A prospective analysis of autograft versus allograft in posterolateral lumbar fusion in the same patient: a minimum of 1 year follow-up in 144 patients. Spine 1994; 18:2048–2053.
5. Kuslich SD, Danielson G, Dowdle JD, Sherman J, Fredrickson B, Yuan H, Griffith SL. Four-year follow-up results of lumbar spine arthrodesis using the Bagby and Kuslich lumbar fusion cage. Spine 2000; 25:2656–2662.

6. Hu R, Bohlman H. Fracture at the iliac bone graft harvest site after fusion of the spine. Clin Orthop 1994; 309:208–213.
7. Younger EM, Chapman MW. Morbidity at bone graft donor sites. J Orthop Trauma 1989; 3:192–195.
8. Fleming J Jr, Cornell CN, Muschler GF. Bone cells and matrices in orthopedic tissue engineering. Orthop Clin North Am 2000; 31:357–374.
9. Brantigan JW. Pseudoarthrosis rate after allograft posterior lumbar interbody fusion with pedicle screw and plate fixation. Spine 1994; 19:1271–1280.
10. Ehrler DM, Vaccaro, AR. The use of allograft bone in lumbar spine surgery. Clin Orthop Rel Res 2000; 371:38–45.
11. Muschler GF, Lane JM, Dawson EG. Science and Techniques: The Biology of Spinal Fusion. In: Cotler JM, Cotler HB, eds. Spinal Fusion. New York: Springer-Verlag 1990:9–21.
12. Muschler GF, Nitto H, Boehm C, Easley K. Age and gender related changes in the cellularity of human bone marrow and the prevalence of osteoblastic progenitors. J Orthop Res 2001; 19:117–125.
13. Wozney JM, Rosen V. Bone morphogenetic protein and bone morphogenetic protein gene family in bone formation and repair. Clin Orthop 1998; 346: 26–37.
14. Muschler GF, Midura RJ. Connective tissue progenitors—practical concepts for clinical applications. Clin Orthop Rel Res 2002; 395:66–80.
15. Maheshwar G, Brown G, Lauffenberger DA, Wells A, Griffith LG. Cell adhesion and motility depend on nanoscale RGD clustering. J Cell Sci 2000; 113:1677–1686.
16. Boden SD, Zdeblick TA, Sandhu HS, Heim SE. The use of rhBMP-2 in interbody fusion cages: definitive evidence of osteoinduction in humans: a preliminary report. Spine 2000; 25:376–381.
17. Mosley JR, Lanyon LE. Strain rate as a controlling influence on adaptive modeling in response to dynamic loading on the ulna in growing male rats. Bone 1998; 23:313–318.
18. Boden SD. The biology of posterolateral lumbar spinal fusion. Orthop Clin North Am 1998; 29:603–619.
19. Fleming J Jr, Muschler GF. The cell biology of bone tissue engineering. Semin Arthroplasty 2002; 13(3) 143–157.
20. Grigoriadis AE, Heersche JNM, Aubin JE. Differentiation of muscle, fat, cartilage, and bone from progenitor cells present in a bone-derived clonal cell population: effect of dexamethasone. J Cell Biol 1988; 106:2139–2151.
21. Bruder SP, Horowitz MP, Haynesworth SE. Monoclonal antibodies selective for human osteogenic cell surface antigens. Bone 1997; 21:225–235.
22. Fleming J Jr, Caplan AI. Monoclonal antibodies against cells of the mesenchymal lineage reveals key events in embryonic bone formation (abstr). Trans Orthop Res Soc 1997; 22:592.
23. Haynesworth SE, Baber MA, Caplan AI. Cell surface antigens on human marrow-derived mesenchymal cells are detected by monoclonal antibodies. Bone 1992; 13:69–80.

24. Lian JB, Stein GS. Concepts of osteoblast growth and differentiation: basis for modulation of bone cell development and tissue formation. Crit Rev Oral Biol Med 1992; 3:269–305.
25. Majors AK, Boehm C, Nitto H, Midura RJ, Muschler GF. Characterization of human bone marrow stromal cells with respect to osteoblastic differentiation. J Orthop Res 1997; 15:546–557.
26. Muschler GF, Boehm C, Easley K. Aspiration to obtain osteoblastic progenitor cells from human bone marrow: the influence of aspiration volume. J Bone Joint Surg (Am) 1997; 79:1699–1709.
27. Muschler GF, Nitto H, Matsukura Y, Boehm C, Valdevit A, Kambic H, Davros W, Powell K, Easley K. Spine fusion using cell matrix composites enriched in bone marrow derived cells. Clin Orthop Rel Res. 2003; 407:102–118.
28. Muschler, GF, Matsukura Y, Nitto H, Boehm C, Kambic H, Valdevit A, Easley K, Powell K. Enhanced spinal fusion using rapid concentration of bone marrow cells in allograft matrix. In press.
29. Healey JH, Zimmerman PA, McDonnell JM, Lane JM. Percutaneous bone marrow grafting of delayed union and nonunion in cancer patients. Clin Orthop Rel Res 1997; 256:280–285.
30. Connolly JF, Guse R, Lippiello L, Dehne R. Development of an osteogenic bone-marrow preparation. J Bone Joint Surg 1989; 71A:684–691.
31. Connolly JF, Guse R, Tiedeman J, Dehne R. Autologous marrow injection as a substitute for operative grafting of tibial nonunions. Clin Orthop Rel Res 1991; 266:259–270.
32. Garg NK, Gaur S. Percutaneous autogenous bone-marrow grafting in congenital tibial pseudarthrosis. J Bone Joint Surg (Br) 1995; 77:830–831.
33. Brantigan JW. Pseudarthrosis rate after allograft posterior lumbar interbody fusion with pedicle screw and plate fixation. Spine 1994; 19:1271–1280.
34. Skaggs DL, Samuelson MA, Hale JM, Kay RM, Tolo VT. Complications of posterior iliac crest bone grafting in spine surgery in children. Spine 2000; 25:2400–2402.
35. Ahlman E, Patzakis M, Roidis N, Sheperd L, Holtom P. Comparison of anterior and posterior iliac crest bone grafts in terms of harvest-site morbidity and functional outcomes. J Bone Joint Surg 2002; 84:716–720.
36. McLain RF. Transpedicular fixation. In: Bradford DS ed. Master Techniques in Orthopaedic Surgery: The Spine. Philadelphia: Lippincott, Williams, and Wilkins, 1997:97–111.
37. Weinstein JN, Rydevik BL, Rauschning W. Anatomic and technical considerations of pedicle screw fixation. Clin Orthop Rel Res 1992; 284:34–46.

5

Molecular Genetic Methods for Evaluating Engineered Tissue

Matthew L. Warman

Case Western Reserve University School of Medicine, Cleveland, Ohio, U.S.A.

I. INTRODUCTION

A goal of tissue engineering is to recapitulate the normal function of damaged or lost tissue. Tissues often have multiple functions. Therefore, several criteria need to be employed when assessing whether an engineered tissue has recapitulated the function of its endogenous predecessor. For example, an artificial skin graft that prevents denuded tissue from becoming further damaged by desiccation and infection restores two essential skin functions. However, the graft would not recapitulate all functions of its predecessor unless skin texture, elasticity, sweat production, and sun protection were also restored. Multiple measures (e.g., histological, physiological, mechanical, etc.) are needed when comparing engineered and endogenous tissue. This chapter addresses how molecular genetic tools are employed to assist in this comparison.

II. GENOMICS

The "genome" contains the entirety of an organism's DNA. Genomics is the study of that DNA complement. The nuclear genome in humans comprises nearly 6 billion basepairs of DNA packaged into 23 pairs of chromosomes. Within an individual, the DNA complement is identical between different cells, even when those cells originate from different tissue sources and have different biological functions. Therefore, genomic DNA cannot be used to assess whether an engineered tissue resembles its endogenous predecessor. Comparisons at the level of RNA (Lockhart & Winzeler, 2000) or protein expression (Tyers & Mann, 2003) must be used when comparing engineered and endogenous tissue. This is because the biological processes that distinguish tissues arise from differences in the transcription of genomic DNA to produce diverse repertoires of RNAs, which in turn are translated into diverse repertoires of proteins.

The Human Genome Project (Wolfsberg et al., 2002) and related projects in model organisms provide essential information for comparing engineered and endogenous tissue. Having a nearly complete genomic DNA sequence permits traditional (i.e., comparison of genomic sequence with mRNA transcript sequences or purified protein sequences) and computational (i.e., using algorithms to predict new genes by identifying likely regulatory regions, such as promoters, and coding sequences, such as exons) approaches to be employed in the discovery of all an organism's expressed genes. Just as the "genome" represents the entirety of an organism's DNA, the "transcriptome" represents the entirety of an organism's expressed genes. In striking contrast to the "genome," which is invariant between an individual's tissues, "transcriptomes" are highly variable. Transcriptomes vary between tissue types, between cells from a single tissue type, and between otherwise identical cells that have been exposed to different environments. Information from the Human Genome Project now permits "transcriptomes" of engineered and endogenous tissues to be compared.

Comparing mRNA expression profiles in normal and engineered tissues is not a new concept. However, in the past only limited numbers of mRNA transcripts could be compared, since most human genes were still unknown and the principal tool for monitoring mRNA expression, the northern blot, was labor and reagent intensive. Northern blots are comprised of RNA species, typically recovered from cells or tissues, which have been size-separated by gel electrophoresis and then transferred and immobilized on stable membranes (Alwine et al., 1977). These membranes can then be probed with fluorescently labeled or radioactively labeled DNA probes to detect the presence and abundance of a specific RNA species on the membrane. Moderate and abundant mRNA species can be detected on northern blots made from 2–5 µg of total cellular RNA. Although an individual northern blot may require a relatively small amount of RNA, it can be probed only a few times before losing sensitivity Also, it cannot be simultaneously studied using large numbers of DNA probes, and it cannot be used to detect low-abundance mRNA species. Reverse-transcriptase PCR-based methods can be employed to quantify the expression levels of low-abundance RNA transcripts (Wang et al., 1989). These assays require small amounts of starting RNA, but, like northern blots, are not easily amenable for studying the expression of thousands of different RNA species. RNAase protection assays are another means of quantifying transcript abundance, but the number of expressed genes that can be queried simultaneously also limits their usefulness (Mittmann et al., 1998).

New technologies have emerged that permit high-throughput measurements of gene expression by querying thousands of genes with amounts of starting material that are comparable to that used in a northern blot (Lockhart & Winzeler, 2000, Holloway et al., 2002). These technologies permit more comprehensive comparisons of mRNA expression patterns between engineered and endogenous tissues. Three commonly employed techniques, RNA microarray (Lipshutz et al., 1999), competitive hybridization (Schena etal., 1995), and sequence-based analyses of gene expression (Velculescu et al., 1995), are described below.

In RNA microarray hybridization, DNA fragments representing known and predicted genes are immobilized, or synthesized, onto stable membranes (Gress et al., 1992; Lockhart et al., 1996). The copy number of each DNA fragment (representing a specific gene) that is attached to the membrane is uniform, as is the density at which DNA fragments representing different genes are arrayed. Since the array density is very high, DNA fragments representing thousands of different genes can be tested simultaneously. The spotted DNA fragments are allowed to hybridize with labeled probes made from total RNA that has been recovered from the tissue of interest. The ability of any particular RNA species within the total recovered RNA to be labeled and, during the hybridization procedure, to bind to its cognate DNA sequence in the array is dependent upon that RNA species' transcript abundance. High-abundance transcripts will give stronger signals in the array than moderate-abundance transcripts. The strength of the RNA microarray approach is that it uses a small amount of starting RNA but is able to measure the abundance of thousands of different RNA species in a single experiment. Similar to traditional northern blots, low-abundance transcripts remain difficult to detect since their low concentration limits their ability to incorporate label and to hybridize to their cognate DNA sequences in the array. Another limitation of microarrays is that they can be probed only once. Therefore, comparisons between microarray experiments are affected by interexperiment variations in RNA labeling efficiency, hybridization, and washing conditions. To improve the reliability of interarray comparisons, many types of internal controls are incorporated throughout the experimental process (Hill et al., 2001; Dudley et al., 2002).

Competitive hybridization utilizes the same principal as RNA microarray, but allows for direct comparisons of RNA species' abundance between tissues (Schena et al., 1995). This is accomplished by labeling total RNA obtained from different tissues with different fluorophores. For example, RNA recovered from endogenous tissue can be labeled with the fluorophore Cy3, and RNA recovered from engineered tissue can be labeled with the fluorophore Cy5. The relative abundance of RNA species in the two tissues (endogenous and engineered) can be directly compared by mixing the differently labeled RNAs and then having them compete when hybridizing to the arrayed DNAs. For any arrayed DNA, the intensity of Cy3- versus Cy5-labeled probe that has hybridized to it will reflect the relative abundance of that specific RNA species between the two tissue sources. Therefore, competitive hybridization allows for direct comparison of abundance for thousands of RNA species that are recoverable from different RNA sources. Internal controls and other normalization procedures are also included in the design and performance of these experiments to account for differences in labeling of the two RNA sources and differences in fluorescence intensity of the Cy3 and Cy5 fluorophores (Churchill, 2002).

Sequence-based analyses of gene expression employ high-through-put sequencing strategies to assess the diversity and abundance of RNA species within a cell or tissue type. One of the early goals of this approach was to determine the entire repertoire of expressed sequences present within a tissue, which meant finding low-abundance transcripts that would not be detectable by northern blot or not represented in tradition-ally constructed cDNA libraries. To make these rare RNA transcripts detectable, "normalized" cDNA libraries were created using methods that specifically decreased the abundance of common RNA species and increased the abundance of rare RNA species (Soares et al., 1994). High-throughput sequencing of these "normalized" libraries from a large variety of cell and tissue sources led to the identification of many pre-viously undiscovered genes (Hillier et al., 1996). An alternate high-throughput sequence-based approach was employed to quantify mRNA species from a single source (Velculescu et al., 1995). This approach fragments RNA into small pieces, randomly ligates the small pieces into concatamers, and sequences the concatamers. The frequency that an expressed gene will have a portion of its sequence present among the concatamers is related to the length of the original RNA species and the abundance of the species in the starting RNA mixture. Computer algo-rithms have been written that analyze the sequence information, assign sequence fragments to known genes, and employ statistical methods to compute the abundance of that gene's transcript in the original starting RNA.

III. COMPARING APPROACHES

Each of the aforementioned approaches can be used to compare RNA expression profiles between engineered and endogenous tissues. Ulti-mately, engineered tissues that completely recapitulate their endogenous predecessors will have transcriptomes that are identical to those of their predecessors. As these tissues are being developed, differences between engineered and endogenous tissues' transcriptomes can guide scientists when exploring how an engineered tissue differs from its endogenous coun-terpart and to decide which other approaches (e.g., physiological, histo-logical) could be used to determine whether these differences are functionally relevant to the engineered tissue's intended use (Barry et al., 2001; St-Amand et al., 2001; Winter et al., 2003).

High-throughput expression profiling is a new technique that is continuously being improved at the hardware and software levels (Holloway et al., 2002). Several areas of hardware-related transcript profiling that will benefit from continued improvement include improving interassay reliability, decreasing the amount of RNA required for individual experiments, and designing arrays that query all expressed genes and their various spliceforms (Phillips & Eberwine, 1996; Hill et al., 2001; Churchill, 2002; Dudley et al., 2002). Ongoing software-related improvements in analyzing and presenting the myriad of accumulated data in a manner that will be meaningful to "mere mortals" will also be required (Ermolaeva et al., 1998; Bassett et al., 1999).

In addition to evaluating engineered tissues at the level of their transcriptome, tissues could also be evaluated at the level of their proteome (i.e., the entirety of protein products). However, expression of a core polypeptide sequence from a transcribed mRNA may be insufficient for restoring normal function to an engineered tissue, if enzymes essential to that protein's posttranslational processing are not coordinately expressed in the tissue. Similar to transcriptome profiling, high-throughput methodologies are being developed to characterize broad repertoires of expressed protein sequences and their posttranslational modifications from small amounts of engineered or endogenous tissue (Shevchenko et al., 1996; Aebersold & Mann, 2003; Tyers & Mann, 2003).

High-throughput approaches that survey the entirety of expressed RNA transcripts or proteins and then analyze and present results in a meaningful manner are increasingly becoming important new methods for studying biology and disease. Obtaining and comparing expression profiles of engineered tissues to the endogenous tissues they are intended to replace will be similarly important.

REFERENCES

Aebersold R, Mann M. Mass-spectrometry-based proteomics. Nature 2003; 422:198–207.

Alwine JC, Kemp DJ, Stark GR. Method for detection of specific RNAs in agarose gels by transfer to diazobenzyloxymethyl-paper and hybridization with DNA probes. Proc Natl Acad Sci USA 1977; 74:5350–5354.

Barry F, Boynton RE, Liu B, Murphy JM. Chondrogenic differentiation of mesenchymal stem cells from bone marrow: differentiation-dependent gene expression of matrix components. Exp Cell Res 2001; 268:189–200.

Bassett DE Jr, Eisen MB, Boguski MS. Gene expression informatics—it's all in your mine. Nat Genet 1999; 21:51–55.

Churchill GA. Fundamentals of experimental design for cDNA microarrays. Nat Genet 2002; 32(suppl):490–495.

Dudley AM, Aach J, Steffen MA, Church GM. Measuring absolute expression with microarrays with a calibrated reference sample and an extended signal intensity range. Proc Natl Acad Sci USA 2002; 99:7554–7559.

Ermolaeva O, Rastogi M, Pruitt KD, Schuler GD, Bittner ML, Chen Y, Simon R, Meltzer P, Trent JM, Boguski MS. Data management and analysis for gene expression arrays. Nat Genet 1998; 20: 19–23.

Gress TM, Hoheisel JD, Lennon GG, Zehetner G, Lehrach H. Hybridization fingerprinting of high-density cDNA-library arrays with cDNA pools derived from whole tissues. Mamm Genome 1992; 3:609–619.

Hill AA, Brown EL, Whitley MZ, Tucker-Kellogg G, Hunter CP, Slonim DK. Evaluation of normalization procedures for oligonucleotide array data based on spiked cRNA controls. Genome Biol 2001; 2:RESEARCH0055.

Hillier LD, Lennon G, Becker M, Bonaldo MF, Chiapelli B, Chissoe S, Dietrich N, et al. Generation and analysis of 280,000 human expressed sequence tags. Genome Res 1996; 6:807–828.

Holloway AJ, van Laar RK, Tothill RW, Bowtell DD. Options available—from start to finish—for obtaining data from DNA microarrays II. Nat Genet 2002; 32(suppl):481–489.

Lipshutz RJ, Fodor SP, Gingeras TR, Lockhart DJ. High density synthetic oligonucleotide arrays. Nat Genet 1999; 21:20–24.

Lockhart DJ, Dong H, Byrne MC, Follettie MT, Gallo MV, Chee MS, Mittmann M, Wang C, Kobayashi M, Horton H, Brown EL. Expression monitoring by hybridization to high-density oligonucleotide arrays. Nat Biotechnol 1996; 14:1675–1680.

Lockhart DJ, Winzeler EA. Genomics, gene expression and DNA arrays. Nature 2000; 405:827–836.

Mittmann C, Munstermann U, Weil J, Bohm M, Herzig S, Nienaber C, Eschenhagen T. Analysis of gene expression patterns in small amounts of human ventricular myocardium by a multiplex RNase protection assay. J Mol Med 1998; 76:133–140.

Phillips J, Eberwine JH. Antisense RNA amplification: a linear amplification method for analyzing the mRNA population from single living cells. Methods 1996; 10:283–288.

Schena M, Shalon D, Davis RW, Brown PO. Quantitative monitoring of gene expression patterns with a complementary DNA microarray. Science 1995; 270:467–470.

Shevchenko A, Jensen ON, Podtelejnikov AV, Sagliocco F, Wilm M, Vorm O, Mortensen P, Boucherie H, Mann M. Linking genome and proteome by mass spectrometry: large-scale identification of yeast proteins from two dimensional gels. Proc Natl Acad Sci USA 1996; 93:14440–14445.

Soares MB, Bonaldo MF, Jelene P, Su L, Lawton L, Efstratiadis A. Construction and characterization of a normalized cDNA library. Proc Natl Acad Sci USA 1994; 91:9228–9232.

St-Amand J, Okamura K, Matsumoto K, Shimizu S, Sogawa Y. Characterization of control and immobilized skeletal muscle: an overview from genetic engineering. FASEB J 2001; 15:684–692.

Tyers M, Mann M. From genomics to proteomics. Nature 2003; 422: 193–197.

Velculescu VE, Zhang L, Vogelstein B, Kinzler KW. Serial analysis of gene expression. Science 1995; 270:484–487.

Wang AM, Doyle MV, Mark DF. Quantitation of mRNA by the polymerase chain reaction. Proc Natl Acad Sci USA 1989; 86: 9717–9721.

Winter A, Breit S, Parsch D, Benz K, Steck E, Hauner H, Weber RM, Ewerbeck V, Richter W. Cartilage-like gene expression in differentiated human stem cell spheroids: a comparison of bone marrow-derived and adipose tissue-derived stromal cells. Arthritis Rheum 2003; 48:418–429.

Wolfsberg TG, Wetterstrand KA, Guyer MS, Collins FS, Baxevanis AD. A user's guide to the human genome. Nat Genet 2002; 32(suppl): 1–79.

6

Biodegradable Scaffolds

Johnna S. Temenoff, Emily S. Steinbis, and Antonios G. Mikos
Rice University, Houston, Texas, U.S.A.

I. INTRODUCTION

Every year in the United States, over 1 million surgeries are performed to restore lost bone function (1). In addition, 36 million Americans suffer from some form of arthritis (2). Such statistics demonstrate the vast need to treat a variety of maladies in both hard and soft orthopedic tissues. While autogeneic or allogeneic tissues can be transplanted to the site of injury, serious concerns such as the lack of donor tissue for autografts or the fear of disease transmission in allografts limit their use (3). An alternate method that holds promise for full functional replacement of orthopedic tissues is based on the tissue engineering paradigm that involves the introduction of cells and/or bioactive agents (growth factors, hormones, etc.) to the defect through the use of a three-dimensional biodegradable scaffold material.

The scaffold is a key component in orthopedic tissue engineering. In addition to providing a boundary for retention of cells at the defect site, the scaffold is necessary because it acts as a temporary substrate for anchorage-dependent cells that will create the new tissue (4–6).

As mentioned above, it may also act as a carrier for soluble and insoluble factors that modulate local cellular function. How cells attach to the scaffold can affect their behavior: strong cell adhesion and spreading is associated with proliferation, while a rounded cell shape is often required for cell-specific function (7). Besides cell morphology, the spatial relationship of cells within their extracellular matrix (ECM) can be important for continuance of differentiated function (8,9). Therefore, the use of three-dimensional scaffolds can encourage cellular migration and proliferation without sacrificing important functions to dedifferentiation.

Three-dimensional scaffolds can take many forms. Generally, scaffolds are considered either macroporous (> 10-μm pores) or, as in the case of many hydrogels, permeable without the need for large, well-defined pores. In the case of macroporous scaffolds, pores can be created through the use of porogens such as salt or gases (10). Alternatively, the material can be extruded into fibers and the fibers can then be stabilized in three dimensions via weaving or other methods (10,11).

A first step in designing tissue engineering scaffolds for orthopedic applications is to determine whether a preformed or injectable construct is most appropriate. Preformed scaffolds may be more biocompatible because, once fabricated, they can be leached in water for several days (or undergo other processes) to remove any residual toxic chemicals. They also offer the advantage that, when seeded with cells in vitro and allowed to grow in culture, the constructs can produce large sections of tissue prior to implantation (12). However, it may be easier to fill irregularly shaped defects with injectable scaffolds. Injectable materials also present the possibility that the scaffold may be delivered using minimally invasive techniques, thus decreasing patient discomfort and procedure cost.

Throughout this chapter, examples of advances in bone and cartilage tissue engineering will represent current avenues of research in scaffolds for hard and soft orthopedic tissues, respectively. While this chapter will focus on natural and synthetic-based polymers, other scaffold materials, such as ceramics, are included where appropriate. Development of a variety of materials has fulfilled scaffold design criteria for very diverse orthopedic applications. The results are promising and pave the way for a new era in treatment of orthopedic pathologies.

II. SCAFFOLD PROPERTIES

When developing a scaffold material for use in orthopedics, several important requirements must be satisfied:

A. Biocompatibility

Biodegradable materials for orthopedic applications, as for any other application, must first be biocompatible. This means that the material must neither evoke an unresolved inflammatory response nor demonstrate extreme immunogenicity or cytotoxicity. Factors that determine biocompatibility (chemical structure, physical structure, and surface morphology of the polymer) can be affected by synthesis or processing techniques. Residual chemicals involved in these processes, such as stabilizers, initiators, cross-linking agents, organic solvents, or unreacted monomers, may leach out of the scaffold once implanted. In addition, because the scaffold degrades in vivo, not only the intact biomaterial and any leachable components, but also the degradation products, must be biocompatible (4). For example, release of acidic by-products from some scaffold materials may cause tissue necrosis or inflammation due to a drop in local pH (12). Alternatively, particles formed in the degradation process may elicit a deleterious response. It has been demonstrated that polymer microparticles suppress initial rat marrow stromal osteoblast proliferation and differentiation in vitro (13).

B. Mechanical Properties

Initial mechanical properties of the scaffold to be implanted are particularly important in orthopedics. Many mechanical properties should be considered for orthopedic materials, including those in compression, tension, torsion, and bending. These properties must be as similar as possible to those of the tissue that is to be regenerated. As well as providing proper support in the early stages of healing, graded load transfer is needed to encourage creation of replacement tissue similar to the original (14). On a more microscopic scale, the local stiffness of the polymer may affect the mechanical tension generated by a cell's cytoskeleton, which can control cell shape and thus function (7). For example, rigid surfaces may cause the cytoskeleton to induce cell spreading and division (15,16).

C. Promotion of Tissue Formation

Properties such as porosity, permeability, pore size, pore structure, and degradation time should be chosen to encourage tissue growth and vascularization (if appropriate) within the material. In addition, the scaffold degradation rate should be coupled to the rate of tissue formation so that the load-bearing capabilities of the tissue are not compromised (4).

Porous scaffolds with large void volume and large surface-area-to-volume ratio are needed to maximize space for cell seeding, attachment, growth, and ECM production. To attain a high surface area per unit volume, smaller pores are preferable as long as the pore size is greater than the diameter of a cell in suspension (typically 10 μm). However, larger pores may be required for cell migration, growth, and ECM production (12). Interconnected pores facilitate diffusion within the scaffold, improving nutrient supply and waste removal and thus increasing viability of cells at the center of the construct.

For injectable scaffolds, porogens such as sodium chloride can be included in the initial formulation. In an aqueous environment such as is found in the body, the salt is leached out, leaving a scaffold with very high porosity. Since the leaching step occurs in vivo, the possibility of tissue damage due to high osmolarity of the extracellular tissue fluid is a concern. Therefore, the amount and type of porogen incorporated should be optimized to ensure sufficient porosity for diffusion and cell migration while not harming local tissues during the leaching process (12).

In the case of hydrogels, often used for tissue engineering of soft orthopedic tissues, the construct is mainly water, so there is minimal diffusion limitation inside the scaffold and large pores may not be required. However, a high permeability must be maintained throughout tissue regeneration to provide nutrients to cells at the center of the construct.

The degradation rate of a scaffold can be altered by many factors such as the structure and molecular weight of the component materials. Scaffold structure (surface-to-volume ratio, porosity, pore size, pore structure) plays a role, as does scaffold geometry. In vivo, the choice of implantation site, amount of mechanical loading, and rate of metabolism of degradation products also affect the degradation time of the scaffold.

In addition to degradation time, the mechanism by which the scaffold degrades should also be considered. In general, biomaterials are thought to degrade by either surface or bulk degradation. In surface erosion, as the name implies, only superficial layers are degraded and thus, degradation products are released gradually (12,17). In bulk degradation, however, degradation occurs simultaneously throughout the construct and degradation products are released when the molecular weight of the material reaches a critical value (9). Therefore, it can be difficult to maintain high mechanical strength past this critical point. In contrast, while mechanical strength may be maintained to some extent in surface-eroding polymers, the continued renewal of the exterior renders cell attachment and culture on these materials problematic (12).

D. Sterilizability

As with all implanted materials, orthopedic materials must be easily sterilizable to prevent infection. The method of sterilization, however, must not interfere with the bioactivity of the materials or alter its chemical composition, which could affect its biocompatibility or degradation properties (14).

E. Processing/Final Product

Orthopedic tissue engineering scaffolds must be reproducibly manufactured on a large scale, have a long shelf life, and be easily available to surgeons in a sterile operating environment (12,18).

Other important properties, particularly for scaffold materials that are injectable, include the following.

F. Setting Time/Temperature Change

The material should set in several minutes to minimize the length of the procedure while allowing surgeons time for placement before hardening (14). Any temperature change during setting should be minimized to reduce damage to the surrounding tissue.

G. Viscosity/Ease of Handling

Ease of handling, often related to viscosity of the material, is of utmost importance for clinical use of orthopedic biomaterials. Therefore, viscous properties must be balanced between the need for the material to remain at the site of injection and the need for the surgeon to easily manipulate its placement.

III. SCAFFOLD APPLICATIONS

When designing a scaffold for tissue engineering, optimizing the parameters described above often depends on the envisioned application for the construct. Biodegradable scaffolds can be used in a variety of ways. In some cases, the presence of a three-dimensional scaffold is enough to encourage tissue regeneration by promoting migration and proliferation of the desired cell types. It has been shown that a scaffold of poly(propylene fumarate) (PPF) acts in such a manner when implanted in tibial defects in rats, with the outer margins of the material being replaced by bone over 5 weeks (19). Synthetic scaffolds have also been used to enhance cartilage regeneration (20,21). In addition, natural-based hyaluronic acid matrices have been shown to support new cartilage and bone formation in rabbit osteochondral defects (6). In many cases however, implantation of a scaffold alone is not sufficient to fully regenerate orthopedic tissues. Further research has explored the use of scaffolds to deliver ECM, cells, or bioactive factors to improve the quality or amount of tissue formed at the site of injury (see Fig. 1).

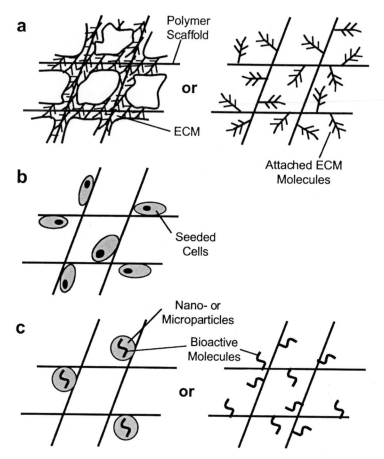

Figure 1 Tissue engineering scaffolds can be employed for delivery of extracellular matrix (ECM) (a), cells (b), or bioactive molecules (c). (a) Use of scaffolds for matrix delivery can involve synthesis of matrix on the scaffold during in vitro preculture or covalently attaching ECM molecules to the scaffold material to form an ECM analog. (b) As cell carriers, scaffolds can encourage attachment, proliferation, and function of both precursor and fully differentiated cells. (c) To facilitate their localized release, bioactive molecules can be encapsulated in nano- or microparticles and entrapped in the scaffold, or covalently bound to the scaffold material.

A. Delivery of Matrix

Strategies that involve the delivery of matrix may be advantageous, as they can be prepared and readily available "off-the-shelf" (1). These approaches involve the delivery of natural ECM or ECM analogs (Fig. 1a). Delivery of natural ECM without the concerns associated with autografts or allografts may be achieved by preculturing scaffolds seeded with autogeneic cells in bioreactors and then transplanting the construct to the injury site. While the cells, particularly at the interior of the scaffold, may die after transplantation owing to poor diffusion throughout the scaffold in the initial stages of tissue regeneration, the matrix left by these cells can induce cell migration from the surrounding tissue to fill the defect. Recently, our laboratory has investigated this method for bone tissue engineering using a flow perfusion bioreactor to stimulate formation of mineralized matrix throughout a titanium mesh scaffold. After 16 days of culture in the flow perfusion system, a greater amount of calcium was found in rat marrow stromal-cell-seeded titanium scaffolds as compared to identically seeded meshes cultured statically. Electron microscopy confirmed that the calcified matrix extended deep within the scaffolds cultured under flow, whereas it formed only a surface layer on the statically cultured samples (22).

In a second matrix delivery strategy, ECM analogs may be created using combinations of natural and synthetic-based materials. Much research in this area has focused on the use of hydrogels, which are less stiff than other types of materials (23,24), and thus may be more appropriate for tissue engineering of cartilage or non-load-bearing bone. In our laboratory, a novel hydrogel system based on oligo[poly(ethylene glycol] fumarate) (OPF) has been created and modified with the peptide sequence Gly-Arg-Gly-Asp (GRGD). The presence of this peptide sequence encourages the attachment of marrow stromal cells (MSCs) seeded on these gels. It has been shown that increased attachment is due to the specific interaction between receptors on the cell's surface and the peptide incorporated in the hydrogel (25). This and other methods provide an effective means to tailor interactions between cells and tissue engineering scaffolds used for matrix delivery.

B. Delivery of Cells

For tissue engineering approaches involving the delivery of cells, a biopsy of cells obtained from a patient may be expanded in culture and seeded onto or within an appropriate scaffold (Fig. 1b). The cell-scaffold construct may be transplanted to the appropriate location in the patient either immediately or after further culture of the cells within the scaffold. Experiments in rats suggest poly(DL-lactic acid-*co*-glycolic acid) (PLGA) scaffolds support proliferation and differentiated function of seeded rat MSCs when implanted in the mesentery for 2 months, resulting in mineralized matrix formation within the scaffolds (26). PPF has also demonstrated an ability to encourage proliferation and differentiation of primary rat MSCs when cultured in vitro for 4 weeks (27). Additionally, healing of cartilage in rabbit femoral condyles has been examined using transplantation of autologous chondrocytes seeded on hyaluronic acid derivatives (28).

C. Delivery of Bioactive Molecules

In another approach to orthopedic tissue engineering, bioactive molecules, including DNA, growth factors, and hormones, can be delivered though the use of scaffolds. The appropriate factors csan be bound to the scaffold material during processing and are released as the material degrades. Another option is to load the molecules into biodegradable microparticles or nanoparticles that are entrapped within the scaffold (Fig. 1c). Work in our laboratory has demonstrated that TGF-β1 encapsulated in blended poly(DL-lactic acid-*co*-glycolic acid)/poly(ethylene glycol) (PLGA/PEG) microparticles was released and promoted proliferation and differentiation of rat marrow stromal cells cultured for 21 days in vitro on PPF substrates (27). Another polymer, poly(ε-caprolactone), has been included as part of an injectable calcium phosphate-based bone substitute as an efficient system for delivery of large molecules (29).

IV. SCAFFOLD MATERIALS

Regardless of the tissue engineering strategy employed, the choice of scaffold material is extremely important to the success of the therapy. The type of scaffold material desired depends on the tissue to be regenerated, whether an injectable or preformed scaffold is needed, and which of the tissue engineering strategies described above is to be used. Usually, scaffold materials can be classified as naturally based, such as collagen, hydroxyapatite, hyaluronic acid, chitosan, and others, or synthetically based, such as poly(L-lactic acid) (PLLA), poly(glycolic acid) (PGA), their copolymer PLGA, and others (30–34).

Naturally derived materials often consist of purified ECM components. An example of such a natural material is collagen. Because collagen can be recognized by cellular enzymes, it can be easily degraded in vivo (35). Many different types of collagen are found in various tissues, and several of these types, particularly types I and II, have formed the basis of scaffolds for orthopedic tissue engineering (36,37).

Polysaccharide-based materials present several options for naturally derived scaffolds. Hyaluronic acid is a glycosaminoglycan (GAG) occurring in human ECM that is degraded enzymatically (11). Chitosan is a polysaccharide found in arthropod exoskeletons and can be degraded by lysozyme (38,39). Agarose is a polysaccharide formed by algae and has shown evidence of degradation in vivo, although the exact degradation mechanism is not known (40,41). Alginate is a polysaccharide derived from seaweed. It has been shown that humans do not produce the enzymes to break down alginate, but through modifications to the molecule, degradable alginate scaffolds can be created (42). Hyaluronic acid and chitosan have been formed into both prefabricated macroporous scaffolds and injectable nonporous formulations, while agarose and alginate have been used primarily as injectable formulations (11,38,41–44).

Natural scaffold materials not based on ECM molecules are the blood-clotting factors of fibrinogen and thrombin, which, when combined, form a fibrin glue. These are degraded by enzymes found in the normal wound healing cascade (45)

While all of these materials have applications in a variety of orthopedic tissues, natural materials specific for bone regeneration are usually ceramics, such as β-tricalcium phosphate, hydroxyapatite, and many others. They are stronger than many other natural materials and can be resorbed as part of the natural turnover process (46).

Although preliminary results are promising for naturally derived polymeric materials, their generally low mechanical properties (11), concerns about the feasibility of finding large amounts of these materials for clinical applications, as well as assurance of pathogen removal, have prompted other researchers to investigate the use of synthetic polymers. These materials can be easily mass-produced and their physical, chemical, mechanical, and degradative properties can be tailored for specific applications. The synthetic materials discussed in this chapter are all degradable polymers, which, like natural materials, allow room for tissue growth in the construct and eliminate the need for a second surgery to remove the implant. However, few of these synthetic-based materials have been FDA-approved for use in humans (4).

Synthetic biomaterials used for orthopedic tissue engineering include poly(esters), poly(anhydrides), poly(acrylamides), and derivatives of poly (ethylene glycols) (12, 31,47–49). The most common biomaterials used for musculoskeletal tissue engineering are poly(esters), particularly the poly(α-hydroxy esters) PLLA, PGA, and PLGA copolymer. These polymers, which undergo bulk degradation via hydrolytic cleavage of the ester bonds, are often chosen for tissue-engineered constructs because they are already FDA-approved for certain uses (4,30,31). Varying the ratios of lactic acid and glycolic acid in the copolymer formulation can alter crystallinity and hydrophobicity of the material, thus affecting the overall degradation time for the scaffold (4).

Other poly(esters) used for orthopedic applications, such as poly(ε-caprolactone) (PCL) and poly(propylene fumarate) (PPF), are also degradable by hydrolysis, although PCL degrades more slowly than the poly (α-hydroxy esters) (31,46,50). The degradation products of PPF include propylene glycol and fumaric acid, a substance that occurs naturally in the Krebs cycle (51). An advantage of PPF over other poly(esters) is its ability to cure in situ, thus facilitating its use for both preformed and injectable scaffolds (46,52,53).

Poly(anhydrides) degrade rapidly by surface erosion and are often used for controlled drug release. Although this type of degradation may result in a more controlled release of by-products, these materials often lack mechanical strength. Moreover, as mentioned previously, surface-eroding polymers may not facilitate cell adhesion in cell-polymer constructs (12).

Poly(acrylamides), such as poly(N-isopropylacrylamide) (PNI-PAAm), and poly(ethylene glycol) (PEG) derivatives have recently been studied as hydrogel scaffolds for cartilage tissue engineering. While the PNIPAAm hydrogels are considered nondegradable, they can be modified to include degradable linkages. Gels with similar characteristics have also been created using copolymers of PEG and poly(propylene oxide) (PPO) (54).

Other PEG derivatives include PEG-dimethacyrate (PEG-DMA), PEG-diacrylate (PEG-DA), and oligo(poly(ethylene glycol) fumarate) (OPF). Networks of PEG-DMA and PEG-DA are considered minimally degradable, but can be copolymerized with poly(lactic acid) to form materials degradable on a clinically relevant time scale (55).

A. Preformed Scaffolds

1. Bone Tissue Engineering

Natural Materials. Because of limitations in strength of natural scaffolds (11), preformed matrices made from these materials are often used in non-load-bearing defects. In particular, collagen has been commonly investigated for a variety of bone tissue engineering applications. When a collagen/hyaluronic acid scaffold was synthesized and implanted into cranial defects in rats for 28 days, generally good biocompatibility was observed and histological scoring revealed there was more bone formation with these scaffolds than with scaffolds of crosslinked collagen or cross-linked hyaluronic acid alone (56).

Collagen matrices have also been used as cell carriers. A preformed collagen scaffold loaded with muscle-derived cells transfected to produce human bone morphogenetic protein-2 (BMP-2) were implanted in skull defects in SCID mice. Treated in this manner, these critical-sized defects demonstrated 95–100% closure at 4 weeks (23).

In a different tissue engineering strategy, collagen scaffolds have been utilized to deliver BMP-2 directly. In one study, collagen sponges with BMP-2 were placed in radial defects in rabbits. After 8 weeks, histological evaluation demonstrated bony tissue bridging the 20-mm defect (57).

Synthetic Materials. The common synthetic scaffold materials, poly(L-lactic acid) (PLLA), poly(glycolic acid) (PGA), and their copolymer, PLGA, are used exclusively for preformed scaffolds. As a matrix-delivery strategy, a modified copolymer of poly(lactic acid), poly(lactic acid-*co*-lysine) has been developed that could provide sites for attachment of specific peptides to modulate cell adhesion and growth (58,59). In a cell-based approach, PLGA has been seeded with different cell types to generate mineralized tissue in rats (5,60).

Unlike PLGA, many synthetic linear polymers may rely on chemical cross-linking to covalently bond the polymer into a three-dimensional structure. The number of these cross-links affects both mechanical strength and degradability of the final scaffold (49). For example, PPF is an unsaturated linear poly(ester) that can be cross-linked through the fumarate double bond (61). Traditional cross-linking agents for this polymer include either methylmethacrylate (MMA) (62,63) or N-vinyl pyrrolidone (NVP) monomers (27). However, the resulting cross-links (PMMA and PNVP) are not biodegradable. Therefore, efforts are underway to produce PPF networks with degradable cross-links such as PPF-diacrylate (51).

Another option is to covalently bond PPF chains to themselves by addition polymerization to form a scaffold without the need for an additional cross-linking agent. It has recently been shown in our laboratory that this is possible by the addition of the photoinitiator bis(2,4,6-trimethyl-benzoyl) phenylphosphine oxide (BAPO) and exposure to ultraviolet (UV) light (52,53). Although, to date, this has been explored for prefabricated scaffolds only, the same techniques could be used to form injectable constructs (see below for discussion of photoinitators for injectable scaffolds). Used as a scaffold alone, cross-linked PPF foams were placed in rabbit cranial defects. At 8 weeks, a mild inflammatory response was seen and a small amount of bone ingrowth was observed (52). However, when these scaffolds were coated and used to deliver transforming growth factor-$\beta1$ (TGF-$\beta1$), significantly more bone ingrowth was evident (53).

2. Cartilage Tissue Engineering

Unlike bone, cartilage does not undergo constant remodeling and often demonstrates poor regenerative capacity (34,64). Thus, most of the constructs implanted to repair cartilage have employed strategies involving delivery of cells or bioactive molecules.

Natural Materials. Of the natural materials investigated for cartilage tissue engineering, the three that have been most extensively studied for preformed scaffolds are collagen, hyaluronic acid, and chitosan. Collagen matrices have been found to contain proper molecular cues to stimulate new collagen production by transplanted bovine chondrocytes as compared with other scaffold types (65). Investigation into what type of collagen was most suitable for cartilage regeneration has shown that more bovine chondrocytes retain their phenotypic morphology in type II than in type I matrices (36). In an effort to further influence cell behavior, type I collagen scaffolds were modified with chondroitin sulfate, a GAG found in cartilaginous ECM. Increased chondrocyte proliferation and retention of proteoglycans in the matrix was observed after 2 weeks when compared with unmodified collagen I matrices (66).

Hyaluronic acid is one of the few materials to be used alone (without cells or additional bioactive molecules) for cartilage tissue engineering. In a recent study, meshes made from two derivatives of hyaluronic acid were implanted in osteochondral defects in rabbits (6). After 12 weeks, there was little inflammatory response and evidence of new bone and cartilage having good integration with surrounding tissue was observed (6).

In another tissue engineering strategy, hyaluronic acid scaffolds have also been used as carriers for progenitor cells or chondrocytes (67–70). When cultured in immunodeficent mice, hyaluronic acid scaffolds or hyaluronic acid/gelatin composite scaffolds seeded with rabbit MSCs were found to produce a combination of cartilage and bone tissue as determined primarily through histological scoring (67,68). When these scaffolds seeded with MSCs were placed in osteochondral defects, there was no observed difference in rate or extent of bone and cartilage formation as compared to unseeded hyaluronic acid scaffolds (69). Hyaluronic acid scaffolds have also been used to culture chondrocytes in vitro with deposition of GAG and collagen II seen over 21 days, indicating maintenance of a differentiated phenotype during this time period (70).

Chitosan scaffolds are also currently being explored as cell carriers. Chitosan is generally well tolerated when implanted in vivo, with little chronic inflammatory response observed (38). Preformed, highly porous chitosan scaffolds can be fabricated with pore sizes ranging from 1 to 250 μm (71). A combination of chitosan and the GAG chondroitin sulfate has demonstrated the ability to maintain the phenotype of bovine chondrocytes when cultured in vitro for 1 week (72).

Synthetic Materials. Much current research has focused on chondrocyte interaction with the synthetic materials PGA, PLLA, and PLGA (65,73–82). Firm hyaline-like cartilage was observed after 6 weeks when undifferentiated perichondrial cells were seeded onto PLLA meshes and implanted in the femoral condyles of rabbits (78,79). Similar cartilage morphology was found using PGA porous nonwoven scaffolds seeded with bovine chondrocytes and cultured in vitro for 12 weeks. In this case, mechanical properties of the constructs, such as aggregate modulus, were the same order of magnitude as normal bovine cartilage (80). Both PGA and PLLA tended to increase proteoglycan synthesis compared to a collagen scaffold (65). Cell growth was approximately twice as high initially (less than 2 months) on PGA than PLLA matrices when seeded with bovine chondrocytes, but after 6 months, total cellularity was found to be similar. Initial differences were attributed to the fact that PLLA degrades much more slowly and so left less space for cell proliferation (76). PLLA has been found to be less toxic to human chondrocytes than PGA in studies maintaining a constant pH over 12 days (81).

B. Injectable Scaffolds

1. Bone Tissue Engineering

Natural Materials. Although some softer natural materials have been used as injectable scaffolds to deliver cells or bioactive molecules to sites of bone injury, a great deal of research has also been done in the area of stronger, naturally based ceramic materials to promote bone formation. Of the softer materials, both alginate and collagen have been explored for bone tissue engineering applications. In a recent study, rat calvarial osteoblasts were encapsulated in poly(aldehyde guluronate), a molecule derived from alginate, and implanted in the backs of nude mice. After 9 weeks, mineralized tissue, as visualized by von Kossa staining of histological sections, was evident (83). In strategies involving delivery of bioactive agents, collagen gels have been used as injectable carriers of BMP-2 (84) and plasmid DNA for fragments of other growth factors (85) to defect sites in rabbits and rats, respectively, with bone formation seen in both models.

In contrast to other injectable natural materials, ceramic-based materials are generally implanted alone, but their use can be considered a matrix delivery strategy as it is believed that the ceramic is bioactive and promotes bone ingrowth into the material (46). Ceramics are also unique in that they do not need a highly porous or permeable structure, because it is thought that osteoclasts resorb the ceramic materials and allow for new bone formation in the implant as part of the natural remodeling process (46). The most common types of calcium phosphate ceramics, hydroxyapatite (HA,

$Ca_{10}(PO_4)_6(OH)_2$) and tricalcium phosphate (TCP, $Ca_3(PO_4)_2$), have different characteristics in vivo, although both forms have Ca/P ratios within the range known to promote bone ingrowth (1.50–1.67). In general, HA was found to be more osteogenic while TCP degraded more quickly (86,87).

The injectable ceramic pastes currently under investigation undergo nonexothermic setting after several minutes to form materials with high compressive strength (88–92). These calcium phosphates can be divided into four types, depending on what is precipitated during setting: dicalcium phosphate dihydrate (DCDP, $CaHPO_4·2H_2O$), calcium magnesium phosphate (CMP, $Ca_4Mg_5(PO_4)_6$), octacalcium phosphate (OCP, $Ca_8(HPO_4)_2(PO_4)_4·5H_2O$), or calcium-deficient hydroxyapatite (CDHA, $Ca_9(HPO_4)(PO_4)_5OH$) (93). Of these, the two types that have been studied most extensively are DCPD (88,89,94) and CDHA (90–92,95–99). Although the DCPD cements have acceptable mechanical properties in compression and are quickly replaced by bone, they have been found to turn acidic during setting, potentially inducing inflammation around the implantation site (93).

In contrast to the DCPD cements, CDHA cements remain neutral after setting (93). Materials of this type are under development by several investigators (90–92,95–104). A CDHA cement has been observed to cause bone replacement in canine proximal tibial metaphyseal and distal femoral metaphyseal defects (100). Because of its properties, this cement has been FDA approved for use in fixation of distal radial fractures (100–105). Clinical trials using the cement in conjunction with screw fixation for hip fractures improved load transfer and reduced screw cutout (103). However, it must be noted that in canines, full cement resorption did not occur during the 78-week experimentation period (100). Despite work on other calcium phosphate materials that are quickly resorbed (106), many existing ceramic-based materials degrade very slowly (95,100), possibly leading to decreased bone regeneration at the site of the implant due to stress shielding. And, while these cements exhibit good biocompatibility (95,100) and perform well in compression (88,90,101), tensile strengths are still below those found in natural bone (101).

Synthetic Materials. Synthetic materials under investigation as injectable scaffolds for bone tissue engineering include poly(anhydrides) cured with visible light, and the poly(ester) PPF cured without the need for a light source (19,24,107–109). Although, as discussed previously, preformed poly(anhydride) scaffolds often lack sufficient mechanical strength, a group of photopolymerizable poly(anhydrides) has been developed that are suitable for use in orthopedics (24,107–109). These materials are polymers of sebacic acid (SA), copolymers of SA and 1,3-bis(p-carbophenoxy) propane (CPP), or copolymers of SA and 1,6-bis(p-carboxyphe-noxy) hexane (CPH). An effective means of polymerization for these applications utilizes the photoinitiation system of camphorquinone (CQ) and ethyl-4-N,N-dimethyl aminobenzoate (4EDMAB) with blue light. This polymerization method, used widely in dentistry, allows greater light penetration depths than many UV systems because of the tendency of CQ to quickly photobleach (107,108).

Both the mechanical properties and degradation times of these materials can be altered depending on the choice of monomer(s) (24,108). Because these polymers are surface-eroding, they maintain their bulk mechanical properties during the degradation process (24). In saline, PSA degrades in a few days, while PCPH degrades much more slowly (estimated 1 year). Thus, copolymers with different combinations of SA with CPH can be synthesized to tailor degradation properties for specific applications (24,108). To further modulate degradation time and mechanical properties, the materials have been photopolymerized with particles or linear polymers within them, making interpenetrating networks (IPNs). In this case, the choice of additive in the IPN provides another means to change the physical properties of the scaffold material (24).

Minimal inflammatory response to a SA/CPP IPN has been observed in rodent trials (109). Implanted without the addition of cells or extrinsic growth factors, a 12-week study using defects in rabbit femurs showed good tolerance of the nonporous SA/CPP material and osseous tissue formation in the outer zone of some implants (109).

While this family of photopolymerizable polymers has many useful qualities for use in bone tissue engineering, polymerization that depends on light may be impractical for repair of deep crevices that can occur in some injuries. In these cases, a combination of photopolymerized and chemically polymerized materials may be required (107). Several studies in the area of chemically cured polymers have focused on PPF. These experiments have so far been conducted with the cross-linking agent NVP and benzoyl peroxide as a radical initiator (19,110,111). While the resulting poly(N-vinyl pyrrolidone) (PNVP) cross-links are not degradable, PNVP is water-soluble and can be excreted through the kidneys (112). Although the curing reaction is exothermic, temperatures remain lower than those seen with poly(methylmethacrylate) (PMMA) bone cements (113).

In studies using the material as a scaffold to encourage bone ingrowth, PPF was combined with ceramic particles such as β-TCP, calcium carbonate, or calcium phosphate (62,63,111,114). Chemically cross-linked PPF does not exhibit a deleterious long-term inflammatory response when implanted subcutaneously in rats. Initially, a mild inflammatory response was observed, and a fibrous capsule formed around the implant at 12 weeks

(113). As mentioned above, a PPF/β-TCP composite was implanted in rat tibiae for up to 5 weeks. At this time, the material was observed to be gradually replaced by bone from the perimeter inward (19).

To explore the idea of cell delivery with PPF, current research involves the addition of osteoblastic cells to the injectable PPF construct (115). Culture of rat MSCs on PPF/β-TCP films has demonstrated that the composite encourages attachment, proliferation, and differentiated osteoblastic function (27). However, the temperature rise during cross-linking and presence of residual, potentially toxic cross-linking agents has resulted in the need to encapsulate cells before inclusion in the injectable formulation (115). Recently in our laboratory, a method for encapsulation of cells has been developed for short-term protection from unfavorable cross-linking conditions. With this technique, cells are encapsulated in gelatin microspheres cross-linked on the surface to prevent premature dissolution (116). It has been shown that MSCs, when encapsulated in this manner and added to cross-linking PPF, exhibit significantly higher initial viability than nonencapsulated cells (117). Additionally, there is evidence that this encapsulation does not affect cellular proliferation and eventual osteoblastic differentiation when cultured up to 28 days in vitro on PPF substrates (118).

2. Cartilage Tissue Engineering

Natural Materials. In addition to preformed scaffolds, collagen and chitosan can also be used as injectable cell carriers for cartilage tissue engineering. It has been found that chondrocytes maintain a differentiated phenotype and produce GAG for 6 weeks in collagen gels (119). Additionally, when rabbit MSCs were seeded into collagen gels and implanted in osteochondral defects in rabbits, both bone and hyaline cartilage were formed, although mechanical properties of the regenerated tissue were significantly less than normal values and there was some evidence of degeneration after 24 weeks (120,121).

A chitosan gel has been developed that is liquid below room temperature and a solid at body temperature. Such thermally stabilized gels provide a means for cell or growth factor delivery while avoiding the potentially toxic initiators and cross-linking agents used for in situ polymerization. Bovine articular chondrocytes were encapsulated within this gel and cultured in vitro and in vivo in athymic mice. In both cases, evidence of maintenance of the chondrocytic phenotype (collagen II and aggregan production over 3 weeks in vivo) was observed (43).

In other cell delivery strategies, an agarose hydrogel has been used with embedded allogeneic rabbit chondrocytes to fill full-thickness cartilage defects. Over 18 months, superior results were obtained with the cell-agarose constructs than with agarose alone. Furthermore, after 18 months, 47% of the implants demonstrated hyaline-like cartilage as determined by histological evaluation (41).

Similar constructs including cells have been created with alginate and bovine articular chondrocytes. When these were injected into nude mice and cross-linked with calcium, histology revealed the architecture of the newly formed tissue to be similar to that of native cartilage, but studies longer than 12 weeks have not been conducted to determine whether there is any long-term tissue degradation (8,122,123). A potential problem with the use of alginate is that some forms have been found to be immunogenic (124). A further concern about the biocompatibility of the material is that there may be a greater inflammatory response to alginate than to injectable synthetic materials (54).

Fibrinogen and thrombin may be combined to form a fibrin gel that can be used to suspend chondrocytes (45,125–127). When fibrin with allogeneic chondrocytes was injected into full-thickness defects in horses, more aggregan and type II collagen were present in the new tissue at 8 months than in defects that were left untreated (126).

Synthetic Materials. A variety of injectable synthetic materials have been used for cartilage tissue engineering. As with other scaffolds for this application, research has focused on delivery and maintenance of cells within a defect. One such cell carrier is the acrylamide-based PNIPAAm. When loaded with bovine chondrocytes and cultured 1–3 months in vitro, tissue with cartilage-like morphology was formed (47). In addition, these gels, like chitosan scaffolds, exploit change in temperature, rather than chemical cross-linking, to form scaffolds in situ, so there is less potential for toxicity when used in conjunction with cells (128).

Other thermally stabilized gels for cartilage tissue engineering have been created using copolymers of PEG and PPO (54). In a comparative study, when seeded with autologous chondrocytes and injected in pigs, the PEG-PPO copolymer was found to produce more cartilage-like tissue than either PGA scaffolds or alginate hydrogels. In this case, however, the chondrocytes were of aural rather than articular origin (54).

Another class of synthetic injectable materials is based on PEG without copolymerization with PPO. When nonmodified PEG was used as a carrier for bovine chondrocytes implanted subcutaneously in nude mice, cartilage that was biochemically similar to natural bovine cartilage had been produced at 12 weeks (129). However, without copolymerization, PEG remains a viscous liquid and does not form a gel-like material in the body. Therefore, functionalized PEG, such as PEG dimethacrylate (PEG-

DMA), that can be photopolymerized in situ has recently been investigated for cartilage tissue engineering (48,55,130,131). Initial results indicate the constructs can be polymerized in 3 min with no harm to embedded chondrocytes. Specimens removed from athymic mice at 2, 4, and 7 weeks show cartilage formation with increasing GAG and collagen content (130). Constructs up to 8 mm thick have been produced using this method, and embedded chondrocytes remain viable at the center of these gels during at least 2 weeks of in vitro culture (48). Over 4–6 weeks in vitro, similar constructs showed production of GAG and collagen II throughout the scaffold (48,55).

An alternate PEG derivative has recently been developed in our laboratory. Oligo[poly(ethylene glycol) fumarate] (OPF) is an oligomer of PEG with fumarate moieties that allow for cross-linking in situ as well as degradation via hydrolysis. Like injectable PPF, a chemical initiation system (ammonium persulfate and ascorbic acid) has been used to form gels without the need for light. It has been found that this material has the ability to form laminated structures with no evidence that lamination decreases mechanical properties of the resulting layered construct (49). In addition to cell delivery applications, this hydrogel could be used in a matrix delivery approach, as it can be modified with peptides to encourage specific cell attachment. Using the model peptide sequence GRGD, it has been demonstrated not only that peptide modification promotes specific interactions between MSC surface receptors and the OPF (discussed previously), but that material properties such as distance between cross-links and PEG spacer length play an important role in controlling the interaction between cells and the hydrogel. Such a system provides great flexibility in guiding tissue growth through formation of surfaces that promote generation of a specific tissue (25).

V. SUMMARY

Although bone and cartilage are very diverse tissues providing different functions within the body, recent work has demonstrated the possibility of creating biodegradable scaffolds with promise to repair both tissues. Like the tissues, the materials are also varied; they can be ceramic, naturally derived, or based on synthetic polymers. They can be used alone, or as carriers for ECM, cells, and bioactive molecules. They may be made into preformed scaffolds or injected and cured at the site of the defect. While there are disadvantages to each material, many have been proven to be largely biocompatible and have physical characteristics that promote tissue formation. In time, each material may find its own unique application. Further improvements in these materials will provide an important step toward the ideal of complete regeneration of orthopedic tissues through the use of tissue engineering paradigms.

REFERENCES

1. Bancroft GN, Mikos AG. Bone tissue engineering by cell transplantation. In: Ikada Y, Ohshima N, eds. Tissue Engineering for Therapeutic Use 5. New York: Elsevier Science 2001:151–163.
2. American Academy of Orthopedic Surgeons website. www.aaos.org.
3. Bostrom RD, Mikos AG. Tissue engineering of bone. In: Atala A, Mooney DJ, eds. Synthetic Biodegradable Polymer Scaffolds. Berlin: Birkhaeuser 1997:215–234.
4. Thomson RC, Wake MC, Yaszemski MJ, Mikos AG. Biodegradable polymer scaffolds to regenerate organs. Adv Polym Sci 1995; 122:245–274.
5. Ishaug SL, Crane GM, Miller MJ, Yasko AW, Yaszemski MJ, Mikos AG. Bone formation by three-dimensional stromal osteoblast culture in biodegradable polymer scaffolds. J Biomed Mater Res 1997; 36:17–28.
6. Solchaga LA, Yoo JU, Lundberg M, Dennis JE, Huibregtse BA, Goldberg VM, Caplan AI. Hyaluronan-based polymers in the treatment of osteochondral defects. J Orthop Res 2000; 18:773–780.
7. Chicurel ME, Chen CS, Ingber DE. Cellular control lies in the balance of forces. Curr Opin Cell Biol 1998; 10:232–239.
8. Rodriguez AM, Vacanti CA. Tissue engineering of cartilage. In: Patrick Jr CW, Mikos AG, McIntire LV, eds. Frontiers in Tissue Engineering. New York: Elsevier Science 1998:400–411.
9. Lu L, Temenoff JS, Tessmar JK, Mikos AG. Synthetic bioresorbable polymer scaffolds. In: Ratner BD, Hoffman AS, Schoen FJ, Lemons JE, eds. Biomaterials Science. 2d ed. New York: Elsevier, in press.
10. Temenoff JS, Mikos AG. Formation of highly porous biodegradable scaffolds for tissue engineering. Electron J Biotechnol 2000;3:http://www.ejb.org/content/vol3/issue2/full/5/index.html
11. Campoccia D, Doherty P, Radice M, Brun P, Abatangelo G, Williams DF. Semisynthetic resorbable materials from hyaluronan esterification. Biomaterials 1998; 19:2101–2127.
12. Temenoff JS, Lu L, Mikos AG. Bone-tissue engineering using synthetic biodegradable polymer scaffolds. In: Davies JE, ed. Bone Engineering. Toronto: em squared, 2000:454–460.
13. Wake MC, Gerecht PD, Lu L, Mikos AG. Effects of biodegradable polymer particles on rat marrow derived stromal osteoblasts in vitro. Biomaterials 1998; 19:1255–1268.
14. Yaszemski MJ, Payne RG, Hayes WC, Langer R, Mikos AG. In vitro degradation of a poly(propylene fumarate)-based composite material. Biomaterials 1996; 17:2127–2130.
15. Boyan BD, Hummert TW, Dean DD, Schwartz Z. Role of material surfaces in regulating bone and cartilage cell response. Biomaterials 1996; 17:137–146.

16. Moghe PV. Soft-tissue analogue design and tissue engineering of liver. Mater Res Soc Bull 1996; 21:52–54.

17. Pachence JM, Kohn J. Biodegradable polymers for tissue engineering. In: Lanza R, Langer R, Chick W, eds. Principles of Tissue Engineering. 1st ed. New York: R.G. Landes Co., 1997:273–293.

18. Peter SJ, Miller MJ, Yasko AW, Yaszemski MJ, Mikos AG. Polymer concepts in tissue engineering. J Biomed Mater Res (Appl Biomater) 1998; 43:422–427.

19. Yaszemski MJ, Payne RG, Hayes WC, Langer RS, Aufdemorte TB, Mikos AG. The ingrowth of new bone tissue and initial mechanical properties of a degradable polymeric composite scaffold. Tissue Eng 1995; 1:41–52.

20. von Schroeder HP, Kwan M, Amiel D, Coutts RD. The use of polylactic acid matrix and periosteal grafts for the reconstruction of rabbit knee articular defects. J Biomed Mater Res 1991; 25:329–339.

21. Athanasiou K, Korvick D, Schenck R. Biodegradable implants for the treatment of osteochondral defects in a goat model. Tissue Eng 1997; 3:363–373.

22. Bancroft GN, Sikavitsas VI, van den Dolder J, Sheffield TL, Ambrose CG, Jansen JA, Mikos AG. Fluid flow increases mineralized matrix deposition in 30 perfusion culture of marrow stromal osteoblasts in a dose-dependent manner. Proc. Nat. Acad. Sci USA 2002; 99:12600–12605.

23. Lee KY, Alsberg E, Mooney DJ. Degradable and injectable poly(aldehyde guluronate) hydrogels for bone tissue engineering. J Biomed Mater Res 2001; 56:228–233.

24. Muggli DS, Burkoth AK, Anseth KS. Crosslinked polyanhydrides for use in orthopedic applications: degradation behavior and mechanics. J Biomed Mater Res 1999; 46:271–278.

25. Shin H, Jo S, Mikos AG. Modulation of marrow stromal osteoblast adhesion on biomimetic oligo(poly(ethylene glycol) fumarate) hydrogels modified with Arg-Gly-Asp peptides and a poly(ethylene glycol) spacer. J Biomed Mat Res. 2002; 61:169–179.

26. Ishaug-Riley SL, Crane GM, Gurlek A, Miller MJ, Yasko AW, Yaszemski MJ, Mikos AG. Ectopic bone formation by marrow stromal osteoblast transplantation using poly(DL-lactic-co-glycolic acid) foams implanted into the rat mesentery. J Biomed Mater Res 1997; 36:1–8.

27. Peter SJ, Lu L, Kim DJ, Mikos AG. Marrow stromal osteoblast function on a poly(propylene fumarate)/β-tricalcium phosphate biodegradable orthopaedic composite. Biomaterials 2000; 21:1207–1213.

28. Grigolo B, Roseti L, Fiorini M, Fini M, Giavaresi G, Aldini NN, Giardino R, Facchini A. Transplantation of chondrocytes seeded on a hyaluronan derivative (Hyaff-11) into cartilage defects in rabbits. Biomaterials 2001; 22:2417–2424.

29. Iooss P, Le Ray A-M, Grimandi G, Daculsi G, Merle C. A new injectable bone substitute combining poly(ε-caprolactone) microparticles with biphasic calcium phosphate granules. Biomaterials 2001; 22:2785–2794.

30. Hutmacher DW. Scaffolds in tissue engineering bone and cartilage. Biomaterials 2000; 21:2529–2543.

31. Agrawal CM, Ray RB. Biodegradable polymeric scaffolds for musculoskeletal tissue engineering. J Biomed Mater Res 2001; 55:141–150.

32. Wirth CJ, Rudert M. Techniques of cartilage growth enhancement: a review of the literature. Arthroscopy 1996; 12:300–308.

33. Hunziker EB. Articular Cartilage Repair: Are the intrinsic biological constraints undermining this process insuperable? Osteoarthr Cartil 1999; 7:15–28.

34. Buckwalter JA. Articular cartilage: injuries and potential for healing. J Orthop Sports Phys Ther 1998; 28:192–202.

35. Speer DP, Chvapil M, Volz RG, Holmes MD. Enhancement of healing in osteochondral defects by collagen sponge implants. Clin Orthop Rel Res 1979; 144:326–335.

36. Nehrer S, Breinan HH, Ashkar S, Shortkroff S, Minas T, Sledge CB, Yannas IV, Spector M. Characteristics of articular chondrocytes seeded in collagen matrices in vitro. Tissue Eng 1998; 4:175–183.

37. Wakitani S, Goto T, Young RG, Mansour JM, Goldberg VM, Caplan AI. Repair of large full-thickness articular cartilage defects with allograft articular chondrocytes embedded in a collagen gel. Tissue Eng 1998; 4:429–444.

38. Suh J-KF, Matthew HWT. Application of chitosan-based polysaccharide biomaterials in cartilage tissue engineering: a review. Biomaterials 2000; 21:2589–2598.

39. Hedberg EL, Mikos AG. Biological polymers for controlled drug delivery technologies. In: Mrsny RJ, Lee VHL, Robinson JR, eds. Controlled Drug Delivery: Fundamentals and Applications. New York: Marcel Deker. In press.

40. Agarose. In: Sigma Catalog, 1999.

41. Rahfoth B, Weisser J, Sternkopf F, Aigner T, Von der Mark K, Braeuer R. Transplantation of allograft chondrocytes embedded in agarose gel into cartilage defects of rabbits. Osteoarthr Cartil 1998; 6:50–65.

42. Bouhadir KH, Mooney DJ. Synthesis of hydrogels: alginate hydrogels. In: Atala A, Lanza RP, eds. Methods of Tissue Engineering. San Diego, CA: Academic Press, 2002.

43. Chenite A, Chaput C, Wang D, Combes C, Buschmann MD, Hoemann CD, Leroux JC, Atkinson BL, Binette F, Selmani A. Novel injectable neutral solutions form biodegradable gels in situ. Biomaterials 2000; 21:2155–2161.

44. Radomsky ML, Thompson AY, Spiro RC, Poser JW. Potential role of fibroblast growth factor in enhancement of fracture healing. Clin Orthop Rel Res 1998; 355S:S283–S293.

45. Sims CD, Butler PEM, Cao YL, Casanova R, Randolph MA, Black A, Vacanti CA, Yaremchuk MJ. Tissue engineered neocartilage using plasma derived polymer substrates and chondrocytes. Plast Reconstr Surg 1998; 101:1580–1585.

46. Temenoff JS, Mikos AG. Injectable biodegradable materials for orthopedic tissue engineering. Biomaterials 2000; 21:2405–2412.

47. Stile RA, Burghardt WR, Healy KE. Synthesis and characterization of injectable poly(N-isopropylacrylamide)-based hydrogels that support tissue formation in vitro. Macromolecules 1999; 1999:7370–7379.

48. Bryant SJ, Anseth KS. The effects of scaffold thickness on tissue engineered cartilage in photocrosslinked poly(ethylene oxide) hydrogels. Biomaterials 2001; 22:619–626.

49. Temenoff JS, Athanasiou KA, LeBaron RG, Mikos AG. Effect of poly(ethylene glycol) molecular weight on tensile and swelling properties of oligo (poly(ethylene glycol) fumarate) hydrogels for cartilage tissue engineering. J Biomed Mater Res 2002; 59:429–437.

50. Corden TJ, Jones IA, Rudd CD, Christian P, Downes S, McDougall KE. Physical and biocompatibility properties of poly-ε-caprolactone produced using in situ polymerisation: a novel manufacturing technique for long-fibre composite materials. Biomaterials 2000; 21:713–724.

51. He S, Timmer MD, Yaszemski MJ, Yasko AW, Engel PS, Mikos AG. Synthesis of biodegradable poly(propylene fumarate) networks with poly(propylene fumarate)-diacrylate monomers as cross-linking agents and characterization of their degradation products. Polymer 2001; 42:1251–1260.

52. Fisher JP, Vehof JWM, Dean D, van der Waerden JPCM, Holland TA, Mikos AG, Jansen JA. Soft and hard tissue response to photocrosslinked poly(propylene fumarate) scaffolds in a rabbit model. J Biomed Mater Res 2002; 59:547–556.

53. Vehof JWM, Fisher JP, Dean D, van der Waerden JPCM, Spauwen PHM, Mikos AG, Jansen JA. Bone formation in transforming growth factor-β-1-coated porous poly(propylene fumarate) scaffolds. J Biomed Mater Res 2002; 60:241–251.

54. Cao Y, Rodriguez A, Vacanti M, Ibarra C, Arevalo C, Vacanti C. Comparative study of the use of poly(glycolic acid), calcium alginate and pluronics in the engineering of autologous porcine cartilage. J Biomater Sci Polym Edn 1998; 9:475–487.

55. Bryant SJ, Anseth KS. Hydrogel properties influence ECM production by chondrocytes photoencapsulated in poly(ethylene glycol) hydrogels. J Biomed Mater Res 2001; 59:63–72.

56. Liu L-S, Thompson AY, Heidaran MA, Poser JW, Spiro RC. An osteoconductive collagen/hyaluronate matrix for bone regeneration. Biomaterials 1999; 20:1097–1108.

57. Hollinger JO, Schmitt JM, Buck DC, Shannon R, Joh S-P, Zegzula HD, Wozney J. Recombinant human bone morphogenetic protein-2 and collagen for bone regeneration. J Biomed Mater Res 1998; 43:356–364.

58. Barrera D, Zylstra E, Lansbury P, Langer R. Copolymerization and degradation of poly(lactic-co-lysine). Macromolecules 1995; 28:425–432.

59. Cook AD, Hrkach JS, Gao NN, Johnson IM, Pajvani UB, Cannizzaro SM, Langer R. Characterization and development of RGD-peptide-modified poly(lactic acid-co-lysine) as an interactive, resorbable biomaterial. J Biomed Mater Res 1997; 35:513–523.

60. Ishaug-Riley SL, Crane-Kruger GM, Yaszemski MJ, Mikos AG. Three-dimensional culture of rat calvarial osteoblasts in porous biodegradable polymers. Biomaterials 1998; 19:1405–1412.

61. Peter SJ, Miller MJ, Yaszemski MJ, Mikos AG. Poly(propylene fumarate). In: Domb AJ, Kost J, Wiseman DM, eds. Handbook of Biodegradable Polymers. Amsterdam: Harwood Academic1997:87–97.

62. Frazier DD, Lathi VK, Gerhart TN, Altobelli DE, Hayes W, C. In vivo degradation of a poly(propylene fumarate) biodegradable, particulate composite bone cement. Mater Res Soc Symp Proc 1995; 394:15–19.

63. Frazier DD, Lathi VK, Gerhart TN, Hayes W, C. Ex vivo degradation of a poly(propylene glycol-fumarate) biodegradable particulate bone cement. J Biomed Mater Res 1997; 35:383–389.

64. Coutts RD, Sah RL, Amiel D. Effect of growth factors on cartilage repair. AAOS Inst Course Lect 1997; 46:481–494.

65. Grande DA, Halberstadt C, Naughton G, Schwartz R, Manji R. Evaluation of matrix scaffolds for tissue engineering of articular cartilage grafts. J Biomed Mat Res 1997; 34:211–220.

66. van Susante JLC, Pieper J, Buma P, van Kuppevelt TH, van Beuningen H, van der Kraan PM, Veerkamp JH, van den Berg WB, Veth RPH. Linkage of chondroitin-sulfate to type I collagen scaffolds stimulates the bioactivity of seeded chondrocytes in vitro. Biomaterials 2001; 22:2359–2369.

67. Solchaga LA, Dennis JE, Goldberg VM, Caplan AI. Hyaluronic acid-based polymers as cell carriers for tissue-engineered repair of bone and cartilage. J Orthop Res 1999; 17:205–213.

68. Angele P, Kujat R, Nerlich M, Yoo J, Goldberg V, Johnstone B. Engineering of osteochondral tissue with bone marrow mesenchymal progenitor cells in a derivatized hyaluronan-gelatin composite sponge. Tissue Eng 1999; 5:545–553.

69. Radice M, Brun P, Cortivo R, Scapinelli R, Battaliard C, Abatangelo G. Hyaluronan-based biopolymers as delivery vehicles for bone-marrow-derived mesenchymal progenitors. J Biomed Mater Res 2000; 50:101–109.

70. Brun P, Abatangelo G, Radice M, Zacchi V, Guidolin D, Gordini DD, Cortivo R. Chondrocyte aggregation and reorganization into three-dimensional scaffolds. J Biomed Mater Res 1999; 46:337–346.

71. Madihally SV, Matthew HWT. Porous chitosan scaffolds for tissue engineering. Biomaterials 1999; 20:1133–1142.

72. Sechriest VF, Miao YJ, Niyibizi C, Westerhausen-Larson A, Matthew HW, Evans CH, Fu FH, Suh J-K. GAG-augmented polysaccharide hydrogel: A novel biocompatible and biodegradable material to support chondrogenesis. J Biomed Mater Res 2000; 49:534–541.

73. Grande DA, Southerland SS, Manji R, Pate DW, Schwartz RE, Lucas PA. Repair of articular cartilage defects using mesenchymal stem cells. Tissue Eng 1995; 1:345–353.

74. Vacanti CA, Kim W, Schloo B, Upton J, Vacanti JP. Joint resurfacing with cartilage grown in situ from cell-polymer structures. Am J Sports Med 1994; 22:485–488.

75. Vacanti CA, Upton J. Tissue-engineered morphogenesis of cartilage and bone by means of cell transplantation using synthetic biodegradable polymer matrices. Clin Plast Surg 1994; 21:445–462.

76. Freed LE, Marquis JC, Nohria A, Emmanual J, Mikos AG, Langer R. Neocartilage formation in vitro and in vivo using cells cultured on synthetic biodegradable polymers. J Biomed Mater Res 1993; 27:11–23.
77. Freed LE, Grande DA, Lingbin Z, Emmanual J, Marquis JC, Langer R. Joint resurfacing using allograft chondrocytes and synthetic biodegradable polymer scaffolds. J Biomed Mater Res 1994; 28:891–899.
78. Chu CR, Coutts RD, Yoshioka M, Harwood FL, Monosov AZ, Amiel D. Articular cartilage repair using allogeneic perichondrocyte-seeded biodegradable porous polylactic acid (PLA): a tissue-engineering study. J Biomed Mater Res 1995; 29:1147–1154.
79. Chu CR, Monosov AZ, Amiel D. In situ assessment of cell viability within biodegradable polylactic acid polymer matrices. Biomaterials 1995; 16: 1381–1384.
80. Ma PX, Schloo B, Mooney D, Langer R. Development of biomechanical properties and morphogenesis of in vitro tissue engineered cartilage. J Biomed Mater Res 1995; 29:1587–1595.
81. Sittinger M, Reitzel D, Dauner M, Hierlemann H, Hammer C, Kastenbauer E, Planck H, Burmester GR, Bujia J. Resorbable polyesters in cartilage engineering: affinity and biocompatibility of polymer fiber structures to chondrocytes. J Biomed Mater Res 1996; 33:57–63.
82. Gugala Z, Gogolewski S. In vitro growth and activity of primary chondrocytes on a resorbable polylactide three-dimensional scaffold. J Biomed Mater Res 2000; 49:183–191.
83. Lee JY, Musgrave D, Pelinkovic D, Fukushima K, Cummins J, Usas A, Robbins P, Fu FH, Huard J. Effect of bone morphogenetic protein-2-expressing muscle-derived cells on healing of critical-sized bone defects in mice. J Bone Joint Surg 2001; 83-A:1032–1039.
84. Hollinger JO, Winn SR, Hu Y, Sipe R, Buck DC, Xi G. Assembling a bone-regeneration therapy. In: Davies JE, ed. Bone Engineering. Toronto: em squared, 2000:435–440.
85. Fang J, Zhu Y-Y, Smiley E, Bonadio J, Rouleau JP, Goldstein SA, McCauley LK, Davidson BL, Roessler BJ. Stimulation of new bone formation by direct transfer of osteogenic plasmid genes. Proc Natl Acad Sci USA 1996; 93:5753–5758.
86. Klein CPAT, Dreissen AA, de Groot K. Biodegradation behavior of various calcium phosphate materials in bone tissue. J Biomed Mater Res 1983; 17:769–784.
87. Daculsi G, LeGros RZ, Nery E, Lynch K, Kerebel B. Transformation of biphasic calcium phosphate ceramics in vivo: ultrastructural and physicochemical characterization. J Biomed Mater Res 1989; 23:883–894.
88. Ikenaga M, Hardouin P, Lemaitre J, Andrianjatovo H, Flautre B. Biomechanical characterization of a biodegradable calcium phosphate hydraulic cement: a comparison with porous biphasic calcium phosphate ceramics. J Biomed Mater Res 1998; 40:139–144.
89. Munting E, Mirtchi AA, Lemaitre J. Bone repair of defects filled with a phospho-calcic hydraulic cement: an in vivo study. J Mater Sci Mater Med 1993:337–344.

90. Miyamoto Y, Ishikawa K, Fukao H, Sawada M, Nagayama M, Kon M, Asaoka K. In vivo setting behaviour of fast-setting calcium phosphate cement. Biomaterials 1995; 16:855–860.
91. Miyamoto Y, Ishikawa K, Takechi M, Toh T, Yuasa T, Nagayama M, Suzuki K. Basic properties of calcium phosphate cement containing atelocollagen in its liquid or powder phases. Biomaterials 1998; 19:707–715.
92. Ishikawa K, Asaoka K. Estimation of ideal mechanical strength and critical porosity of calcium phosphate cement. J Biomed Mater Res 1995; 29:1537–1543.
93. Driessens FCM, Boltong MG, Bermudez O, Planell JA, Ginebra MP, Fernandez E. Effective formulations for the preparation of calcium phosphate bone cements. J Mater Sci Mater Med 1994; 5:164–170.
94. Ohura K, Bohner M, Hardouin P, Lemaitre J, Pasquier G, Flautre B. Resorption of, and bone formation from, new β-tricalcium phosphate-monocalcium phosphate cements: an in vivo study. J Biomed Mater Res 1996; 30:193–200.
95. Miyamoto Y, Ishikawa K, Takechi M, Toh T, Yoshida Y, Nagayama M, Kon M, Asaoka K. Tissue response to fast-setting calcium phosphate cement in bone. J Biomed Mater Res 1997; 37:457–464.
96. Miyamoto Y, Ishikawa K, Takechi M, Toh T, Yuasa T, Nagayama M, Suzuki K. Histological and compositional evaluations of three types of calcium phosphate cements when implanted in subcutaneous tissue immediately after mixing. J Biomed Mater Res Appl Biomater 1999; 48:36–42.
97. Ishikawa K, Miyamoto Y, Kon M, Nagayama M, Asaoka K. Non-decay type fast-setting calcium phosphate cement: composite with sodium alginate. Biomaterials 1995; 16:527–532.
98. Ishikawa K, Miyamoto Y, Takechi M, Toh T, Kon M, Nagayama M, Asaoka K. Non-decay type fast-setting calcium phosphate cement: hydroxyapatite putty containing an increased amount of sodium alginate. J Biomed Mater Res 1997; 36:393–399.
99. Takechi M, Miyamoto Y, Ishikawa K, Toh T, Yuasa T, Nagayama M, Suzuki K. Initial histological evaluation of anti-washout type fast-setting calcium phosphate cement following subcutaneous implantation. Biomaterials 1998; 19:2057–2063.
100. Frankenburg EP, Goldstein SA, Bauer TW, Harris SA, Poser RD. Biomechanical and histological evaluation of a calcium phosphate cement. J Bone Joint Surg 1998; 80-A:1112–1124.
101. Constanz BR, Ison IC, Fulmer MT, Poser RD, Smith ST, Van Wagoner M, Ross J, Goldstein SA, Jupiter JB, Rosenthal DI. Skeletal repair by in situ formation of the mineral phase of bone. Science 1995; 267:1796–1799.
102. Constanz BR, Barr BM, Ison IC, Fulmer MT, Baker J, McKinney L, Goodman SB, Gunasekaren S, Delaney DC, Ross J, Poser RD. Histological, chemical, and crystallographic analysis of four calcium phosphate cements in different rabbit osseous sites. J Biomed Mater Res Appl Biomater 1998; 43:451–461.
103. Goodman SB, Bauer TW, Carter D, Casteleyn PP, Goldstein SA, Kyle RF, Larsson S, Stakewich CJ, Swiontkowski MF, Tencer AF, Yetkinler DN,

Poser RD. Norian SRS cement augmentation in hip fracture treatment. Clin Orthop Rel Res 1998; 348:42–50.

104. Kopylov P, Jonsson K, K.G T, Aspenberg P. Injectable calcium phosphate in the treatment of distal radial fractures. J Hand Surg 1996; 21B:768–771.

105. Food and Drug Administration (USA) website, www.fda.gov

106. Knaack D, Goad MEP, Aiolova M, Rey C, Tofighi A, Chakravarthy P, Lee DD. Resorbable calcium phosphate bone substitute. J Biomed Mater Res Appl Biomater 1998; 43:399–409.

107. Muggli DS, Burkoth AK, Keyser SA, Lee HR, Anseth KS. Reaction behavior of biodegradable, photo-cross-linkable polyanhydrides. Macromolecules 1998; 31:4120–4125.

108. Anseth KS, Shastri VR, Langer R. Photopolymerizable degradable poly-anhydrides with osteocompatibility. Nature Biotech 1999; 17:156–159.

109. Shastri VR, Marini RP, Padera RF, Kirchain S, Tarcha P, Langer R. Osteo-compatibility of photopolymerizable anhydride networks. Mater Res Soc Symp Proc 1998; 530:93–98.

110. Gresser JD, Hsu S-H, Nagaoka H, Lyons CM, Nieratko DP, Wise DL, Barabino GA, Trantolo DJ. Analysis of a vinyl pyrrolidone/poly(propylene fumarate) resorbable bone cement. J Biomed Mater Res 1995; 29:1241–1247.

111. Kharas GB, Kamenetsky M, Simantirakis J, Beinlich KC, Rizzo A-MT, Caywood GA, Watson K. Synthesis and characterization of fumarate-based polyesters for use in bioresorbable bone cement composites. J Appl Polym Sci 1997; 66:1123–1137.

112. Robinson BV, Sullivan FM, Borzelleca JF, Schwartz SL. . PVP: A Critical Review of the Kinetics and Toxicology of Polyvinylpyrrolidone (Povidone). Chelsea, MI: Lewis, 1990.

113. Peter SJ, Miller ST, Zhu G, Yasko AW, Mikos AG. In vivo degradation of a poly(propylene fumarate)/β-tricalcium phosphate injectable composite scaffold. J Biomed Mater Res 1998; 41:1–7.

114. Peter SJ, Nolley JA, Widmer MS, Merwin JE, Yaszemski MJ, Yasko AW, Engel PS, Mikos AG. In vitro degradation of a poly(propylene fumarate)/β-tricalcium phosphate composite orthopedic scaffold. Tissue Eng 1997; 3:207–215.

115. Payne RG. Development of an injectable, in situ crosslinkable, degradable polymeric carrier for osteogenic populations. Ph.D. thesis, Houston, TX: Department of Chemical Engineering, Rice University, 2001.

116. Payne RG, Yaszemski MJ, Yasko AW, Mikos AG. Development of an inject-able, in situ crosslinkable, degradable polymeric carrier for osteogenic cell populations. Part 1. Encapsulation of marrow stromal osteoblasts in surface crosslinked gelatin microparticles. Biomaterials 2002; 23:4359–4371.

117. Payne RG, McGonigle JS, Yaszemski MJ, Yasko AW, Mikos AG. Develop-ment of an injectable, in situ crosslinkable, degradable polymeric carrier for osteogenic cell populations: Part 2. Viability of encapsulated marrow stromal osteoblasts cultured on crosslinking poly(propylene fumarate). Biomaterials 2002; 23:4373–4380.

118. Payne RG, McGonigle JS, Yaszemski MJ, Yasko AW, Mikos AG. Development of an injectable, in situ crosslinkable, degradable polymeric carrier for osteogenic cell populations: Part 3. Proliferation and differentiation of encapsulated marrow stromal osteoblasts cultured on crosslinking poly(propylene fumarate). Biomaterials 2002; 23:4381–4387.

119. Kimura T, Yasui N, Ohsawa S, Ono K. Chondrocytes embedded in collagen gels maintain cartilage phenotype during long-term cultures. Clin Orthop Rel Res 1984; 186:231–239.

120. Wakitani S, Goto T, Pineda SJ, Young RG, Mansour JM, Caplan AI, Goldberg VM. Mesenchymal cell-based repair of large, full-thickness defects of articular cartilage. J Bone Joint Surg 1994; 76-A·579–592.

121. Caplan AI, Elyaderani M, Mochizuki Y, Wakitani S, Goldberg VM. Principles of cartilage repair and regeneration. Clin Orthop Rel Res 1997; 342:254–269.

122. Paige KT, Cima LG, Yaremchuk MJ, Vacanti JP, Vacanti CA. Injectable cartilage. Plast Reconstr Surg 1995; 96:1390–1400.

123. Paige KT, Cima LG, Yaremchuk MJ, Schloo BL, Vacanti JP, Vacanti CA. De novo cartilage generation using calcium alginate-chondrocyte constructs. Plast Reconstr Surg 1996; 97:168–180.

124. Kulseng B, Skjak-Braek G, Ryan L, Andersson A, King A, Faxvaag A, Espevik T. Transplantation of alginate microcapsules. Transplantation 1999; 67:978–984.

125. Ting V, Sims CD, Brecht LE, McCarthy JG, Kasabian AK, Connelly PR, Elisseeff J, Gittes GK, Longaker MT. In vitro prefabrication of human cartilage shapes using fibrin glue and human chondrocytes. Ann Plast Surg 1998; 40:413–421.

126. Hendrickson DA, Nixon AJ, Grande DA, Todhunter RJ, Minor RM, Erb H, Lust G. Chondrocyte-fibrin matrix transplants for resurfacing extensive articular cartilage defects. J Orthop Res 1994; 12:485–497.

127. van Susante JLC, Buma P, Schuman L, Homminga GN, van den Berg WB, Veth RPH. Resurfacing potential of heterologous chondrocytes suspended in fibrin glue in large full-thickness defects of femoral articular cartilage: an experimental study in the goat. Biomaterials 1999; 20:1167–1175.

128. Stile RA, Healy KE. Synthesis of hydrogels: environmentally sensitive hydrogels based on N-isopropylacrylamide. In: Atala A, Lanza RP, eds. Methods of Tissue Engineering. San Diego, CA: Academic Press, 2002.

129. Sims CD, Butler PEM, Casanova R, Lee BT, Randolph MA, Lee WPA, Vacanti CA, Yaremchuk MJ. Injectable cartilage using polyethylene oxide polymer substrates. Plast Reconstr Surg 1996; 98:843–850.

130. Elisseeff J, Anseth K, Sims D, McIntosh W, Randolph M, Langer R. Transdermal photopolymerization for minimally invasive implantation. Proc Natl Acad Sci USA 1999; 96:3104–3107.

131. Elisseeff J, McIntosh W, Anseth K, Riley S, Ragan P, Langer R. Photoencapsulation of chondrocytes in poly(ethylene-oxide)-based semi-interpenetrating networks. J Biomed Mater Res 2000; 51:164–171.

7

Biomechanical Factors in Tissue Engineering of Articular Cartilage

Farshid Guilak

Duke University Medical Center,
Durham, North Carolina, U.S.A.

I. INTRODUCTION

Articular cartilage is the connective tissue that serves as the load-bearing material lining the ends of long bones in diarthrodial joints. The primary functions of this tissue are to support and transmit forces generated during joint loading while providing a lubricated surface that prevents wear and degeneration of the joint (1). The composition and architecture of this tissue, which give it its unique mechanical properties, are maintained through a balance of the anabolic and catabolic activities of the chondrocytes. Chondrocytes are the only cell type present in cartilage and comprise a small fraction of the tissue volume. However, articular cartilage possesses limited capacity for intrinsic repair, and even minor lesions or injuries may lead to progressive damage and joint degeneration.

The poor repair response of articular cartilage is attributed to several factors, including the low cell density, the lack of a blood supply, and the lack of a source of undifferentiated cells that can promote tissue repair. For these reasons, many surgeons have used different means of penetrating the subchondral bone to induce bleeding in a repair site in the cartilage. These techniques have included drilling, abrasion, and microfracture of the subchondral bone in a manner that often penetrates to the marrow cavity (2–5). These methods generally lead to the formation of a fibrocartilaginous repair tissue, which in some cases is satisfactory and decreases pain and disability. In general, however, fibrocartilaginous repair tissue differs in its mechanical properties in comparison with normal articular cartilage (6) and may not function effectively as a long-term replacement for normal cartilage (7). Other techniques have included the transplantation of allograft or autograft cartilage in an effort to restore tissue function. The long-term efficacy of such methods remains unproven, and recent evidence has shown that significant morbidity may be associated with the donor site of autograft cartilage in the joint (8).

In recent years, the field of "tissue engineering" has introduced technologies for cartilage repair that involve the implantation of cells, biomaterials, and biologically active molecules (9–17). At this writing, there is one clinically approved cell-based therapy for cartilage repair (Carticel procedure, Genzyme Biosurgery, Cambridge MA). This technique involve the isolation and amplification of autologous chondrocytes, which are then implanted into the cartilage defect and covered with a flap of autologous periosteum (18–20). The long-term success of this technique has not been shown in an animal model (21), although clinical outcomes have been good to excellent (22).

Despite some early successes and rapid advances in the field, however, tissue engineering has faced significant challenges in the successful long-term repair of mechanically functional tissues such as articular cartilage. The precise reasons for failure are not fully understood, but include a combination of biomechanical and biochemical factors that lead to the breakdown of repair cartilage under physiological loading conditions. A new and evolving discipline termed "functional tissue engineering" seeks to address these challenges by developing guidelines for rationally investigating the role of biomechanical factors in engineered repairs. A series of formal goals for functional tissue engineering have been proposed in a generalized format (23) as well as with specific reference to articular cartilage (24). Here, we review several of the issues involved in the interaction of biomechanical factors in the outcome of tissue-engineered cartilage repair. Presumably, many of the issues discussed in this chapter will be relevant to other tissues and organs of the body that serve some biomechanical functions and are targets for engineered tissue replacement (e.g., bone, muscle, blood vessels).

II. DEVELOPING STANDARDS OF SUCCESS FOR CARTILAGE REPAIR

The primary objectives in cartilage repair procedures are generally acknowledged to be the elimination of pain and the restoration of joint function. Often, a secondary consideration is that the repair procedure serves to prevent or slow the onset and progression of degenerative arthritis in the joint. However, few quantitative surgical outcome measures are available to guide the use of different repair procedures. What constitutes success after cartilage repair will depend not only on the functional efficacy of the procedure, but also on numerous other factors. For example, the cost of the procedure, comorbidities and age of the patient, the duration that a specific treatment may last, and the invasiveness and difficulty of the procedure (e.g., arthroscopic vs. open arthrotomy) may factor into its perceived success. In this respect, controlled, prospective outcome studies and cost analyses will be critical in defining the actual goals of a successful repair procedure and will assist in developing clear guidelines on the cost-benefit ratio of different cartilage repair procedures.

From a functional standpoint, however, the assessment of whether a repair procedure has successfully restored the biomechanical characteristics of the joint will require the development of more quantitative measures of outcome at the clinical level (e.g., pain, range of motion, gait, joint forces) (25,26) as well as the joint and tissue levels (e.g., tissue biomechanical properties, engraftment, structure, and composition). Most previous studies have used histological, morphological, and compositional assessment of repair cartilage as measures of success (19,13–17,27). In recent years, these definitions of success have been advanced through the development of standardized guidelines for quantitative assessment, such as those established by the International Cartilage Repair Society (ICRS) (28). With respect to the biomechanical properties and function of repair cartilage, however, no such guidelines are available. In the future, the emphasis on the functional behavior of grafts and repair tissues will require the ability to quantify and report outcome measures directly related to tissue function, namely the material properties, ultrastructure, and morphology of repair tissues. However, an important gap still remains in the scientific knowledge with respect to a full understanding of the relationships between cartilage structure, composition, and biomechanical properties. In particular, little or no such information is available for repair or regenerated tissues. While several studies have shown some correlation between matrix composition and specific mechanical properties in native cartilage (29), these relationships are not present in all species and sites of cartilage (30).

The development of new minimally invasive methodologies for the assessment of tissue properties may improve our understanding of structure-function-composition relationships in native and repair cartilage. For example, biological markers, or "biomarkers" of tissue metabolism (31–33), arthroscopic biomechanical probes (34), or imaging techniques such as magnetic resonance imaging , computed tomography, ultrasound, or dual x-ray absorptiometry (35,36) are being investigated for their quantitative and predictive abilities to assess tissue function with cartilage injury or disease, but have not been applied extensively to the study of cartilage repair. These methods may be particularly important in longitudinal studies of tissue-engineered repair in the clinical setting. A more thorough understanding of the relationships between the function, structure, and composition of normal and repair cartilage will ultimately contribute to the success of these minimally invasive techniques.

III. THE BIOMECHANICAL PROPERTIES OF NATIVE AND REPAIR ARTICULAR CARTILAGE

The unique biomechanical and frictional properties of cartilage are attributed to the complex structure and composition of extracellular tissue matrix (1). The material properties of cartilage are viscoelastic (dependent on rate or time), nonlinear (stress-strain relationships are not linear), anisotropic (dependent on direction), and inhomogeneous (dependent on site). It now is well accepted that the primary mechanism of viscoelasticity in cartilage results from frictional interactions between the solid and fluid phases (37), although the solid matrix also exhibits intrinsic viscoelastic behavior (38,39). Cartilage also exhibits highly nonlinear mechanical properties such as strain-dependent moduli (40), strain-dependent hydraulic permeability (41), and a difference of nearly two orders of magnitude in tensile and compressive moduli (29,37). This nonlinear behavior serves to enhance the mechanisms of fluid load support in the tissue (42). These properties also are anisotropic and vary significantly with site (distance from the tissue surface and location on the joint surface) (29). Other mechanical behaviors include the presence of internal swelling pressures that give rise to inhomogeneous residual stresses within the tissue (43,44). In addition to these material properties, cartilage also possesses important geometrical characteristics that provide for unique frictional properties (45). The low coefficient of friction of cartilage-on-cartilage surfaces, coupled with fluid-dependent mechanisms of load support, allows for minimal tissue wear under very high mechanical stresses.

The fundamental physical mechanisms governing these behaviors are the topic of numerous investigations, and researchers are still uncovering new information on the load-bearing and lubrication properties of cartilage. It remains to be determined which aspects of the mechanical properties of articular cartilage are essential for normal tissue function, as well as for successful tissue-engineered replacements. Despite the well-accepted biomechanical requirements of articular cartilage, there have been relatively few reports of the biomechanical properties of engineered or repair cartilage (6,17,46–50).

To effectively develop new techniques for cartilage repair or regeneration, it is important to understand both the subfailure and failure characteristics of the native tissues as well as those of engineered repair. The subfailure properties represent the tissue characteristics within the bounds of normal, expected loading conditions. However, since biomechanical failure is often a problem with newly implanted grafts, knowledge of the failure properties of native tissues may provide crucial information on "safety factors" that are required for engineered repairs (23). A safety factor is defined as the ratio of the failure stress to the peak stress that is experienced during normal activities. Failure testing can provide information on the structural and material properties of the tissue to be replaced. Structural properties allow comparison of tissues or constructs to a baseline functional level, and incorporate the role of morphological parameters, such as tissue geometry. Material properties are valuable in that they may be determined in simplified loading configurations and represent the intrinsic properties of the tissue, irrespective of size or geometry. Material properties are of particular value in that they may be used to describe the mechanical response of the tissue to any loading history, when combined with physiologically relevant theoretical models.

IV. MECHANICAL PROPERTIES AS DESIGN PARAMETERS IN CARTILAGE REPAIR

The biomechanical design parameters for engineered cartilage are not well defined, and it is often proposed that repair tissues must match the biomechanical properties of the adjacent native articular cartilage to function properly. Unfortunately, there is little direct evidence to either support or refute this premise. Realistically, it will be difficult, if not impossible, to match all of the material properties and structure of native cartilage with tissue-engineered constructs or surgical repair procedures over the lifetime of a graft. To further complicate this issue, native tissues also may show signs of disease or degeneration, raising the question of whether the goal is to match the properties of healthy tissue or those of adjacent tissues, regardless of their state. Currently, little is known about the relative importance of different material properties in the long-term success of an engineered repair.

An important next step in improving engineered repair will be the prioritization of the multitude of complex tissue properties as design parameters.

There have been few reports of the material properties of tissue engineered cartilage grafts, either prior to implantation (51–54) or at sacrifice (47,55). In most studies, focus has been placed on the compressive aggregate or Young's modulus and the hydraulic permeability of cartilage (46,47,52,56). These properties are likely to be the most logical starting points; however, the relative importance of recreating the tissue's compressive properties in comparison with the tensile, shear, failure, wear, frictional, or other properties (23) is not yet known.

Many questions also remain regarding the relative importance of recreating the native tissue and joint architecture. For example, attempts at articular cartilage regeneration have sought to promote complete integration between host and repair tissues (51,57,58). Indeed, complete graft integration has been used as a gold standard of cartilage repair, yet neither the short-term nor the long-term implications of either complete or incomplete integrative repair are known. Similarly, the importance of restoring cartilage thickness, geometry, and joint congruence is not well understood, and these factors may have an important influence on the stress environment within the joint (59,60). Currently, however, few tissue engineering or cartilage repair approaches have the ability to precisely control the structure and geometry of newly formed tissues, and in many cases, the repair of osteochondral defects is characterized either by hypertrophy or by incomplete filling of the defect site (22).

As it is unlikely that all of these complex material and structural issues are simultaneously addressed, it becomes critical to prioritize their relative influence on the overall success of a given procedure. Furthermore, most surgical or engineered repair procedures involve remodeling or degradation of biological or artificial scaffolds over time as new tissues are synthesized and assembled. Thus, the functional properties of an engineered graft will be expected to change in a controlled manner subsequent to implantation. Unfortunately, there is a dearth of information on the biomechanical properties of various biomaterials that are used as matrices for cartilage repair, and few are able to replicate any aspects of native cartilage biomechanical properties (reviewed in Ref. 61). Furthermore, tissue-engineered constructs must be capable of retaining their mechanical, structural, and biological integrity during large-scale production, packaging, storage, and, eventually, surgical implantation. In defining rational design criteria for cartilage repair, it will be essential to understand biomechanical requirements of a tissue-engineered product from the time of production, to delivery to the operating room, during surgical implantation, and throughout its life span within the body.

In attempting to define such design parameters for the biomechanical function of repair tissues, it will be critical to understand the mechanical history that normal and repair tissues may encounter for different in vivo activities. These measurements can establish the patterns of activity and the safety factors that need to be designed into each material property. In certain tissues of the body, such as blood vessels, bone, or tendon/ligament, there is considerable quantitative information on the in vivo stress-strains environment (62–68). For articular cartilage, however, little information is available on in vivo stresses or strains. Peak stresses in articular cartilage, measured against an instrumented prosthesis, have been shown to reach 18 MPa (69), while experiments using pressure-sensitive films have shown that stresses within a normal joint may range from 5 to 10 MPa (70–72). Additionally, the presence of a cartilage defect may significantly alter the stress field within the defect or the surrounding tissue (73). Similarly, there is little information on the magnitude of in situ strains in articular cartilage. In one study, sequential planar radiography showed that cartilage deforms no more than 15–20% under physiological conditions (74). More recently, magnetic resonance imaging studies have shown that cartilage height and volume may decrease by approximately 5% after exercise (75).

Because of the inherent difficulties involved in experimental measurements of in situ loads and deformations of cartilage, several investigators have used theoretical models of joint contact to predict the distribution of these parameters within native and repair articular cartilage (42,76,77). The accuracy of these models has increased significantly in recent years with increasing computational capabilities and the development of minimally invasive methods for measuring joint and tissue geometry.

V. BIOMECHANICAL FACTORS AND THE REGULATION OF CELLULAR ACTIVITY

Chondrocytes are able to perceive and respond to signals generated by the normal load-bearing activities of daily living (78). Under abnormal conditions, however, mechanical factors may be responsible for initiating inflammatory and degradative processes that ultimately may lead to progressive joint degeneration. The physical mechanisms involved in the process of mechanical signaling potentially involve a variety of mechanical, chemical, and electrical signals that are generated secondary to joint loading. Physiological loading of the joint produces deformation of the articular cartilage and associated changes in the stress-strain environment of the cell within the extracellular matrix (1). In addition, the presence of interstitial water containing mobile ions, and a high density of negatively charged proteoglycans in the solid matrix (i.e., fixed charge density), gives rise to coupled electrical and chemical phenomena during tissue loading (43,79). The ability of the chondrocytes to regulate their metabolic activity in response to such biophysical signals provides a means by which articular cartilage can alter its structure and composition to the physical demands of the body. In this sense, the mechanical environment of the cells is believed to play an important role in the health and function of the diarthrodial joint. Therefore, it is presumed that the long-term success of cell-based repairs may require similar capabilities for cells to remodel—and potentially repair—the tissue in response to functional demands.

In this light, it would be important to characterize the diverse array of physical signals that cells may experience within an engineered repair in vivo and to understand their biological response to such stimuli. Cellular responsiveness to physical stimuli may be an additional factor that contributes to the long-term capabilities of engineered constructs to maintain the proper cellular phenotype. In native tissue, a number of different model systems have been used to investigate the role of physical stimuli in regulating cartilage and chondrocyte activity, ranging from in vivo studies to experiments at the cell and molecular level (see reviews in Refs. 78,80–82). Each type of study provides important advantages and disadvantages that often involve a trade-off between the physiological relevance of the model and the ability to maximally control the test conditions. For example, in vivo animal studies based on emulating the physiological relevant loading conditions provide a means to study long-term (i.e., weeks to years) changes associated with repair, remodeling, or disease (83,84), but are limited by difficulties in determining the precise loading history of the tissue as well as the effect of systemic factors. In tissue models, in vitro studies of cartilage explants or isolated cells grown in three-dimensional matrices can provide model systems where both the applied loading and biochemical environment can be better controlled. Such systems can provide information on the relationships between matrix loading and cellular metabolic activity. It is important to note that the loading of an explant or artificial matrix in a controlled and isolated manner in vitro will not completely reproduce the in vivo environment of the chondrocytes, making it difficult to relate in vitro findings directly to physiologically relevant situations that are characteristic of daily living in an intact joint.

Because of intrinsic coupling between the mechanical and physicochemical properties of articular cartilage, it is often difficult to separate the influence of various biophysical factors on cellular activity. For example, compressive loading of articular cartilage or engineered tissues can expose the cells to spatially and time-varying stress, strain, fluid flow and pressure, osmotic pressure, and electric fields (43,85,86). A fundamental step in determining the role of various factors in regulating chondrocyte activity is to characterize the mechanical environment within the tissue under physiological conditions of mechanical loading. This characterization would facilitate the reproduction of specific aspects of this environment in different model systems. For example, several novel microscopy techniques have provided important measurements of the in situ deformation behavior (i.e., shape and volume changes) of living chondrocytes or organelles in situ, showing that chondrocyte deformation is coordinated with that of the extracellular matrix (87–91). In other studies, similar techniques have investigated chondrocyte deformation within artificial matrices, generally consisting of hydrogels (92–95). An important finding of these studies is that the mechanical environment of the chondrocyte within the native extracellular matrix may differ significantly from that in an artificial gel matrix. For example, chondrocytes undergo significant volume loss with compression of the native extracellular matrix (88–91), but little or no change in volume when compressed in artificial gel matrices such as agarose (92–95).

Much of the information currently available on chondrocyte response to mechanical stress has been realized from tissue explant culture experiments, which provide a more controlled mechanical and biochemical environment than the in vivo condition. The great majority of such studies has been performed using chondrocytes embedded within their native extracellular matrix (reviewed in Ref. 80). However, several experiments examining the response of chondrocytes in artificial matrices or engineered constructs suggest that cellular response to mechanical loading may be altered significantly in the absence of the native extracellular matrix. A comparison of the biological response of chondrocytes to compression within their native extracellular matrices to that within artificial matrices such as agarose reveals several important and distinct differences. For example, chondrocytes embedded within agarose show little metabolic response to compression until a newly synthesized matrix has accumulated within the agarose (96). This phenomenon has been attributed to alterations in the biomechanical and physicochemical microenvironment of the chondrocytes secondary to the increase in the local fixed-charge density of the matrix. Within such a model system, chondrocytes undergo significant deformation until a new pericellular matrix has been synthesized (94). Furthermore, dynamic compression of chondrocytes within the native extracellular matrix significant increases the production of nitric oxide, an important inflammatory mediator (97); within an agarose matrix, similar regimens of compression suppress nitric oxide synthesis. As nitric oxide is an important regulator of both anabolic and catabolic activities in cartilage

(98), alteration of the "normal" response of the cells to mechanical stimuli may influence the balance between synthesis and degradation of the extracellular matrix.

Other studies have revealed important characteristics of the response of repair cartilage to mechanical stress using in vitro models (51,99,100). For example, static compression of chondrocytes transplanted onto articular cartilage significantly decreases proteoglycan synthesis rates (99) and cell proliferation (100), and thus may affect subsequent integrative cartilage repair in vivo. Together, these findings suggest that various aspects of the repair process, including cellular proliferation, matrix biosynthesis, and tissue integration, may be influenced directly or indirectly by mechanical factors.

VI. THE USE OF BIOPHYSICAL FACTORS TO PROMOTE CARTILAGE REGENERATION IN VITRO

Mechanical stress is an important modulator of cell physiology, and there is significant evidence that controlled application of biophysical stimuli within "bioreactors" may be used to improve or accelerate tissue regeneration and repair in vitro. For example, early studies showed that cyclical mechanical stretch of skeletal myofibers increased the alignment of myotubes that assembled into organoids in culture (101,102). In other studies, mechanical stimulation has been shown to increase cellular alignment, proliferation, and matrix synthesis in many different cell types (103–106). Recent studies have shown improved success of tissue-engineered systems such as blood vessels and smooth muscle by pre-conditioning grafts with pulsatile fluid flow and pressure (107–109).

Specific to articular cartilage, there is growing evidence that mechanical stimuli can increase matrix deposition in tissue-engineered cartilage in vitro. Although the specific biophysical signals are not fully understood, a variety of stimuli have been shown to increase matrix synthesis and accumulation. In particular, increased fluid flow and perfusion within constructs has a stimulatory effect on matrix synthesis and accumulation (110,111), presumably owing to increased shear stresses, nutrient transport, and metabolite exchange. Cyclical compression of chondrocytes bioartificial matrices may also increase matrix synthesis (56,96) through a mechanism that potentially involves increased localized fluid flow. However, other stimuli such as hypogravity (52) also influence chondrogenesis, indicating a more complex relationship between mechanical stimuli and cell activity within bioreactors.

There is also increasing evidence that biomechanical stimuli can promote the differentiation of progenitor, or "stem" cells, into a chondrogenic phenotype. Dynamic fluid pressure has been shown to increase the proliferation of periosteal cells (112), potentially through a paracrine signaling mechanism between the cells in cambium and fibrous layers. In other studies, cyclical compression of chick limb mesenchymal cells in an agarose extracellular matrix was found to double the number of cartilage nodules and the rate of proteoglycan synthesis, whereas static compression had little effect on cellular differentiation (113).

These findings indicate a potentially important role for biomechanical and biophysical factors in stimulating cellular differentiation, gene expression, macromolecular synthesis, and matrix assembly in tissue engineering systems. The use of mechanical stimuli in place of or in combination with biochemical factors may provide means to facilitate the development of functional tissues in vitro, prior to implantation in the body. A more thorough understanding of the response of native and engineered cartilage to mechanical stress, and the mechanisms involved in these responses, will improve the success of tissue-engineered cartilage repair.

VII. FUTURE DIRECTIONS

It is now well accepted that mechanical factors play an important role in the health and maintenance of native articular cartilage. Mechanical signals, along with local and systemic biochemical factors, appear to contribute to the regulatory pathways used by chondrocytes to maintain a homeostatic balance of anabolic and catabolic activities. Once implanted within the joint, engineered tissues will be exposed to mechanical factors whose characteristics may differ from the native state. A better understanding of the in vivo mechanical environment, as well as the interaction of mechanical factors with cells in engineered tissues, may serve to improve the chances for success. It is important to note that other rapidly evolving technologies may have a significant impact on functional tissue engineering and cartilage repair, and these guidelines must be considered in light of the role of novel growth factors, new biomaterials, progenitor cells, gene therapy, and other new technologies.

ACKNOWLEDGMENTS

The author thanks Drs. David Butler, Steve Goldstein, David Mooney, and Lori Setton for many important discussions on the topics outlined in this chapter. This work was supported in part by grants from the National Institutes of Health AG15768, AR49294, AR48182 and the North Carolina Biotechnology Center.

REFERENCES

1. Mow VC, Ratcliffe A, Poole AR. Cartilage and diarthrodial joints as paradigms for hierarchical materials and structures. Biomaterials 1992; 13:67–97.
2. Akizuki S, Yasukawa Y, Takizawa T. Does arthroscopic abrasion arthroplasty promote cartilage regeneration in osteoarthritic knees with eburnation? A prospective study of high tibial osteotomy with abrasion arthroplasty versus high tibial osteotomy alone. Arthroscopy 1997; 13:9–17.
3. Blevins FT, Steadman JR, Rodrigo JJ, Silliman J. Treatment of articular cartilage defects in athletes: an analysis of functional outcome and lesion appearance. Orthopedics 1998; 21:761–767.
4. Frisbie DD, Trotter GW, Powers BE, et al. Arthroscopic subchondral bone plate microfracture technique augments healing of large chondral defects in the radial carpal bone and medial femoral condyle of horses. Vet Surg 1999; 28:242–255.
5. Ghivizzani SC, Oligino TJ, Robbins PD, Evans CH. Cartilage injury and repair. Phys Med Rehab Clin North Am 2000; 11:289–307, vi.
6. Hale JE, Rudert MJ, Brown TD. Indentation assessment of biphasic mechanical property deficits in size-dependent osteochondral defect repair. J Biomech 1993; 26:1319–1325.
7. Nehrer S, Spector M, Minas T. Histologic analysis of tissue after failed cartilage repair procedures. Clin Orthop 1999; 365:149–162.
8. Lee CR, Grodzinsky AJ, Hsu HP, Martin SD, Spector M. Effects of harvest and selected cartilage repair procedures on the physical and biochemical properties of articular cartilage in the canine knee. J Orthop Res 2000; 18:790–799.
9. Coutts RD, Woo SL, Amiel D, von Schroeder HP, Kwan MK. Rib perichondrial autografts in full-thickness articular cartilage defects in rabbits. Clin Orthop 1992; 275:263–273.
10. Gao J, Dennis JE, Solchaga LA, Awadallah AS, Goldberg VM, Caplan AI. Tissue-engineered fabrication of an osteochondral composite graft using rat bone marrow-derived mesenchymal stem cells. Tissue Eng 2001; 7:363–371.
11. Malemud CJ, Goldberg VM. Future directions for research and treatment of osteoarthritis. Frontiers Biosci 1999; 4:D762–771.
12. Goldberg VM, Caplan AI. Biological resurfacing: an alternative to total joint arthroplasty. Orthopedics 1994; 17:819–821.
13. Grande DA, Pitman MI, Peterson L, Menche D, Klein M. The repair of experimentally produced defects in rabbit articular cartilage by autologous chondrocyte transplantation. J Orthop Res 1989; 7:208–218.
14. O'Driscoll SW, Keeley FW, Salter RB. The chondrogenic potential of free autogenous periosteal grafts for biological resurfacing of major full-thickness defects in joint surfaces under the influence of continuous passive motion: an experimental investigation in the rabbit. J Bone Joint Surg 1986; 68A:1017–1035.
15. Sams AE, Nixon AJ. Chondrocyte-laden collagen scaffolds for resurfacing extensive articular cartilage defects. Osteoarthritis Cartilage 1995; 3:47–59.

16. Temenoff JS, Mikos AG. Review: tissue engineering for regeneration of articular cartilage. Biomaterials 2000; 21:431–440.
17. Wakitani S, Goto T, Pineda SJ, et al. Mesenchymal cell-based repair of large, full-thickness defects of articular cartilage. J Bone Joint Surg 1994; 76A:579–592.
18. Brittberg M, Lindahl A, Nilsson A, Ohlsson C, Isaksson O, Peterson L. Treatment of deep cartilage defects in the knee with autologous chondrocyte transplantation. N Engl J Med 1994; 331:889–895.
19. Gillogly SD, Voight M, Blackburn T. Treatment of articular cartilage defects of the knee with autologous chondrocyte implantation. J Orthop Sports Phys Ther 1998; 28:241–251.
20. Minas T, Nehrer S. Current concepts in the treatment of articular cartilage defects. Orthopedics 1997; 20:525–538.
21. Breinan HA, Minas T, Hsu HP, Nehrer S, Sledge CB, Spector M. Effect of cultured autologous chondrocytes on repair of chondral defects in a canine model. J Bone Joint Surg 1997; 79A:1439–1451.
22. Peterson L, Minas T, Brittberg M, Nilsson A, Sjogren-Jansson E, Lindahl A. Two- to 9-year outcome after autologous chondrocyte transplantation of the knee. Clin Orthop 2000; 374:212–234.
23. Butler D, Goldstein SA, Guilak F. Functional tissue engineering: the role of biomechanics. J Biomech Eng 2000; 122:570–575.
24. Guilak F, Butler DL, Goldstein SA. Functional tissue engineering - The role of biomechanics in articular cartilage repair. Clin Orthop 2001; 391:S295–S305.
25. Andriacchi TP, Alexander EJ. Studies of human locomotion: past, present and future. J Biomech 2000; 33:1217–1224.
26. Wimmer MA, Andriacchi TP. Tractive forces during rolling motion of the knee: implications for wear in total knee replacement. J Biomech 1997; 30:131–137.
27. Pineda S, Pollack A, Stevenson S, Goldberg V, Caplan A. A semiquantitative scale for histologic grading of articular cartilage repair. Acta Anatomica 1992; 143:335–340.
28. http://www.cartilage.org, 2001.
29. Kempson GE, Freeman MA, Swanson SA. Tensile properties of articular cartilage. Nature 1968; 220:1127–1128.
30. Guilak F, Ratcliffe A, Lane N, Rosenwasser MP, Mow VC. Mechanical and biochemical changes in the superficial zone of articular cartilage in canine experimental osteoarthritis. J Orthop Res 1994; 12:474–484.
31. Heinegård D, Saxne T. Macromolecular markers in joint disease. J Rheumatol 1991; 27:27–29.
32. Lindhorst E, Vail TP, Guilak F, et al. Longitudinal characterization of synovial fluid biomarkers in the canine meniscectomy model of osteoarthritis. J Orthop Res 2000; 18:269–280.
33. Lohmander LS, Felson DT. Defining the role of molecular markers to monitor disease, intervention, and cartilage breakdown in osteoarthritis. J Rheumatol 1997; 24:782–785.

34. Lyyra T, Jurvelin J, Pitkanen P, Vaatainen U, Kiviranta I. Indentation instrument for the measurement of cartilage stiffness under arthroscopic control. Med Eng Phys 1995; 17:395–399.

35. Hodler J, Resnick D. Current status of imaging of articular cartilage. Skeletal Radiol 1996; 25:703–709.

36. Karvonen RL, Negendank WG, Fraser SM, Mayes MD, An T, Fernandez-Madrid F. Articular cartilage defects of the knee: correlation between magnetic resonance imaging and gross pathology. Ann Rheum Dis 1990; 49:672–675.

37. Mow VC, Kuei SC, Lai WM, Armstrong CG. Biphasic creep and stress relaxation of articular cartilage in compression: theory and experiments. J Biomech Eng 1980; 102:73–84.

38. Mak AF. The apparent viscoelastic behavior of articular cartilage–the contributions from the intrinsic matrix viscoelasticity and interstitial fluid flows. J Biomech Eng 1986; 108:123–130.

39. Setton LA, Zhu W, Mow VC. The biphasic poroviscoelastic behavior of articular cartilage: role of the surface zone in governing the compressive behavior. J Biomech 1993; 26:581–592.

40. Ateshian GA, Warden WH, Kim JJ, Grelsamer RP, Mow VC. Finite deformation biphasic material properties of bovine articular cartilage from confined compression experiments. J Biomech 1997; 30:1157–1164.

41. Lai WM, Mow VC. Drag-induced compression of articular cartilage during a permeation experiment. Biorheology 1980; 17:111–123.

42. Donzelli PS, Spilker RL, Ateshian GA, Mow VC. Contact analysis of biphasic transversely isotropic cartilage layers and correlations with tissue failure. J Biomech 1999; 32:1037–1047.

43. Lai WM, Hou JS, Mow VC. A triphasic theory for the swelling and deformation behaviors of articular cartilage. J Biomech Eng 1991; 113:245–258.

44. Narmoneva DA, Wang JY, Setton LA. Nonuniform swelling-induced residual strains in articular cartilage. J Biomech 1999; 32:401–408.

45. Wang H, Ateshian GA. The normal stress effect and equilibrium friction coefficient of articular cartilage under steady frictional shear. J Biomech 1997; 30:771–776.

46. Kwan MK, Coutts RD, Woo SL, Field FP. Morphological and biomechanical evaluations of neocartilage from the repair of full-thickness articular cartilage defects using rib perichondrium autografts: a long-term study. J Biomech 1989; 22:921–930.

47. Mow VC, Ratcliffe A, Rosenwasser MP, Buckwalter JA. Experimental studies on repair of large osteochondral defects at a high weight bearing area of the knee joint: a tissue engineering study. J Biomech Eng 1991; 113:198–207.

48. Suzuki Y. Studies on the repair tissue of injured articular cartilage–biochemical and biomechanical properties. J Jpn Orthop Assoc 1983; 57:741–752.

49. Wayne JS, Woo SL, Kwan MK. Finite element analyses of repaired articular surfaces. Proceedings of the Institution of Mechanical Engineers Part H. J Eng Med 1991; 205:155–162.

50. Woo SL, Kwan MK, Lee TQ, Field FP, Kleiner JB, Coutts RD. Perichondrial autograft for articular cartilage. Shear modulus of neocartilage studied in rabbits. Acta Orthop Scand 1987; 58:510–515.
51. Ahsan T, Sah RL. Biomechanics of integrative cartilage repair. Osteoarthritis Cartilage 1999; 7:29–40.
52. Freed LE, Langer R, Martin I, Pellis NR, Vunjak-Novakovic G. Tissue engineering of cartilage in space. Proc Natl Acad Sci USA 1997; 94:13885–13890.
53. Ma PX, Langer R. Morphology and mechanical function of long-term in vitro engineered cartilage. J Biomed Mater Res 1999; 44:217–221.
54. Peretti GM, Bonassar LJ, Caruso EM, Randolph MA, Trahan CA, Zaleske DJ. Biomechanical analysis of a chondrocyte-based repair model of articular cartilage. Tissue Eng 1999; 5:317–326.
55. Wakitani S, Goto T, Young RG, Mansour JM, Goldberg VM, Caplan AI. Repair of large full-thickness articular cartilage defects with allograft articular chondrocytes embedded in a collagen gel. Tissue Eng 1998; 4:429–444.
56. Mauck RL, Soltz MA, Wang CC, et al. Functional tissue engineering of articular cartilage through dynamic loading of chondrocyte-seeded agarose gels. J Biomech Eng 2000; 122:252–260.
57. Hunziker EB, Rosenberg LC. Repair of partial-thickness defects in articular cartilage: cell recruitment from the synovial membrane. J Bone Joint Surg 1996; 78A:721–733.
58. Solchaga LA, Yoo JU, Lundberg M, et al. Hyaluronan-based polymers in the treatment of osteochondral defects. J Orthop Res 2000; 18:773–780.
59. Ateshian GA, Rosenwasser MP, Mow VC. Curvature characteristics and congruence of the thumb carpometacarpal joint: Differences between female and male joints. J Biomech 1992; 25:591–607.
60. Merz B, Eckstein F, Hillebrand S, Putz R. Mechanical implications of humero-ulnar incongruity–finite element analysis and experiment. J Biomech 1997; 30:713–721.
61. Awad H, Erickson GR, Guilak F. Biomaterials for cartilage tissue engineering. In: al Le, ed. Tissue Engineering and Biodegradable Equivalents. New York: Marcel Dekker, 2002:267–299.
62. Biewener AA. Safety factors in bone strength. Calcif Tiss Int 1993; 53: S68–74.
63. Chuong CJ, Fung YC. Three-dimensional stress distribution in arteries. J Biomech Eng 1983; 105:268–274.
64. Han HC, Fung YC. Longitudinal strain of canine and porcine aortas. J Biomech 1995; 28:637–641.
65. Korvick DL, Cummings JF, Grood ES, Holden JP, Feder SM, Butler DL. The use of an implantable force transducer to measure patellar tendon forces in goats. J Biomech 1996; 29:557–561.
66. Malaviya P, Butler DL, Korvick DL, Proch FS. In vivo tendon forces correlate with activity level and remain bounded: evidence in a rabbit flexor tendon model. J Biomech 1998; 31:1043–1049.

67. Milgrom C, Finestone A, Simkin A, et al. In-vivo strain measurements to evaluate the strengthening potential of exercises on the tibial bone. J Bone Joint Surg 2000; 82B:591–594.

68. Woo SL, Debski RE, Wong EK, Yagi M, Tarinelli D. Use of robotic technology for diathrodial joint research. J Sci Med Sport 1999; 2:283–297.

69. Hodge WA, Carlson KL, Fijan RS, et al. Contact pressures from an instrumented hip endoprosthesis. J Bone Joint Surg 1989; 71A:1378–1386.

70. Brown TD, Shaw DT. In vitro contact stress distributions in the natural human hip. J Biomech 1983; 16:373–384.

71. Ronsky JL, Herzog W, Brown TD, Pedersen DR, Grood ES, Butler DL. In vivo quantification of the cat patellofemoral joint contact stresses and areas. J Biomech 1995; 28:977–983.

72. von Eisenhart R, Adam C, Steinlechner M, Muller-Gerbl M, Eckstein F. Quantitative determination of joint incongruity and pressure distribution during simulated gait and cartilage thickness in the human hip joint. J Orthop Res 1999; 17:532–539.

73. Brown TD, Pope DF, Hale JE, Buckwalter JA, Brand RA. Effects of osteo-chondral defect size on cartilage contact stress. J Orthop Res 1991; 9:559–567.

74. Armstrong CG, Bahrani AS, Gardner DL. In vitro measurement of articular cartilage deformations in the intact human hip joint under load. J Bone Joint Surg 1979; 61A:744–755.

75. Eckstein F, Lemberger B, Stammberger T, Englmeier KH, Reiser M. Patellar cartilage deformation in vivo after static versus dynamic loading. J Biomech 2000; 33:819–825.

76. Ateshian GA, Wang H. A theoretical solution for the frictionless rolling contact of cylindrical biphasic articular cartilage layers. J Biomech 1995; 28:1341–1355.

77. Blankevoort L, Kuiper JH, Huiskes R, Grootenboer HJ. Articular contact in a three-dimensional model of the knee. J Biomech 1991; 24:1019–1031.

78. Helminen HJ, Jurvelin J, Kiviranta I, Paukkonen K, Saamanen AM, Tammi M. Joint loading effects on articular cartilage: a historical review. In: Helminen HJ, Kiviranta I, Tammi M, Saamanen AM, Jurvelin J, eds. Joint Loading: Biology and Health of Articular Structures. Bristol: Wright & Sons, 1987:1–46.

79. Grodzinsky AJ. Electromechanical and physicochemical properties of con-nective tissue. Crit Rev Biomed Eng 1983; 9:133–199.

80. Guilak F, Sah RL, Setton LA. Physical Regulation of Cartilage Metabolism. In: VC Mow, WC Hayes, eds. Basic Orthopedic Biomechanics. Philadelphia: Lippincott-Raven, 1997:179–207.

81. Stockwell RA. Structure and function of the chondrocyte under mechanical stress. In: Helminen HJ, Kiviranta I, Tammi M, Saamanen AM, Jurvelin J, eds. Joint Loading: Biology and Health of Articular Structures. Bristol: Wright & Sons, 1987:126–148.

82. van Campen GPJ, van de Stadt RJ. Cartilage and chondrocytes responses to mechanical loading in vitro. In: Helminen HJ, Kiviranta I, Tammi M, Saamanen AM, Jurvelin J, eds. Joint Loading: Biology and Health of Articular Structures. Bristol: Wright & Sons, 1987:112–125.

83. Moskowitz RW. Experimental models of osteoarthritis. In: Moskowitz RW, Howell DS, Goldberg VM, Mankin HJ, eds. Osteoarthritis: Diagnosis and Medical/Surgical Management. Philadelphia: WB Saunders, 1992:213–232.

84. Pritzker KPH. Animal models for osteoarthritis: processes, problems and prospects. Ann Rheum Dis 1994; 53:406–420.

85. Maroudas A. Physicochemical properties of articular cartilage. In: Freeman M, ed. Adult Articular Cartilage. Tunbridge Wells. Pitman Medical, 1979: 215–290.

86. Mow VC, Bachrach N, Setton LA, Guilak F. Stress, strain, pressure, and flow fields in articular cartilage. In: Mow VC, Guilak F, Tran-Son-Tay R, Hochmuth R, eds. Cell Mechanics and Cellular Engineering. New York: Springer Verlag, 1994:345–379.

87. Broom ND, Myers DB. A study of the structural response of wet hyaline cartilage to various loading situations. Connect Tissue Res 1980; 7:227–237.

88. Buschmann MD, Hunziker EB, Kim YJ, Grodzinsky AJ. Altered aggrecan synthesis correlates with cell and nucleus structure in statically compressed cartilage. J Cell Sci 1996; 109:499–508.

89. Guilak F, Ratcliffe A, Mow VC. Chondrocyte deformation and local tissue strain in articular cartilage: a confocal microscopy study. J Orthop Res 1995; 13:410–421.

90. Guilak F. Compression-induced changes in the shape and volume of the chondrocyte nucleus. J Biomech 1995; 28:1529–1542.

91. Wong M, Wuethrich P, Buschmann MD, Eggli P, Hunziker E. Chondrocyte biosynthesis correlates with local tissue strain in statically compressed adult articular cartilage. J Orthop Res 1997; 15:189–196.

92. Freeman PM, Natarjan RN, Kimura JH, Andriacchi TP. Chondrocyte cells respond mechanically to compressive loads. J Orthop Res 1994; 12:311–320.

93. Knight MM, Lee DA, Bolton JF, Bader DL. Cell and nucleus deformation in compressed chondrocyte-agarose constructs- implications for mechanotransduction. Trans Orthop Res Soc 1999; 24:710.

94. Knight MM, Ghori SA, Lee DA, Bader DL. Measurement of the deformation of isolated chondrocytes in agarose subjected to cyclic compression. Med Eng Phys 1998; 20:684–688.

95. Lee DA, Knight MM, Bolton JF, Idowu BD, Kayser MV, Bader DL. Chondrocyte deformation within compressed agarose constructs at the cellular and sub-cellular levels. J Biomech 2000; 33:81–95.

96. Buschmann MD, Gluzband YA, Grodzinsky AJ, Hunziker EB. Mechanical compression modulates matrix biosynthesis in chondrocyte/agarose culture. J Cell Sci 1995; 108:1497–1508.

97. Fermor B, Weinberg JB, Pisetsky DS, Misukonis MA, Banes AJ, Guilak F. The effects of static and intermittent compression on nitric oxide production in articular cartilage explants. J Orthop Res 2001; 19:729–737.

98. Stefanovic-Racic M, Morales TI, Taskiran D, McIntyre LA, Evans CH. The role of nitric oxide in proteoglycan turnover by bovine articular cartilage organ cultures. J Immunol 1996; 156:1213–1220.

99. Chen AC, Sah RL. Effect of static compression on proteoglycan biosynthesis by chondrocytes transplanted to articular cartilage in vitro. J Orthop Res 1998; 16:542–550.

100. Li KW, Falcovitz YH, Nagrampa JP, et al. Mechanical compression modulates proliferation of transplanted chondrocytes. J Orthop Res 2000; 18: 374–382.

101. Vandenburgh H, Kaufman S. In vitro model for stretch-induced hypertrophy of skeletal muscle. Science 1979; 203:265–268.

102. Vandenburgh HH. Dynamic mechanical orientation of skeletal myofibers in vitro. Dev Biol (Orlando) 1982; 93:438–443.

103. Banes AJ. Mechanical strain and the mammalian cell. In: Frangos J, ed. Physical Forces and the Mammalian Cell. Orlando, FL: Academic Press, 1993.

104. Ives CL, Eskin SG, McIntire LV. Mechanical effects on endothelial cell morphology: in vitro assessment. In Vitro Cell Dev Biol 1986; 22:500–507.

105. Lee RC, Rich JB, Kelley KM, Weiman DS, Mathews MB. A comparison of in vitro cellular responses to mechanical and electrical stimulation. Am Surg 1982; 48:567–574.

106. Thoumine O, Ziegler T, Girard PR, Nerem RM. Elongation of confluent endothelial cells in culture: the importance of fields of force in the associated alterations of their cytoskeletal structure. Exp Cell Res 1995; 219:427–441.

107. Kim BS, Nikolovski J, Bonadio J, Mooney DJ. Cyclic mechanical strain regulates the development of engineered smooth muscle tissue. Nature Biotechnol 1999; 17:979–983.

108. Niklason LE, Gao J, Abbott WM, et al. Functional arteries grown in vitro. Science 1999; 284:489–493.

109. Seliktar D, Black RA, Vito RP, Nerem RM. Dynamic mechanical conditioning of collagen-gel blood vessel constructs induces remodeling in vitro. Ann Biomed Engng 2000; 28:351–362.

110. Freed LE, Martin I, Vunjak-Novakovic G. Frontiers in tissue engineering. In vitro modulation of chondrogenesis. Clin Orthop 1999; 367:S46–58.

111. Pazzano D, Mercier KA, Moran JM, et al. Comparison of chondrogensis in static and perfused bioreactor culture. Biotechnol Prog 2000; 16:893–896.

112. Saris DB, Sanyal A, An KN, Fitzsimmons JS, O'Driscoll SW. Periosteum responds to dynamic fluid pressure by proliferating in vitro. J Orthop Res 1999; 17:668–677.

113. Elder SH, Kimura JH, Soslowsky LJ, Lavagnino M, Goldstein SA. Effect of compressive loading on chondrocyte differentiation in agarose cultures of chick limb-bud cells. J Orthop Res 2000; 18:78–86.

8

Bioreactors for Orthopedic Tissue Engineering

G. Vunjak-Novakovic

Harvard-MIT Division of Health Sciences and Technology,
Massachusetts Institute of Technology,
Cambridge, Massachusetts, U.S.A.

B. Obradovic

University of Belgrade,
Belgrade, Yugoslavia

H. Madry

Saarland University, Homburg-Saar,
Germany

G. Altman and D. L. Kaplan

Tufts University, Medford,
Massachusetts, U.S.A.

I. INTRODUCTION

Tissue engineering can potentially address the clinical problem of tissue failure by implanting an engineered graft that has the capacity to induce orderly and mechanically competent tissue regeneration, develop site- and scale-specific structural and mechanical properties, and integrate firmly and completely to the adjacent host tissues. It is thought that these goals

123

can be met if the engineered construct has the ability to support and mediate matrix remodeling in a fashion similar to that present in immature tissue. Functional constructs can also serve as physiologically relevant models for in vitro studies of tissue development and help distinguish the effects of specific environmental signals (cell derived, biochemical, and physical) from the complex milieu of factors present in vivo (1). In a general case, the utility of engineered tissues critically depends upon our ability to direct cells to form specialized tissues with characteristic properties across different hierarchical scales.

Cells, biomaterial scaffolds, and biochemical and physical regulatory signals can be utilized in a variety of ways to engineer tissues, in vitro (using bioreactors) and in vivo (following implantation). In all cases, the goal of tissue engineering is to recapitulate aspects of the environment present in vivo during tissue development and thereby stimulate the cells to regenerate functional tissues. This generally involves the presence of reparative cells, facilitated transport of chemical species, and the use of physical regulatory signals. Tissue engineering of cartilage, bone, and ligaments has been studied in vitro by using: (1) cells that were selected and/or expanded as required and in some cases transfected to overexpress the genes of interest, (2) scaffolds that provide a structural and logistic template for tissue development and biodegrade at a controlled rate, and (3) bioreactors that provide an in vitro environment for the development of functional tissues.

Bioreactors are designed to perform one or more of the following functions: (1) establish spatially uniform concentrations of cells within biomaterial scaffolds, (2) control conditions in culture medium (e.g., temperature, pH, osmolality, levels of oxygen, nutrients, metabolites, regulatory molecules), (3) facilitate mass transfer between the cells and the culture environment, and (4) provide physiologically relevant physical signals (e.g., interstitial fluid flow, shear, pressure, compression/stretch, torsion). In this chapter, we discuss the design and operation of representative bioreactors for orthopedic tissue engineering, and review three examples of controlled in vitro studies. We focus on cartilage and ligaments, as two distinctly different clinically useful tissues that have been successfully engineered and extensively studied in vitro.

II. BIOREACTORS FOR CARTILAGE TISSUE ENGINEERING

One approach to tissue engineering of cartilage involves an in vitro model system (1–3) in which the scaffold provides a framework for tissue regeneration (4,5) and the bioreactor provides control over cell seeding and tissue culture (6,7) (Fig. 1a).

Seeding of three-dimensional scaffolds with isolated chondrogenic cells (e.g., chondrocytes, bone-marrow derived progenitors) is the first step in bioreactor cultivation of engineered cartilage. Seeding requirements include (1) high cell yield (to maximize cell utilization), (2) high kinetic rate of cell attachment (to minimize the time in suspension for anchorage-dependent cells), and (3) high and spatially uniform distribution of attached cells (to promote rapid and spatially uniform tissue development) (3,6). For engineered cartilage based on highly porous scaffolds (e.g., fibrous meshes with large interconnected pores and 98% void volume) these requirements are best met in mixed flasks containing scaffolds that are fixed in place and seeded in a well-mixed suspension of isolated cells (typically, up to 12 scaffolds per flask in 120 mL of cell suspension containing 5×10^5 cells/cm^3 and magnetically stirred at 50–80 rpm). Under these conditions, magnetic stirring maintains the uniformity of cell suspension and provides relative velocity between the cells and the scaffolds. Essentially all cells attach throughout the scaffold volume in less than 24 h and maintain their spherical shape (6). The kinetics and possible mechanisms of cell seeding were rationalized using a simple mathematical model, which can be used to select seeding conditions for specific scaffold sizes and cell seeding densities (6).

The seeding requirements can also be met using rotating vessels in which scaffold settling provides convective mixing of cell suspension and relative velocity between the cells and scaffolds (8). Most recently, rapid gel-cell inoculation into collagen sponges was used in conjunction with direct medium perfusion through the seeded scaffold to further increase the rate and spatial uniformity of cell seeding (9). In this system, cells were "locked" into the scaffold during a short (10 min) gelation period, and evenly distributed by direct perfusion of culture medium. As a result, high cell yields and spatially uniform cell distributions were achieved within seeding times of only 1.5–4.5 h.

Cultivation of cell-polymer constructs for cartilage tissue engineering is routinely done in static flasks, mixed flasks, and rotating vessels (Fig. 1a, h). All culture vessels are operated in incubators (to maintain the temperature and pH), with continuous gas exchange and periodic medium replacement. Flasks contain constructs that are fixed in place (up to 12 constructs, 5–10 mm in diameter, 2–5 mm thick, in 120 cm^3 culture medium) and cultured either statically or with magnetic stirring (in most cases at 50–80 rpm). Medium is exchanged periodically and partially (usually at a rate of 3 cm^3 per construct per day), to replenish nutrients and regulatory molecules while maintaining the presence of cell-secreted factors. Gas exchange is by surface aeration (7,10). Rotating vessels contain constructs that are cultured without external fixation (up to 12 constructs, 5–10 mm

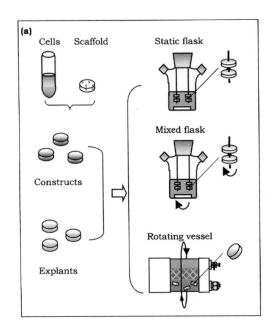

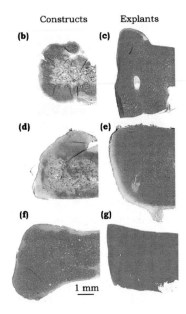

(h) Cultivation parameter	Static flask	Mixed flask	Rotating vessel
Vessel diameter (cm)	6.5	6.5	14.6/5.1
Medium volume (cm³)	120	120	110
Tissue constructs or explants (5 mm dia x 2 mm thick discs)	Fixed in place; n Š 12 per vessel	Fixed in place; n Š 12 per vessel	Freely settling; n Š 12 per vessel
Medium exchange	Batch-wise (3 cm3 per construct per day)	Batch-wise (3 cm3 per construct per day)	Batch-wise (3 cm3 per construct per day)
Gas exchange	Continuous, via surface aeration	Continuous, via surface aeration	Continuous, via an internal membrane
Stirring/rotation rate (s⁻¹)	0	0.83 - 1.25	0.25 - 0.67
Flow conditions	Static fluid	Turbulent [1]	Laminar [2]
Mixing mechanism	None	Magnetic stirring	Settling in rotational flow
Mass transfer in bulk medium	Molecular diffusion	Convection (due to medium stirring)	Convection (due to tissue settling)
Fluid shear at construct surfaces	None	Steady, turbulent	Dynamic, laminar
References	(107, 108, 160, 174, 175, 198, 243)	(107, 108, 115, 159, 160, 174, 175, 198, 242, 243)	(107, 108, 110, 115, 160, 174, 175, 177, 198, 243)

(1) The smallest turbulent eddies had a diameter of 250 µm and velocity of 0.4 cm/s (239, 242)
(2) Tissues were settling in a laminar tumble-slide regimen in a rotational field (177, 240, 241)

in diameter, 2–5 mm thick, in 110 cm^3 culture medium). Two concentric cylinders are rotated in a horizontal plane to provide viscous coupling that suspends the construct in rotating flow (11), and the rotational speed is adjusted (usually 12–40 rpm) to maintain the dynamic equilibrium between the gravitational, centrifugal, and drag forces as the construct increases in size and weight. Medium is exchanged at the same rate as in flasks. Gas exchange with culture medium is through the inner cylinder membrane.

III. IN VITRO CHONDROGENESIS IN CARTILAGE CONSTRUCTS AND EXPLANTS

Hydrodynamic factors in bioreactors can modulate chondrogenesis in at least two ways: via associated effects on mass transport of biochemical factors between the developing tissue and culture medium and by direct physical stimulation of the cells. The effects of three different in vitro environments—static flasks (tissues fixed in place, static medium), mixed flasks (tissues fixed in place, unidirectional turbulent flow) and rotating bioreactors (tissues dynamically suspended in laminar flow)—were studied for engineered cartilage constructs and native cartilage explants (Fig. 1b–g). After 6 weeks of culture in static flasks, cartilaginous matrix accumulated mostly at the periphery of constructs and explants (Fig. 1b and c, respectively), in contrast to constructs and explants cultured in mixed flasks (Fig. 1d and e, respectively) where cartilaginous matrix accumulated in the inner tissue phase but was surrounded by a thick fibrous capsule (~ 450 μm after 6 weeks of culture) (15). Only in rotating vessels, constructs and explants were uniformly cartilaginous throughout their entire cross sections and had normal tissue morphology except for the lack of zonal

---

FIGURE 1 **Representative bioreactors for cartilage tissue engineering (a) Model system.** Articular bovine chondrocytes were seeded on biodegradable scaffolds (5-mm diameter × 2-mm-thick mesh) in mixed flasks (6). The resulting cell-polymer constructs and 5-mm-diameter × 2-mm-thick explants of native bovine cartilage were cultured for 6 weeks in static flasks (tissues fixed in place, static medium), mixed flasks (tissues fixed in place, unidirectional turbulent flow), and rotating bioreactor vessels (tissues dynamically suspended in dynamic laminar flow) (7). **(b–g) Histological sections:** engineered constructs (**b, d, f**) and cartilage explants (**c, e, g**) cultured in static flasks (**b, c**), mixed flasks (**d, e**), and rotating vessels (**f, g**). Safranin-O-stained cross sections were bisected, and one representative half is shown for each group (58). **(h) Operating conditions:** hydrodynamic and mass transfer conditions in static flasks, mixed flasks and rotating vessels (58).

Constructs

Explants

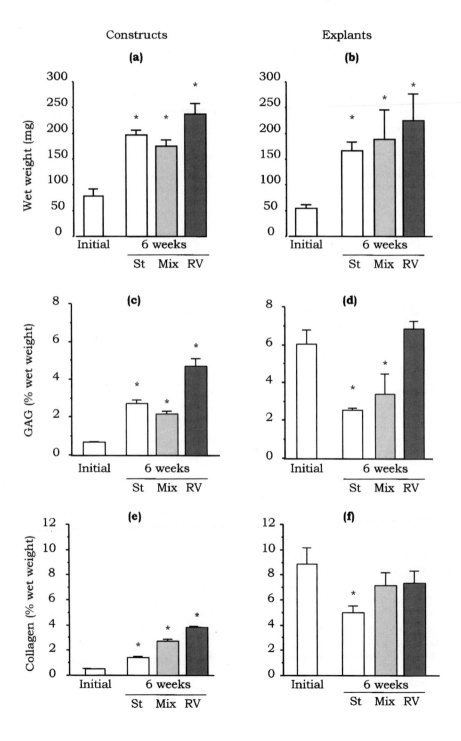

organization and cell columnarization (Fig. 1f, g). The gradients in GAG level at the tissue surfaces were consistent with the measured fractional release of newly synthesized GAG into the culture medium (16): 10–30% for constructs and explants cultured in static flasks and rotating vessels, and 40–60% for constructs and explants cultured in mixed flasks.

The differences in tissue morphology (Fig. 1b–g) could be related to the respective differences in flow and mass transport conditions (Fig. 1h). In static flasks, mass transport between culture medium and tissue constructs is slow as it occurs by molecular diffusion only and there is no hydrodynamic shear at construct surfaces (therefore tissue formation on the construct periphery). In mixed flasks, magnetic stirring generates convective motion that enhances the rates of mass transport but also generates turbulent shear (therefore capsule formation at construct surfaces). The smallest turbulent eddies have diameters of $\sim$250 µm and velocities of $\sim$0.4 cm/s, values that are below levels reported to cause cell damage, but apparently sufficient to affect cell shape and function, and tissue development (10). In rotating vessels, construct settling generates dynamic fluctuations in laminar fluid flow that enhance mass transport at construct surfaces (therefore spatially uniform chondrogenesis throughout the construct). Under conditions commonly used to engineer cartilage (Fig. 1h), constructs settle in a laminar tumble-slide regimen associated with dynamic fluctuations in fluid shear, pressure, and velocity (11–13), efficient mixing in bulk medium (14), and low hydrodynamic shear at construct surfaces ($<$1 dyn/cm^2) (12).

Over 6 weeks of in vitro culture, the wet weights of cartilage constructs and explants increased 4–5-fold (Fig. 2a and b, respectively), owing to the progressive accumulation of newly synthesized glycosaminoglycans and collagen. In constructs from rotating vessels, the fractions of glycosaminoglycans (Fig. 2c) and total collagen (Fig. 2e) were 5 times as high as in the initial constructs, and markedly higher than in either static or mixed flasks. In explants from rotating vessels, the fractions of glycosaminoglycans (Fig. 2d) and total collagen (Fig. 2f) were maintained at their initial levels,

---

FIGURE 2 **In vitro chondrogenesis in engineered constructs (a, c, e) and cartilage explants (b, d, f). (a, b) Tissue wet weight** (mg). **(c, d) Glycosaminoglycans** (% wet weight). **(e, f) Total collagen** (% wet weight). Data represent the average $\pm$ SD for $n = 3$–6 samples per group at time zero (initial) and after 6 weeks of culture. St, Mix, and RV, respectively, refer to static flasks, mixed flasks, and rotating bioreactor vessels. (*) significantly different level of a given variable among groups, as assessed by ANOVA in conjunction with Tukey's HSD test ($p < 0.05$) (58).

in contrast to static and mixed flasks where both fractions decreased to ~50–70% of initial. The changes in biomechanical construct properties correlated with the respective changes in biochemical construct compositions (Table 1a). The zero-strain compressive modulus of 6-week constructs from static flasks, mixed flasks, and rotating vessels was 53, 51, and 172 kPa, respectively, as compared to 270 kPa measured for the articular surface and 710 kPa measured for the deep zone of bovine articular cartilage (17). The dynamic stiffness of constructs from rotating vessels was also approximately 3 times as high as in either static or mixed flasks. Consistently, the hydraulic permeability decreased from static and mixed flasks to rotating vessels.

A recent related study (18) showed that mechanical behavior of engineered constructs, cultured explants, and fresh cartilage in confined axial

TABLE 1   Tissue-engineered Cartilage: Biochemical Composition and Mechanical Properties

(a) Effects of bioreactor vessel (6 weeks of culture)

Culture vessel	Static flask	Mixed flask	Rotating vessel	Explants
GAG (% wet weight)	2.73±0.2	2.19±0.17	4.71±0.41	6.06±0.29
Collagen (% wet weight)	1.41±0.08	2.94±0.16	3.79±0.05	8.84±1.34
Equilibrium modulus (kPa)	53.3±11.8	50.8±4.6	172.4±35.5	928.4±30.2
Permeability ($\times 10^{-15} m^4/Ns$)	47.82±21.6	21.28±17.4	10.43±5.0	2.14±0.5
Dynamic stiffness (Mpa, 1 Hz)	0.88±0.33	1.09±0.22	2.91±0.97	16.8±1.1

(b) Effects of cultivation time (rotating bioreactor vessel)

Cultivation time	3 days	6 weeks	7 months	Explants
GAG (% wet weight)	0.71±0.03	4.71±0.41	8.83±0.93	6.06±0.29
Collagen (% wet weight)	0.48±0.08	3.79±0.05	3.68±0.27	8.84±1.34
Equilibrium modulus (kPa)	Not measurable	172.4±35.5	932.0+49	928.4±30.2
Permeability ($\times 10^{-15} m^4/Ns$)	Not measurable	10.43±5.0	3.72±0.17	2.14±0.5
Dynamic stiffness (Mpa, 1 Hz)	Not measurable	2.91±0.97	7.75±0.30	16.8±1.1

compression and osmotic swelling was consistent with the model of pre-stressed collagen fibers balanced by swelling pressure of proteoglycans. Constructs and explants contained comparable amounts of proteoglycans (50% and 65% of normal, respectively), whereas the volumetric fractions of collagen in constructs were only one half of those in explants (34% and 68% of normal, respectively); the collagen fiber stiffness decreased from cartilage to explants and constructs. The aggregate, lateral, and shear moduli all decreased from cartilage to explants and constructs, decreased with an increase in saline bath concentration, and correlated with wet weight fractions of proteoglycans and collagen

IV. TISSUE-ENGINEERED CARTILAGE: DURATION OF CULTURE AND REGULATORY FACTORS

For engineered cartilage, the optimal duration of in vitro cultivation (or even the need for in vitro cultivation) has not been determined. Implantations were done as early as within 2 h of cell seeding, with functional tissue development required to occur in vivo (19–21), and using cartilaginous constructs engineered in vitro that were already functional at the time of implantation (22).

With increasing cultivation time, the constructs more closely approximated articular cartilage both structurally and functionally (7,23). The wet weight fraction of glycosaminoglycans increased progressively from very low at 3 days to significantly higher than physiological at 7 months, whereas the fraction of total collagen increased during the first 6 weeks but remained at this level for the duration of culture (Table 1b). Constructs cultivated for 6 weeks had 75% as much glycosaminoglycans and 40% as much collagen per unit wet weight, equilibrium moduli of approximately 175 kPa, and hydraulic permeabilities that were fourfold higher than those for native cartilage (Table 1b). The collagen network of 6-week constructs had normal fibril density and diameter, and the fractions of collagen types II, IX, and X, but the number of pyridinium cross-links per collagen molecule was only one third of normal (24). In 7-month constructs, both the equilibrium modulus and the hydraulic permeability became comparable with those measured in native cartilage (Table 1b).

Importantly, the compositions and mechanical properties of 6-week constructs were in the range of values measured for fetal cartilage (25,26), suggesting that bioreactors yield engineered constructs resembling immature rather than mature native cartilage, even after prolonged cultivation. It is likely that the functional deficiencies present in constructs grown in vitro are due to the absence of specific biochemical and physical factors normally present in vivo. Following implantation, engineered cartilage remodeled into physiologically stiff cartilage and new subchondral bone (21,27), in response to local and systemic regulatory factors (28,29). Notably, columnar cells and a tidemark at an appropriate depth were observed in engineered cartilage following in vivo exposure to physiological loading (27), but not in vitro.

The composition, morphology, and mechanical properties of engineered cartilage grown in mechanically active environments were generally better than those grown in static environments. In particular, the hydrodynamic stresses acting at the surfaces of constructs cultured in dynamic laminar flow of rotating bioreactors yielded cartilaginous constructs with markedly improved compositions and mechanical properties as compared to constructs cultured either statically or in mixed flasks (7,30). In vivo, mass transfer within articular cartilage is largely enhanced by tissue loading which involves a combination of diffusion and convective flow driven by gradients in concentrations of chemical and ionic species, hydrodynamic pressure, and fluid content. In vitro, direct perfusion through cultured tissue constructs at physiological interstitial flow velocities ($\sim$1 μm/s) stimulated chondrogenesis, presumably owing to combined effects of enhanced mass transport, pH regulation, and fluid shear in the cell microenvironment (31–33). It is possible that the observed effects of dynamic mechanical compression in vitro (34,35) and in vivo (36) were also due in part to the increased fluid flow within cultured tissue constructs. Physical stimuli (pressure, shear) conveyed by the flow of culture medium, although different in nature and intensity from physical signals associated with joint loading, can be utilized to promote in vitro synthesis and functional assembly of cartilaginous matrix (37).

Mechanically active environments were shown to mediate the effects of biomaterial scaffolds (5) and regulatory molecules (38,39) on chondrogenesis in vitro. The interactive effects of the insulin-like growth factor-I (IGF-I) and mechanical environment (static and orbitally mixed dishes, static and mixed flasks, rotating vessels) on structure, biochemical composition, and mechanical properties of engineered cartilage were studied using bioreactor cultures of engineered constructs (40). The IGF-I and flow modulated tissue properties in a manner consistent with previous studies, and interacted to produce tissues superior to those obtained by utilizing the two factors independently. The study also confirmed that there is a positive correlation between tissue composition and mechanical function. After 4 weeks of culture, the best constructs had wet weight fractions of glycosaminoglycans and collagen and equlibrium moduli that were approximately 50% of values measured for the middle zone of native articular cartilage.

Related studies by other investigators have shown enhanced chondro-genesis in engineered and native cartilage exposed to dynamic compression (34,35).

V. BIOREACTORS FOR LIGAMENT TISSUE ENGINEERING

One approach to tissue engineering of anterior cruciate ligaments involves biophysical regulation of mesenchymal progenitor cells cultured on collagen or silk scaffolds in advanced bioreactor systems providing multi-dimensional mechanical strains (axial tension/compression and torsion) (41,42,59). Two bioreactor units are shown in Figure 3a. Each unit is computer-controlled and consists of (1) 12 individual cartridges (19 mm in diameter, 75 mm long) containing tissue constructs (4–12 mm in diameter, 3 cm long), each within a separate perfusion loop, (2) gas exchanger to control medium pH and oxygen levels, (3) a 12-channel peristaltic pump, and (4) a motion control system for mechanical stimulation of cultured constructs. The oxygen and pH in culture medium are maintained at set levels by gas exchange, and varied within ranges normally found in native tissues (10–150 mmHg; pH 6.7–7.4). Culture medium (10–30 mL per loop) is exchanged at a desired rate (e.g., 1–5 mL/cartridge/day). Biomaterial scaffold (collagen gel, fibrous silk) is anchored between the top and bottom mounts in each cartridge and seeded with cells (e.g., 3–4×10^6 cells per scaffold) (Fig. 3b). The bottom platen is fixed in place, and the top platen is connected to gear trains driven by motors. The bioreactor provides independent but concurrent control over axial and torsional strains imparted to the growing tissue. Axial strain (5–10%) and torsional strain ($< 90°$) can be applied via top platen at frequencies of 0.01–1 Hz, with periods of loading and rest (e.g., 20 min of mechanical stimulation every 8 h) (41).

Mechanical stimulation in vitro, without supplementation of ligament-selective exogenous growth and differentiation factors, induced the differentiation of bone-marrow-derived mesenchymal progenitor cells into a ligament cell lineage in preference to alternative paths (i.e., bone or cartilage cell lineages). A total of 24 engineered ligaments based on human cells were cultured for up to 21 days with 90° rotational and 10% axial strain at 0.0167 Hz. Mechanical stimulation up-regulated collagen types I and III and tenascin-C, fostered cell alignment in the direction of the resulting force (compare Fig. 3c and 3d), and resulted in the formation of oriented collagen fibers, all features characteristic of ligament cells. On collagen matrices, helically organized collagen fibers (20-μm-diameter bundles) with characteristic collagen-banding patterns were formed in the direction of the applied load at the periphery of the mechanically stimulated ligaments, a feature absent in the controls. On silk matrices, the expression of

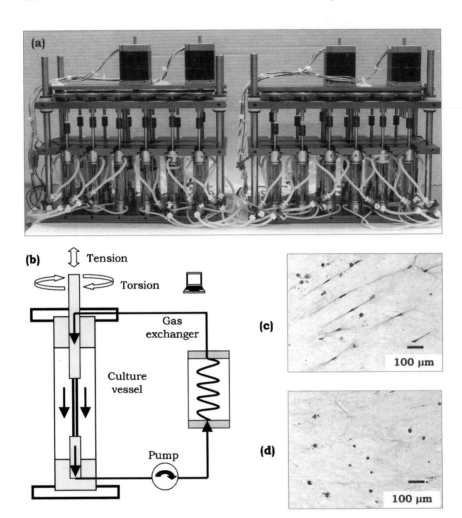

FIGURE 3 **Bioreactor for tissue engineering o f ligaments**. The bioreactor system with medium perfusion and mechanical loading was used to engineer
anterior cruciate ligaments starting from human bone-marrow-derived cells
cultured on collagen or silk scaffolds. **(a) Bioreactor system:** two computer-
controlled units are shown, each containing 12 individual cartridges within
separate perfusion loops (41). **(b) Cartridge:** cell-seeded scaffold is anchored
between the bottom platen (fixed in place) and the top platen (connected to
gear trains), and subjected to axial strains (5–10%) and torsional strains
($<90°$) applied at frequencies of 0.01–1 Hz and with periods of loading and
rest. **(c, d) H&E stains** of mechanically stimulated **(c)** and control **(d)** ligaments cultured for 3 weeks. Mechanical stimulation caused cell alignment
in the direction of the resultant force ($45°$).

collagen types I and III and tenascin-C was observed; the ratio of collagen type I expression to collagen type III was 8.9:1, consistent with that of native cruciate ligaments. At the same time, no up-regulation of bone or cartilage-specific cell markers was observed. We recently utilized a similar bioreactor design to apply axial dynamic compression to demineralized bone seeded with human MPC, which resulted in osteogenic differentiation (43,44). These studies support the notion that advanced bioreactors providing physiologically relevant mechanical loading are essential for meeting the complex requirements of in vitro engineering of functional skeletal tissues.

VI. CASE STUDY I: TEMPOROSPATIAL PROFILES OF CARTILAGE DEVELOPMENT

Bioreactors have been used to study chondrogenesis (30), and to establish structure-function relationships for engineered cartilage constructs (7). The temporospatial changes in local concentrations of the cells and cartilaginous matrix are shown in Figure 4A, B for three selected time points during cultivation (3 days, 10 days, 6 weeks). Cells at the construct periphery proliferated more rapidly during the first 3 days of culture (Fig. 4d) and initiated chondrogenesis (Fig. 4a), which progressed appositionally, both inward toward the construct center and outward from its surface (Fig. 4a–c). By 6 weeks of culture, self-regulated cell proliferation and ECM deposition yielded constructs that had physiological cell densities and appeared uniformly cartilaginous (Fig. 4c, f). Quantitatively, the development of tissue-engineered cartilage has been modeled using a spatially varying, deterministic continuum model (45). The model accounted for the deposition and diffusion of oxygen and glycosaminoglycan as a function of the spatial position within the construct and the duration of tissue cultivation. Glycosaminoglycan was taken as a marker of chondrogenesis in light of prior association of its deposition with that of collagen type II (30). Oxygen consumption due to energy metabolism and matrix biosynthesis resulted in a gradual decrease of oxygen concentration from the construct surface toward its center (Fig. 4C). Model predictions for concentration profiles of glycosaminoglycans (Fig. 4D, lines) were qualitatively and quantitatively consistent with those measured via high-resolution (40 μm) image processing of tissue samples (15) (Fig. 4D, data points).

Models of this kind can be used to rationalize experimental data for chondrogenesis in engineered constructs, and to relate these data to earlier observations of the dependence of global construct properties on cultivation conditions (the domain of focus in each case being limited by available

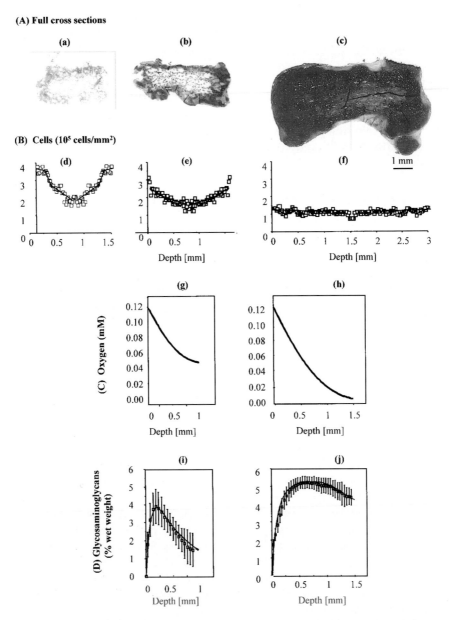

(A) Full cross sections

(a)   **(b)**   **(c)**

(B) Cells (10^5 cells/mm^2)

(d)   **(e)**   **(f)**

1 mm

Depth [mm]   Depth [mm]

(g)   **(h)**

(C) Oxygen (mM)

Depth [mm]   Depth [mm]

(i)   **(j)**

(D) Glycosaminoglycans (% wet weight)

Depth [mm]   Depth [mm]

FIGURE 4 **Case study I: in vitro chondrogenesis**. (**A**) Full cross sections of tissue constructs after (**a**) 3 days, (**b**) 10 days, and (**c**) 6 weeks of culture. Stain: safranin-O/fast green. Scale bar: 1 mm. (**B**) Spatial profiles of cell distribution after (**d**) 3 days, (**e**) 10 days, and (**f**) 6 weeks of culture (measured by image

analytical tools). Construct function has been correlated with overall construct composition, which itself depended on the conditions of bioreactor cultivation (7). Empirical relationships like these are fundamentally instructive. However, Fig. 4a–h shows clearly that the spatial distributions of cells and ECM are highly nonuniform during most of the cultivation period. Therefore, the spatial averaging intrinsic to measurement of overall construct properties can filter out potentially significant information regarding internal gradients and associated mass transfer limitations upon cell metabolism and tissue growth. Additional quantitative models are needed to describe structure-function relationships for engineered constructs and the repair tissue, and obtain predictive tools for the design of tissue-engineered cartilage repair (44,46,47).

VII. CASE STUDY II: INTEGRATION OF ENGINEERED AND NATIVE CARTILAGE

Incomplete integration with host tissues has been a serious problem of cartilage repair (25,28,44,48,49). In particular, poor bonding with adjacent cartilage suggests that mature cartilage, either native or engineered, may not have sufficient capacity for integration (50). Controlled bioreactor studies demonstrated a trade-off between the stiffness of engineered cartilage and its integration potential (51). Disc-shaped constructs cultured for 5 days or 5 weeks, or cartilage explants (intact or trypsin-treated), were sutured into cartilage rings made of cartilage (intact or trypsin-treated), cultured for 1–8 weeks, and evaluated structurally and functionally (compressive stiffness of the central disc, adhesive strength of the integration interface). Immature constructs integrated better than either more mature constructs or cartilage explants. In a related in vitro study, bonding of engineered cartilage and bone was also better for immature constructs (52). Integration of immature constructs involved cell proliferation and the progressive formation of cartilaginous tissue (Fig. 5a–d), in contrast to the integration of more mature constructs or native cartilage, which involved only the secretion of extracellular matrix components. Integration patterns correlated with the adhesive strength of the disc-ring interface. The compressive stiffness increased from immature constructs to more

---

processing). (**C**) Spatial profiles of oxygen distribution after (**g**) 10 days and (**h**) 6 weeks of culture (model predictions). (**D**) Spatial profiles of glycosaminoglycan distribution after (**i**) 10 days and (**j**) 6 weeks of culture (data points: measured by image processing; lines: model predictions). (Based on data reported in Ref. 45).

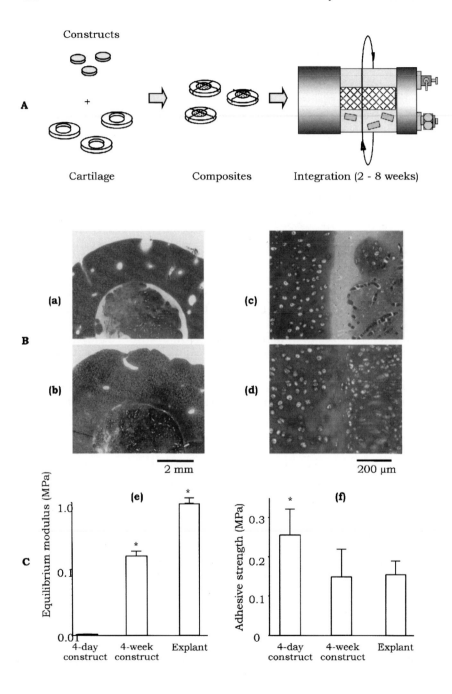

A

Constructs

+

Cartilage   Composites   Integration (2 - 8 weeks)

B

(a)   (c)

(b)   (d)

2 mm   200 µm

C

(e)   (f)

mature constructs and cartilage explants (Fig. 5e), whereas the adhesive stiffness at disc-ring interface was markedly higher for immature constructs than for either more mature constructs or cartilage explants (Fig. 5f). Trypsin treatment of the adjacent cartilage further enhanced the integration of immature constructs (51), as previously shown for cartilage repair in vivo (53). The adhesive strength of the integration interface correlated with collagen biosynthesis and deposition (54). Ideally, the duration of in vitro cultivation should be selected for each application such that constructs have certain minimal mechanical functionality along with certain minimal capacity for integration.

Large osteochondral defects in adult rabbits were repaired using composites based on in vitro–engineered cartilage (27). Articular chondrocytes were expanded, seeded on PGA scaffolds in bioreactors, cultured for 4–6 weeks, sutured to an osteoconductive support, implanted, and evaluated histologically, biochemically, and biomechanically. At the time of implantation, constructs had wet weight fractions of gycosaminoglycans and collagen that were respectively two thirds and one third those in adult cartilage, and equilibrium moduli that were one fifth that of adult cartilage. Engineered cartilage allowed handling, withstood physiological loading immediately following implantation, and remodeled into osteochondral tissue with physiological composition and mechanical properties. After 6 months, defects implanted with engineered constructs were repaired with cartilage that had normal thickness and characteristic architectural features including the tidemark and columnar arrangement of chondrocytes, and new subchondral bone. In contrast, defects implanted with cell-free scaffolds or left untreated repaired with fibrocartilage. Repair tissues based on engineered cartilage composites had Young's moduli comparable to native articular cartilage. Integration with subchondral bone was excellent, whereas integration with cartilage was not consistently good. These results suggest that functional engineered cartilage can provide a mechanically

---

FIGURE 5 **Case study II: integration of engineered cartilage**. (A) **Model system**: Discs of engineered cartilage (5 mm diameter × 2 mm thick) were sutured into rings of native cartilage (10/5 mm diameter × 2 mm thick) and cultured in bioreactors for 1–8 weeks. (B) **Integration patterns**: Face sections of composites are shown after (**a, b**) 2 weeks of culture and (**c, d**) 4 weeks of culture; disc is in the center (a, c) and on the right (b, d). Stain: safranin-O/fast green. (C) **Functional evaluation**: (**e**) Confined-compression equilibrium modulus of the discs at the time of construct preparation, and (**f**) adhesive strength of the integration interface. (Data from Ref. 51).

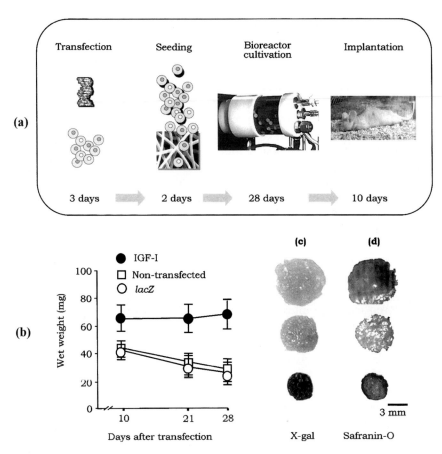

FIGURE 6 **Case study III: gene transfer for cartilage tissue engineering. (a) Model system.** Bovine articular chondrocytes were expanded in vitro, transfected with the cDNA encoding for the human insulin-like growth factor-I (IGF-I), and dynamically seeded onto biodegradable polymer scaffolds. The resulting constructs were transferred to rotating bioreactors and cultured for 28 days in basal medium, followed by an additional 10 days in vivo (in nude mice) or in vitro (in bioreactors). **(b) Wet weights** of constructs based on chondrocytes transfected with *lacZ* (○), the human IGF-I (●), or nontransfected chondrocytes (□) over 28 days of in vitro cultivation. Data represent the average ± SD of $n = 10$ samples per group. **(c) X-gal staining** and **(d) safranin O staining** of representative construct sections (top: IGF-I; middle: nontransfected; bottom: *lac Z*) on day 28 posttransfection (55).

stable tissue-like template that remodels in vivo into osteochondral tissue with physiologically thick and stiff cartilage.

VIII. CASE STUDY III: GENE TRANSFER FOR CARTILAGE TISSUE ENGINEERING

Two novel approaches to cartilage formation, gene transfer and tissue engineering, have been limited by short-term transgene expression in transplanted chondrocytes (60) and inability to deliver regulatory signals according to specific temporal and spatial patterns. We recently used controlled bioreactor studies to test the hypothesis that gene transfer can provide sustained gene expression in cell-polymer constructs in vitro and in vivo and enhance the structural and functional properties of tissue-engineered cartilage (55). The human insulin-like growth factor-I (IGF-I) gene served as a model to demonstrate the potential benefits of gene transfer for tissue engineering. Calf articular chondrocytes (unmodified, genetically modified to overexpress the *Escherichia coli* ß-galactosidase gene or the human IGF-I gene) were cultured on fibrous polyglycolic acid scaffolds in bioreactors and evaluated structurally and functionally, in vitro and in vivo (Fig. 6a).

The initial wet weight and size of IGF-I constructs were maintained throughout the period of bioreactor cultivation and after 28 days were significantly higher than for either control (Fig. 6b). Transgene expression was maintained throughout the duration of the study, over 4 weeks in vitro followed by an additional 10 days either in vitro or in vivo (Fig. 6c). The corresponding IGF-I constructs stained more intensely with safranin O than either control (Fig. 6d), contained markedly larger amounts of glycosaminoglycans and collagen, and had fourfold higher equilibrium moduli as compared to nontransfected or *lacZ* constructs. The amounts of glycosaminoglycans and collagen per unit DNA in IGF-I constructs were markedly higher than in either constructs cultured in serum-supplemented medium or native cartilage.

The observed enhancement of in vitro chondrogenesis by spatially defined overexpression of human IGF-I suggested that cartilage tissue engineering based on genetically modified chondrocytes may be advantageous compared to either gene transfer or tissue engineering alone. The enhancement of the per cell production of extracellular matrix components by the sustained overexpression of IGF-I may not have been fully utilized owing to the low construct cellularity, which in turn may be caused by the lack of specific serum components in the serum-free culture medium. Recent studies have demonstrated that multiple factors, rather than a single growth factor at a time, are required to achieve rapid chondrogenesis in this model of cartilage tissue engineering (38–40,56,57). Also, because the environment of the joint differs from that in a bioreactor and may contribute to the properties of the tissue, the application of such constructs to in vivo models may further modulate their properties. Genetically modified cartilaginous constructs may be applied for the repair of articular cartilage lesions and for controlled studies of factors and mechanisms involved in the regulation of chondrogenesis. One intriguing possibility is that the effects of growth factors overexpressed by genetically modified cells can be further enhanced by physical regulatory signals in a manner similar to that observed for supplemental growth factors.

IX. SUMMARY

Functional tissue constructs for scientific studies and tissue repair can be engineered in vitro by using differentiated or progenitor cells, biomaterial scaffolds, and bioreactors. We have discussed the design and operation of representative bioreactors that have been used to engineer articular cartilage and anterior cruciate ligament, two distinctly different orthopedic tissues. For cartilage, we focused on the paradigm of tissue-engineered repair that is based on the in vitro engineering of immature cartilaginous constructs, and the subsequent remodeling and maturation of these constructs following in vivo implantation. For ligament, we focused on biophysical regulation of mesenchymal progenitor cell differentiation. In both cases, tissue structure and function were discussed with respect to the conditions and duration of bioreactor cultivation. Three case studies were presented to illustrate the usefulness of bioreactor-cultured engineered tissues as physiologically relevant models for controlled in vitro studies: (1) temporospatial profiles of cartilage development, (2) integration of engineered and native cartilage, and (3) gene transfer for cartilage tissue engineering. Overall, bioreactors can provide a powerful tool for engineering functional tissues, conducting basic studies of cell function and tissue development, and optimizing the properties of engineered grafts for each specific application.

ACKNOWLEDGMENTS

Much of the work presented in this chapter has been supported by the National Aeronautics and Space Administration and the National Institutes of Health. The authors thank Sue Kangiser for her help with the manuscript preparation.

REFERENCES

1. Freed LE, Martin I, Vunjak-Novakovic G. Frontiers in tissue engineering: in vitro modulation of chondrogenesis. Clin Orthop 1999; 367S:S46–S58.
2. Freed LE, Vunjak-Novakovic G. Tissue engineering of cartilage. In: Bronzino JD, eds. The Biomedical Engineering Handbook. 2d Boca Raton, FL: CRC Press, 2000:124–126.
3. Freed LE, Vunjak-Novakovic G. Tissue engineering bioreactors. In: Lanza RP, Langer R, Vacanti J, eds. Principles of Tissue Engineering. 2 San Diego: Academic Press, 2000:143–156.
4. Freed LE, Vunjak Novakovic G, Biron R, Eagles D, Lesnoy D, Barlow S, Langer R. Biodegradable polymer scaffolds for tissue engineering. Bio/Technology 1994; 12:689–693.
5. Pei M, Solchaga LA, Seidel J, Zeng L, Vunjak-Novakovic G, Caplan AI, Freed LE. Bioreactors mediate the effectiveness of tissue engineering scaffolds. FASEB J 2002; 16:1691–1694.
6. Vunjak-Novakovic G, Obradovic B, Bursac P, Martin I, Langer R, Freed LE. Dynamic cell seeding of polymer scaffolds for cartilage tissue engineering. Biotechnol Prog 1998; 14:193–202.
7. Vunjak-Novakovic G, Martin I, Obradovic B, Treppo S, Grodzinsky AJ, Langer R, Freed LE. Bioreactor cultivation conditions modulate the composition and mechanical properties of tissue engineered cartilage. J Orthop Res 1999; 17:130–138.
8. Carrier RL, Papadaki M, Rupnick M, Schoen FJ, Bursac N, Langer R, Freed LE, Vunjak-Novakovic G. Cardiac tissue engineering: cell seeding, cultivation parameters and tissue construct characterization. Biotechnol Bioeng 1999; 64:580–589.
9. Vunjak-Novakovic G, Radisic M. Cell seeding of polymer scaffolds. In: Hollander AP, Hatton P, eds. Biopolymer Methods in Tissue Engineering. Totowa, NJ: Humana Press, In press.
10. Vunjak-Novakovic G, Freed LE, Biron RJ, Langer R. Effects of mixing on the composition and morphology of tissue-engineered cartilage. AIChE J 1996; 42:850–860.
11. Freed LE, Vunjak-Novakovic G. Cultivation of cell-polymer constructs in simulated microgravity. Biotechnol Bioeng 1995; 46:306–313.
12. Neitzel GP, Nerem RM, Sambanis A, Smith MK, Wick TM, Brown JB, Hunter C, Jovanovic IP, Malaviya P, Saini S, Tan S. Cell function and tissue growth in bioreactors: fluid mechanical and chemical environments. J Jpn Soc Microgr Appl 1998; 15:602–607.
13. Clift R, Grace JR, Weber ME. Bubbles, Drops, and Particles. New York: Academic Press, 1978.
14. Freed LE, Vunjak-Novakovic G. Tissue culture bioreactors: chondrogenesis as a model system. In: Langer R, Chick W, eds. Principles of Tissue Engineering: Austin: RG Landes, 1997:150–158.
15. Martin I, Obradovic B, Freed LE, Vunjak-Novakovic G. A method for quantitative analysis of glycosaminoglycan distribution in cultured natural and engineered cartilage. Ann Biomed Eng 1999; 27:656–662.

16. Obradovic B, Martin I, Freed LE, Vunjak-Novakovic G. Bioreactor studies of natural and tissue engineered cartilage. Ortop Traumatol Rehab 2001; 3: 181–189.
17. Chen AC, Bae WC, Schinagl RM, Sah RL. Depth- and strain-dependent mechanical and electromechanical properties of full-thickness bovine articular cartilage in confined compression. J Biomech 2001; 34:1–12.
18. Bursac PM. Collagen network contributions to structure-function relationships in cartilaginous tissues in compression. Ph.D. dissertation, Boston: Boston University, 2001.
19. Wakitani S, Goto T, Young RG, Mansour JM, Goldberg VM, Caplan AI. Repair of large full-thickness articular cartilage defects with allograft articular chondrocytes embedded in a collagen gel. Tissue Eng 1998; 4:429–444.
20. Chu C, Dounchis JS, Yoshioka M, Sah RL, Coutts RD, Amiel D. Osteochondral repair using perichondrial cells: a 1 year study in rabbits. Clin Orthop 1997; 340:220–229.
21. Wakitani S, Goto T, Pineda SJ, Young RG, Mansour JM, Caplan AI, Goldberg VM. Mesenchymal cell-based repair of large, full-thickness defects of articular cartilage. J Bone Joint Surg Am 1994; 76A:579–592.
22. Schaefer D, Martin I, Heberer M, Jundt G, Seidel J, Bergin J, Grodzinsky AJ, Vunjak-Novakovic G, Freed LE. Tissue engineered composites for the repair of large osteochondral defects. Trans Orthop Res Soc 2000; 25:619.
23. Freed LE, Langer R, Martin I, Pellis N, Vunjak-Novakovic G. Tissue engineering of cartilage in space. Proc Natl Acad Sci USA 1997; 94:13885–13890.
24. Riesle J, Hollander AP, Langer R, Freed LE, Vunjak-Novakovic G. Collagen in tissue-engineered cartilage: types, structure and crosslinks. J Cell Biochem 1998; 71:313–327.
25. Vunjak-Novakovic G, Goldstein SA. Biomechanical principles of cartilage and bone tissue engineering. In: Mow VC, Huiskes R, eds. Basic Orthopaedic Biomechanics and Mechanobiology. 3rd ed. : Lippincott-Williams and Wilkens, 2002. In press.
26. Vunjak-Novakovic G. Fundamentals of tissue engineering: scaffolds and bioreactors. In: Caplan AI, ed. Tissue Engineering of Cartilage and Bone. London: John Wiley, 2002. In press.
27. Schaefer D, Martin I, Jundt G, Seidel J, Heberer M, Grodzinsky AJ, Bergin I, Vunjak-Novakovic G, Freed LE. Tissue engineered composites for the repair of large osteochondral defects. Arthritis Rheum 2002; 46:2524–2534.
28. Caplan AI, Elyaderani M, Mochizuki Y, Wakitani S, Goldberg VM. Principles of cartilage repair and regeneration. Clin Orthop 1997; 342:254–269.
29. Sellers RS, Zhang R, Glasson SS, Kim HD, Peluso D, D'Augusta DA, Beckwith K, Morris EA. Repair of articular cartilage defects one year after treatment with recombinant human bone morphogenetic protein-2 (rhBMP-2). J Bone Joint Surg Am 2000; 82:151–160.
30. Freed LE, Hollander AP, Martin I, Barry JR, Langer R, Vunjak-Novakovic G. Chondrogenesis in a cell-polymer-bioreactor system. Exp Cell Res 1998; 240:58–65.

31. Pazzano D, Mercier KA, Moran JM, Fong SS, DiBiasio DD, Rulfs JX, Kohles SS, Bonassar LJ. Comparison of chondrogensis in static and perfused bioreactor culture. Biotechnol Prog 2000; 16:893–896.

32. Sittinger M, Bujia J, Minuth WW, Hammer C, Burmester GR. Engineering of cartilage tissue using bioresorbable polymer carriers in perfusion culture. Biomaterials 1994; 15:451–456.

33. Dunkelman NS, Zimber MP, Lebaron RG, Pavelec R, Kwan M, Purchio AF. Cartilage production by rabbit articular chondrocytes on polyglycolic acid scaffolds in a closed bioreactor system. Biotechnol Bioeng 1995; 46:299–305.

34. Buschmann MD, Gluzband YA, Grodzinsky AJ, Hunziker EB. Mechanical compression modulates matrix biosynthesis in chondrocyte/agarose culture. J Cell Sci 1995; 108:1497–1508.

35. Mauck RL, Soltz MA, Wang CCB, Wong DD, Chao PG, Valhmu WB, Hung CT, Ateshian GA. Functional tissue engineering of articular cartilage through dynamic loading of chondrocyte-seeded agarose gels. J Biomech Eng 2000; 122:252–260.

36. Takahashi I, Nuckolis GH, Takahashi K, Tanaka O, Semba I, Dashner R, Shum L, Slavkin HC. Compressive force promotes Sox9, type II collagen and aggrecan and inhibits IL-1b expression resulting in chondrogenesis in mouse embryonic limb bud mesenchymal cells. J Cell Sci 1998; 111:2067–2076.

37. LeBaron RG, Athanasiou KA. Ex vivo synthesis of articular cartilage. Biomaterials 2000; 21:2575–2587.

38. Gooch KJ, Blunk T, Tennant CJ, Vunjak-Novakovic G, Langer R, Freed LE. Mechanical forces and growth factors utilized in tissue engineering. In: Patrick CW, Mikos AG, McIntire LV, eds. Tissue Engineering Principles and Practices. Oxford: Elsevier. In press.

39. Pei M, Seidel J, Vunjak-Novakovic G, Freed LE. Growth factors for sequential cellular de- and re-differentiation in tissue engineering. Biochem Biophys Res Commun 2002; 294:149–154.

40. Gooch KJ, Blunk T, Courter DL, Sieminski AL, Bursac PM, Vunjak-Novakovic G, Freed LE. IGF-I and mechanical environment interact to modulate engineered cartilage development. Biochem Biophys Res Commun 2001; 286:909–915.

41. Altman GH, Stark P, Lu HH, Horan RL, Calabro T, Martin I, Ryder D, Richmond JC, Vunjak-Novakovic G, Kaplan DL. Bench-top bioreactor for the development of tissue engineered ligaments via multi-dimensional strains. J Biomech Eng 2002; 124:742–749.

42. Altman G, Horan R, Martin I, Farhadi J, Stark P, Volloch V, Vunjak-Novakovic G, Richmond J, Kaplan DL. Cell differentiation by mechanical stress. FASEB J 2002; 16:270–272.

43. Mauney J, Blumberg J, Pirun M, Volloch V, Vunjak-Novakovic G, Kaplan DL. Osteogenic differentiation of human bone marrow stromal cells on 3D partially demineralized bone scaffolds in vitro. J Biomed Mater Res In review.

44. Freed LE, Rupnick MA, Schaefer D, Vunjak-Novakovic G. Engineering functional cartilage and cardiac tissue: in vitro culture parameters.

In: Guilak F, Butler D, Mooney D, Goldstein S, eds. Functional Tissue Engineering: the Role of Biomechanics. Chapter 27, Springer Verlag, 2003:360–376.

45. Obradovic B, Meldon JH, Freed LE, Vunjak-Novakovic G. Glycosaminogly-can deposition in engineered cartilage: experiments and mathematical model. AIChE J 2000; 46:1860–1871.

46. Klisch SM, Chen SS, Sah RL, Hoger A. A growth mixture theory for cartilage with application to growth-related experiments on cartilage explants. J Biomech Eng 2003; 125:169–179.

47. Williamson AK, Chen AC, Sah RL. Compressive properties and function-composition relationships of developing bovine articular cartilage. J Orthop Res 2001; 19:1113–1121.

48. Grande DA, Southerland SS, Manji R, Pate DW, Schwartz RE, Lucas PA. Repair of articular cartilage defects using mesenchymal stem cells. Tissue Eng 1995; 1:345–353.

49. Schreiber RE, Ilten-Kirby BM, Dunkelman NS, Symons KT, Rekettye LM, Willoughby J, Ratcliffe A. Repair of osteochondral defects with alloge-neic tissue-engineered cartilage implants. Clin Orthop 1999; 367S:S382–S395.

50. Grande DA, Breitbart AS, Mason J, Paulino C, Laser J, Schwartz RE. Carti-lage tissue engineering: current limitations and solutions. Clin Orthop 1999; 367 (suppl):S176–S185.

51. Obradovic B, Martin I, Padera RF, Treppo S, Freed LE, Vunjak-Novakovic G. Integration of engineered cartilage. J Orthop Res 2001; 19:1089–1097.

52. Schaefer D, Martin I, Shastri VP, Padera RF, Langer R, Freed LE, Vunjak-Novakovic G. In vitro generation of osteochondral composites. Biomaterials 2000; 21:2599–2606.

53. Hunziker EB, Kapfinger E. Removal of proteoglycans from the surface of defects in articular cartilage transiently enhances coverage by repair cells. J Bone Joint Surg Br 1998; 80B:144–150.

54. DiMicco MA, Sah RL. Integrative cartilage repair: adhesive strength corre-lates with collagen deposition. J Orthop Res 2001; 19:1105–1112.

55. Madry H, Padera R, Seidel J, Langer R, Freed LE, Trippel SB, Vunjak-Novakovic G. Gene transfer of a human insulin-like growth factor I cDNA enhances tissue engineering of cartilage. Hum Gene Ther 2002; 13:1621–1630.

56. Martin I, Suetterlin R, Baschong W, Heberer M, Vunjak-Novakovic G, Freed LE. Enhanced cartilage tissue engineering by sequential exposure of chondro-cytes to FGF-2 during 2D expansion and BMP-2 during 3D cultivation. J Cell Biochem 2001; 83:121–128.

57. Blunk T, Sieminski AL, Gooch KJ, Courter DL, Hollander AP, Nahir AM, Langer R, Vunjak-Novakovic G, Freed LE. Differential effects of growth fac-tors on tissue-engineered cartilage. Tissue Eng 2002; 8:73–84.

58. Vunjak-Novakovic G, Obradovic B, Martin I, Freed LE. Bioreactor studies of native and tissue engineered cartilage. Biorheology 2002; 39:259–268.

59. Altman, G, Horan, R, Lu,H, Moreau,J, Martin I, Richmond J, Kaplan DL. Silk matrix for tissue engineered anterior cruciate ligaments. Biomaterials 2002; 23:4131–4141.

60. Madry H, Trippel SB. Efficient lipid-mediated gene transfer to articular chondrocytes. Gene Ther 2000; 7(4):286–291.

9

Clinically Applicable Animal Models in Tissue Engineering

Ernst B. Hunziker
University of Bern, Bern, Switzerland

I. INTRODUCTION

In orthopedics, tissue engineering is a rapidly growing field of interest. It is also one that holds considerable promise for success, since the tissues implicated are generally of mesodermal origin and thus formed from cells of great versatility with a high potential for repair (1). Moreover, these tissues are characterized by high remodeling activities, which also renders them amenable to engineering. The purpose of tissue engineering is to generate a construct in vitro—using precursor cells and an appropriate carrier system—for implantation in vivo (2,3). Such constructs are destined to replace tissue that has degenerated, been lost or destroyed, and that cannot be replaced naturally owing either to its poor capacity to repair or to excessive demands on its repair potential (as in the case of very large defects). Several different approaches can be adopted to achieve the desired end. Precursor cells for cartilage (4), bone (5,6), tendon (7,8), meniscus (9,10), etc., can be differentiated in vitro and a fully matured tissue construct then implanted within the defect. Alternatively, and this is the more favored approach, precursor cells (with stem cell potential) can be grown within an appropriate carrier system containing the necessary signaling substances to induce tissue formation and maturation after implantation (1,11). Precursor cells can also be transfected with appropriate genes to trigger the signal necessary for tissue maturation following deposition at the orthotopic site (12).

Tissue engineering studies are complex in nature and involve many stages of testing before the experimental construct is ripe for human clinical trials. Biocompatibility questions, toxicological problems, pharmacological aspects, safety issues, and proof of the principle itself represent but a few of the concerns that must be scrutinized.

This chapter deals with the different types of animal experiments that are usually undertaken in tissue engineering studies. During the initial phase, small-animal models are used to screen all potential components of the proposed construct, e.g., carrier materials, cells, and transfection modes. In the second phase, the principle itself is put to the test using an appropriate defect and animal model. The choice of species for this purpose is by no means trivial, many factors having to be considered and special requirements satisfied for meaningful experimentation. Finally, clinically relevant setups are designed in animal models to furnish basic information respecting the construct's suitability and readiness for testing in human trials.

II. PHASE ONE: SCREENING OF A CONSTRUCT'S COMPONENTS

Each of the components comprising a construct needs to be screened in small-animal models to assess its likelihood of eliciting an adverse response in humans. Biocompatibility and biodegradability issues, as well as pharmacological and toxicological effects, are analyzed in various tissue compartments, but usually within the subcutaneous space, of rats or mice (13–15). In some instances, especially in studies involving constructs for bone repair, the orthotopic site itself is used (16,17). This is, of course, the ideal choice, in that the elicitation or absence of a response can be taken to be tissue-specific. For example, titanium-based materials are known to be biocompatible with bony substances but not with subcutaneous tissue (18,19). And in some special cases, testing directly at the orthotopic site is essential, as with constructs destined for the repair of articular cartilage, which is an immunologically privileged tissue and thus governed by a specific biological microenvironment.

With respect to the carrier system itself, the excretory pathway and half-life of each degradation product need to be evaluated in the mammalian body, with special attention being paid to the long-term pharmacological and possible toxicological or carcinogenic effects.

The fate of autologous, and especially of allogenic, precursor cells used in constructs must be very carefully investigated. Aspects such as their bodily distribution, homing preference, and localization, as well as their potential for undesired reactivity and uncontrolled proliferation, need to be evaluated. Some of these cells, such as bone-marrow-derived mesenchymal precursor cells, have proved to be useful in reestablishing the bone marrow space and in enhancing the hemopoietic activities of cancer patients who have undergone chemo- or radiation therapy (20).

III. PHASE TWO: PROOF OF PRINCIPLE

As soon as an engineered tissue construct can be produced and maintained in vitro on a scale that is meaningful in terms of human applications, its functionality needs to be tested in a suitable animal model. In the case of constructs destined for different sites within the musculoskeletal system, the small mammalian species (such as rats and mice) used for the screening of its individual components are not appropriate. The surgical implantation of these constructs requires their being of a minimal size for optimal positioning and fixing in situ under mechanically stable conditions. For this reason, middle-sized animals (such as guinea pigs or rabbits) or even larger ones (such as dogs, sheep, goats, or miniature pigs) have to be employed (18,21,22).

Following the surgical implantation of a construct within a model defect site, such as a bony lesion, its fate is pursued for varying periods of time, and the advantages and drawbacks of the tissue engineering approach over the conventional therapeutic one are assessed. If the evaluation is to be meaningful, then the appropriate control experiments must be set up. These are often larger in number than most investigators realize, or are able to undertake owing to the high costs involved in such a systematic analysis. Strictly, the functionality of each component of the construct should be tested separately. And each of these constituents should also be replaced by an alternative one, either with or without biological activity (when appropriate), to assess its specificity (or nonspecificity) as a contributing factor to the engineered system. This includes the precursor cells utilized (if at all). They should be substituted by a type that is known to be unable to perform the task required of it, to confirm the necessity of the specific one chosen for the engineered construct.

Other important aspects necessitating strict experimental control include the biological and mechanical microenvironments, which, in most instances, contribute significantly to the outcome of tissue repair

(23–26). Despite their importance, such environmental factors are all too often insufficiently considered in experimental designs. For example, following the surgical implantation of a construct within a large full-thickness articular cartilage defect, it has become common practice to prevent its postoperative loss into the joint cavity by securing a periosteal flap over the top of it (27). But such an appendage cannot be considered merely as an inert lid. It is living tissue that may well serve as a source of connective-tissue cells (such as fibroblasts) for repair (21). In the absence of a construct, these cells will probably invade the defect and influence the course of healing (28). The presence of a construct could act as a barrier to the invasion of cells from the periosteal tissue, but this circumstance has yet to be established. Indeed, the point has not even been the subject of investigation; nor has the one relating to the retention rate of such flaps (29). Clearly though, if the periostal flap were to be replaced by an artificial membrane, then one potential source of cells for repair would certainly be eliminated, thus allowing for a better-controlled investigation and at the same time permitting a more reliable assessment of the construct's biological contribution to the repair process (30).

Likewise in studies relating to tendon or ligament repair, sheets of tendonous or ligamentous tissue used in conjunction with an engineered construct have to be considered as potential sources of cells for repair. The integrity of the vascular system running along the surfaces of these sheets must also be duly taken into account (31).

In articular cartilage repair studies, one needs to be especially heedful of a model defect's dimensions relative to its surrounds. When using middle-sized or even large animals, investigators tend to work with full-thickness defects, which embrace the entire depth of the articular cartilage layer and also penetrate the subchondral bone plate. In these models, more than 90% of the lesion void generally lies within the bony compartment (32). But bone, unlike cartilage, is heavily vascularized, and this vascularized tissue serves as a rich source of precursor cells and signaling substances, which will promote a spontaneous repair response (33). If defects are confined to the articular cartilage layer, virtually no spontaneous repair reaction takes place. If it occurs at all, such a response is confined to the defect borders, which lie within the range of weak signaling from the vicinal articular cartilage tissue (34,35). Hence, to obtain useful information concerning the repair potential of an engineered construct in the context of purely cartilaginous lesions in human pathology, these bony sources of cells and signaling substances need to be cut off (see next section).

A careful selection of animal model is important already during this second phase of experimentation, when the principle of the engineered construct is being put to the test. In several reports relating to bone repair, rats have been chosen. But this mammalian species is so small as to render surgically based experiments fraught with difficulties from the onset. The dimensions to be dealt with are far too small to permit precise and adequate control of many surgical factors, such as wound closure and the placement of periosteal flaps or internal fixation devices. This state of affairs gives rise to considerable variations in the biological and mechanical situations pertaining, which will complicate the interpretation of results.

One animal model that is frequently used in orthopedic research is the adult rabbit. It must be emphasized that by the term "adult," a skeletally mature animal is implied. Rabbits attain skeletal maturity when they are about 8 months old. Their age must be known with certainty, since body weight is not a reliable indicator of when puberty has been passed through and adulthood entered. However, if studies relate to articular cartilage, then younger animals can serve as an adult model, since this tissue matures at an earlier date than the epiphyseal plates of the long bones. Growth of articular cartilage peaks and then ceases when rabbits are around 3 or 4 months old, after which time only that of the long bones continues (Hunziker et al., unpublished data). This is a useful point to bear in mind, since systematic experiments with older animals, which are expensive, may be difficult to fund.

It is also worth mentioning that the bones of rabbits are fairly brittle and thus liable to fracture if more than a few defects are produced within any one of these. Moreover, this animal's mode of locomotion—hopping—does not tend to mitigate this risk, since quite a considerable force of impact is generated when the ground is hit during such a movement. If an engineered construct principle is to be tested in a rabbit model, then the number of defects should be restricted to one or maximally two, created preferably at the epiphyseal end of either the proximal tibia or distal femur. Careful and precise surgery is, of course, indispensable to avoid interference with adjacent tissues, such as the periosteum or subcutaneous connective tissue, whose heterogeneous cell pools may otherwise be recruited for repair and thereby complicate the experimental design.

IV. PHASE THREE: CLINICALLY RELEVANT TESTING

A precondition for clinically relevant testing of a tissue engineering strategy in animal models is the detailed definition and establishment of the human pathology and of the treatment mode that need to be developed. Although one would suppose this backdrop to be instituted as a matter of course, it is, in fact, but rarely given due consideration and is, indeed, not so rapidly achieved from a practical point of view.

The tissue to be repaired must first be minutely characterized in terms of its composition, cellularity, and structure. Only then is the investigator in a position to know what must be aimed at therapeutically in a patient and thus simulated in the engineered construct. Human articular cartilage, for example, is characterized by an extraordinarily low cellularity and a highly anisotropic structure (36). If its functionality and mechanical competence are to be assured in the repair tissue, then these architectural features must be re-established. Even if an engineered construct is successfully implanted within an experimental animal, such as a goat or sheep, the cartilage tissue generated will at best be goat-like or sheep-like, but not human-like, unless measures are taken from the onset of the tissue engineering process to simulate the human characteristics. When it comes to the testing phase in an animal model, it is important ultimately to imitate the human scale of the defect to be repaired. The smallest type of human clinical lesion involving articular cartilage is a focal, partial-thickness one. Such defects, which are generated by trauma or during the initial stages of osteoarthritis, would be maximally 2–3 mm in height (i.e., the thickness of the human articular cartilage layer). But a defect of this height, when created in any commonly used animal model, extends far beyond the confines of the cartilaginous compartment into the bony one. The biological environment around the implanted construct (Fig. 1) is thus quite different from that in humans (32). Measures must therefore be taken to generate a microenvironment that is analogous to the human one. This can be achieved by producing a "virtual" partial-thickness defect (Fig. 2). A lesion 2–3 mm in depth would be created in the animal model, but its walls so treated as to become impervious to bleeding, signaling substances, and cell infiltration from the bone marrow space. A fibrin glue (37) containing this polymer at a concentration of 120 mg/mL (compared to one of 2 mg/mL in serum) could be used effectively in this capacity. This imitation of the physiological scenery is important in testing the functionality, survival rate, and durability of a construct destined for clinical use.

Not only the depth of the human clinical defect but also its lateral dimensions must be recreated in the chosen animal model. Partial-thickness articular cartilage lesions of the type described above would, in the human knee joint, typically span 1–2 cm in this direction. The engineered construct thus needs to be quite voluminous and this circumstance in itself is associated with specific problems following implantation. If the construct is required to undergo differentiation in situ rather than in vitro, then the requisite signaling agents must be incorporated; vicinal native cartilage will not furnish these substances in sufficient quantities to sustain the necessary level of activity within such a large volume of engineered tissue (34). Furthermore, it must be remembered that the bone-marrow-derived source

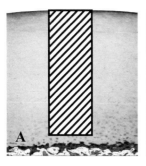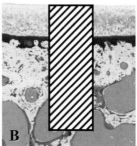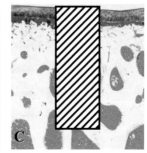

FIGURE 1 Schematic representations of like-sized defects superimposed upon light micrographs of (A) human, (B) goat, and (C) rabbit articular cartilage tissue (together with varying portions of the underlying subchondral bone), represented at the same magnification. Because the thickness of the articular cartilage layer in humans is several times greater than that in goats, and many times more so than that in rabbits, the biological environment surrounding each defect differs. In the human, the defect is a partial-thickness one, and, as such, it is surrounded exclusively by cartilage tissue. In the goat and rabbit, lesions of the same dimensions are full-thickness ones, approximately 85% and 95% of their volumes, respectively, being surrounded by osseous tissue and bone marrow spaces. In these two latter cases, bleeding from the bone marrow spaces will furnish the defects with an abundant supply of signaling substances and cells to which the human partial-thickness one will not be accessible.

of such substances will have been cut off by the "protective" wall of fibrin glue. Signaling activity from the opposite side, namely, from the synovium, is not desirable, since the fluid derived therefrom contains tissue-degrading proteases.

General problems that will be encountered both during and after the implantation of a construct include its mechanical fixation, its integration with neighboring healthy tissue, and interfacial shear forces.

Irrespective of the animal model chosen, the question to be tackled is always the same: How can the human microenvironment, pathology, and repair conditions be most closely imitated such as to obtain convincing evidence for moving forward to human clinical trials?

Careful experimental planning relates not only to the defect model itself and simulation of the human situation, but also to the biomechanical conditions operative during the healing phase. All orthopedic tissues have biomechanical functions, and appropriate stimulation of these during the process of tissue repair is likely to have a considerable bearing on the outcome. For this reason, it is of the utmost importance to instigate

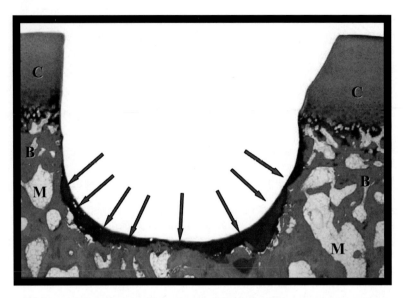

FIGURE 2 Light micrograph of a full-thickness defect in mature bovine articular cartilage. A virtual partial-thickness defect has been created by lining its floor and walls with fibrin glue (arrows), which blocks cell migration and vascular invasion from osseous tissue and the bone marrow spaces into the defect void for a considerable time (up to 1 week). C: articular cartilage; B: bone tissue; M: bone marrow spaces. Thick section, surface-stained with McNeil's Tetrachrome, Toluidine Blue 0, and basic Fuchsine.

well-defined loading protocols (38). In experimental animals, control over the loading conditions cannot be achieved to the desired degree, although the use of appropriate bandages is helpful in defining limited degrees of joint movement. In this respect, modern bandage systems involving very light materials possess great advantages over outdated cast-like ones (29).

Another important postsurgical issue relates to the period of time over which a construct should be tested in an experimental animal and its bearing on the human situation. This is an extremely difficult question to answer. The life expectancy of most experimental animals in their natural environment is much shorter than the human one. Hence, translation of the time span of healing in an animal model into human terms can only be a matter of speculation. An animal with a life expectancy of 15–20 years under laboratory conditions must generally be monitored for up to 1 year before any meaningful statement can be made respecting the possible long-term outcome in human patients.

The foregoing account has of necessity highlighted but a few of the general issues that must be addressed and yet are often overlooked when adopting the tissue engineering approach to repair and its testing in animal experiments. Obviously, each of the orthopedic tissues comprising the musculoskeletal system will pose its unique and specific set of problems that must be minutely dissected and tackled. No single animal model can perfectly simulate the human pathology. But the closest approach to clinical relevance will be achieved if endeavors are made to imitate the human situation in all possible respects at each stage of investigation (e.g., in the composition, cellularity, and structure of the engineered construct; in the defect dimensions; in the biological microenvironment and signaling scenery; in terms of biomechanical factors; and in the time span of healing). The final step from a clinically relevant experimental animal to the human patient will, of course, always be a large one carrying many risks. But by adopting the aforementioned policy, these risks can be reduced considerably, and the information thereby gleaned will furnish a solid basis for making reasonable predictions as to a beneficial outcome in human patients.

REFERENCES

1. Reddi AH. Morphogenesis and tissue engineering of bone and cartilage: inductive signals, stem cells, and biomimetic biomaterials. Tissue Eng 2000; 6:351–359.
2. Jackson DW, Simon TM. Tissue engineering principles in orthopaedic surgery. Clin Orthop 1999:S31–45.
3. Glowacki J. In vitro engineering of cartilage. J Rehabil Res Dev 2000; 37: 171–177.
4. Grande DA, Breitbart AS, Mason J, Paulino C, Laser J, Schwartz RE. Cartilage tissue engineering: current limitations and solutions. Clin Orthop 1999:S176–185.
5. Puelacher WC, Vacanti JP, Ferraro NF, Schloo B, Vacanti CA. Femoral shaft reconstruction using tissue-engineered growth of bone. Int J Oral Maxillofac Surg 1996; 25:223–228.
6. Breitbart AS, Grande DA, Kessler R, Ryaby JT, Fitzsimmons RJ, Grant RT. Tissue engineered bone repair of calvarial defects using-cultured periosteal cells. Plast Reconstr Surg 1998; 101:567–574.
7. Isogai N, Landis W, Kim TH, Gerstenfeld LC, Upton J, Vacanti JP. Formation of phalanges and small joints by tissue-engineering. J Bone Joint Surg Am 1999; 81:306–316.
8. Carpenter JE, Thomopoulos S, Soslowsky LJ. Animal models of tendon and ligament injuries for tissue engineering applications. Clin Orthop 1999:S296–311.

9. Peretti GM, Caruso EM, Randolph MA, Zaleske DJ. Meniscal repair using engineered tissue. J Orthop Res 2001; 19:278–285.

10. Sweigart MA, Athanasiou KA. Toward tissue engineering of the knee meniscus. Tissue Eng 2001; 7:111–129.

11. Hedbom E, Ettinger L, Hauselmann HJ. Culture of articular chondrocytes in alginate gel—a means to generate cartilage-like implantable tissue. Osteoarthritis Cartilage 2001; 9:S123–130.

12. Gelse K, Jiang QJ, Aigner T, Ritter T, Wagner K, Poschl E, von der Mark K, Schneider II. Fibroblast-mediated delivery of growth factor complementary DNA into mouse joints induces chondrogenesis but avoids the disadvantages of direct viral gene transfer. Arthritis Rheum 2001; 44:1943–1953.

13. Festing MF. Genetic variation in outbred rats and mice and its implications for toxicological screening. J Exp Anim Sci 1993; 35:210–220.

14. Vohr HW. Experiences with an advanced screening procedure for the identification of chemicals with an immunotoxic potential in routine toxicology. Toxicology 1995; 104:149–158.

15. Fu ZD, Chen WR, Gu LJ, Gu ZW. The influence of the extent of target organs on sensitivities of methods for screening rodent carcinogens. Mutat Res 1995; 331:99–117.

16. Halloran PF, Ziv I, Lee EH, Langer F, Pritzker KP, Gross AE. Orthotopic bone transplantation in mice. I. Technique and assessment of healing. Transplantation 1979; 27:414–419.

17. Werntz JR, Lane JM, Burstein AH, Justin R, Klein R, Tomin E. Qualitative and quantitative analysis of orthotopic bone regeneration by marrow. J Orthop Res 1996; 14:85–93.

18. Kasemo B. Biocompatibility of titanium implants: surface science aspects. J Prosthet Dent 1983; 49:832–837.

19. Prigent H, Pellen-Mussi P, Cathelineau G, Bonnaure-Mallet M. Evaluation of the biocompatibility of titanium-tantalum alloy versus titanium. J Biomed Mater Res 1998; 39:200–206.

20. Koc ON, Peters C, Aubourg P, Raghavan S, Dyhouse S, DeGasperi R, Kolodny EH, Yoseph YB, Gerson SL, Lazarus HM, Caplan AI, Watkins PA, Krivit W. Bone marrow-derived mesenchymal stem cells remain host-derived despite successful hematopoietic engraftment after allogeneic transplantation in patients with lysosomal and peroxisomal storage diseases. Exp Hematol 1999; 27:1675–1681.

21. Hunziker EB. Articular cartilage repair: are the intrinsic biological constraints undermining this process insuperable? Osteoarthritis Cartilage 1999; 7:15–28.

22. Pritzker KPH. Animal models for osteoarthritis: Processes, problems and prospects. Ann Rheum Dis 1994; 53:406–420.

23. Williams JM, Brandt KD. Temporary immobilisation facilitates repair of chemically induced articular cartilage injury. J Anat 1984; 138:435–446.

24. Shahgaldi BF, Amis AA, Heatley FW, McDowell J, Bentley G. Repair of cartilage lesions using biological implants: a comparative histological and biomechanical study in goats. J Bone Joint Surg (Br) 1991; 73:57–64.

25. Roeddecker K, Muennich U, Nagelschmidt M. Meniscal healing: a biomechanical study. J Surg Res 1994; 56:20–27.
26. Yetkinler DN, Ladd AL, Poser RD, Constantz BR, Carter D. Biomechanical evaluation of fixation of intra-articular fractures of the distal part of the radius in cadavera: Kirschner wires compared with calcium-phosphate bone cement. J Bone Joint Surg Am 1999; 81:391–399.
27. Brittberg M, Lindahl A, Nilsson A, Ohlsson C, Isaksson O, Peterson L. Treatment of deep cartilage defects in the knee with autologous chondrocyte transplantation. N Engl J Med 1994; 331:879–895.
28. O'Driscoll SW, Recklies AD, Poole AR. Chondrogenesis in periosteal explants - An organ culture model for in vitro study. J Bone Joint Surg Am 1994; 76A:1042–1051.
29. Driesang IM, Hunziker EB. Delamination rates of tissue flaps used in articular cartilage repair. J Orthop Res 2000; 18:909–911.
30. Breinan HA, Minas T, Hsu HP, Nehrer S, Sledge CB, Spector M. Effect of cultured autologous chondrocytes on repair of chondral defects in a canine model. J Bone Joint Surg Am 1997; 79A:1439–1451.
31. Woo SL, Buckwalter JA. AAOS/NIH/ORS workshop. Injury and repair of the musculoskeletal soft tissues. Savannah, Georgia, June 18–20, 1987. J Orthop Res 1988; 6:907–931.
32. Hunziker EB. Biologic repair of articular cartilage. Defect models in experimental animals and matrix requirements. Clin Orthop 1999:S135–146.
33. Shapiro F, Koide S, Glimcher MJ. Cell origin and differentiation in the repair of full-thickness defects of articular cartilage. J Bone Joint Surg Am 1993; 75A:532–553.
34. Hunziker EB, Rosenberg LC. Repair of partial-thickness defects in articular cartilage: cell recruitment from the synovial membrane. J Bone Joint Surg Am 1996; 78A(5):721–733.
35. Mitchell N, Lee ER, Shepard N. The clones of osteoarthritic cartilage. J Bone Joint Surg (Br) 1992; 74:33–38.
36. Hunziker EB. Articular cartilage structure in humans and experimental animals. In: Kuettner KE, Schleyerbach R, Peyron JG, Hascall VC, eds. Articular Cartilage and Osteoarthritis. New York: Raven Press1992:183–199.
37. Silver FH, Wang MC, Pins GD. Preparation and use of fibrin glue in surgery. Biomaterials 1995; 16:891–903.
38. Mow V, Rosenwasser M. Articular cartilage: biomechanics. Woo SLY, Buckwalter JA, eds. Injury and Repair of the Musculoskeletal Soft Tissues. Park Ridge, IL: American Academy of Orthopaedic Surgeons1988:427–463.

10

Bone Tissue Engineering: Basic Science and Clinical Concepts

Safdar N. Khan
Hospital for Special Surgery,
New York, New York, U.S.A.

Joseph M. Lane
Weill Medical College of Cornell University and
Hospital for Special Surgery,
New York, U.S.A.

I. INTRODUCTION

Autogenous corticocancellous bone grafting has remained the preferred form of enhancing fracture healing, spinal fusion, and filling osseous defects. Since the procedure of procuring bone graft has been associated at times with inadequate volume and significant morbidity, efforts have been directed toward developing biosynthetic tissue-engineered alternatives to autogenous grafting. Three primary concepts of biosynthetic grafts, the osteoprogenitor cells, the osteoconductive matrix, and the osteoinductive factors, will be discussed in this chapter.

Autogenous grafting provides the components essential for achieving osseous healing. These components include osteoprogenitor stem cells present in the bone marrow elements, an osteoconductive hydroxyapatite collagen matrix, and a series of osteoinductive growth factors, of which the bone morphogenetic proteins (BMP) are the most prominent. The major limitations of using autogenous grafting are the inadequacy of supply and surgical morbidity, including donor site pain, paresthesias, and infection, which can approach 8–10% (1). Allografts, as an alternative to autogenous grafts, are biologically inferior and are associated with infection and inflammation (2). To overcome these deficiencies attempts have been directed to develop synthetic composite grafts that are intended to mimic the natural components required for bone regeneration and repair. Tissue-engineered constructs ideally should contain: (1) osteoprogenitor stem cells with receptors that respond to osteoinductive signals and have the capability of proliferating and differentiating into osteoblasts; (2) sufficient osteoinductive growth factor proteins to stimulate these osteoprogenitor cells; and (3) an osteoconductive matrix to provide a favorable environment and three-dimensional scaffold for the cell growth.

II. BONE MARROW AND OSTEOGENIC CELLS

Autogenous bone marrow contains osteoprogenitor stem cells and has been used alone and in combination with inorganic matrix to promote osteogenesis (3–5). Currently, autogenous bone marrow is being employed clinically to augment both synthetic graft materials and allografts. In addition, it may be used to re-establish normal fracture hematomas following surgical irrigation. Marrow is advantageous because there is essentially no morbidity associated with harvesting.

Bone marrow has been introduced in porous ceramic and used to bring osteoprogenitor cells to deficient grafting beds. Using a rat femoral segmental defect model, bone marrow produced rates of union comparable to those of autogenous cancellous bone (6). This marrow-augmented bone demonstrated biomechanical properties similar to that produced by cancellous grafting. Autogenous bone marrow has been shown to be synergistic when used in combination with recombinant human BMP-2. Therefore, it is hypothesized that bone marrow osteoprogenitor stem cells have BMP receptors (7).

Clinically, bone marrow has been used to successfully treat patients with nonunions (8–10). It should be harvested in aliquots of approximately 2.5 mL/site and used immediately to maintain viability. Although marrow contains osteoprogenitor cells in concentrations ranging from 1/50,000 to 1/2 million nucleated cells, depending on the age of the patient, filtration techniques exist to increase these numbers up to fivefold (11). Mesenchymal stem cells have been expanded by logarithmic-growing marrow in culture and used to heal osseous defects in combination with ceramics and collagen mixtures (12). Use of these expanded stem cell populations for osteogenesis offers many future possibilities.

III. OSTEOCONDUCTIVE MATRICES

Ceramics currently used in the repair of osseous defects may be divided into three categories based on their chemical reactivity following implantation: (1) *bioabsorbable* ceramics, (2) *bioactive* ceramics, and (3) *bioinert* ceramics (13). Bioabsorbable and bioactive substances are able to directly bond physically to the host bed, whereas bioinert substances never actually bond to bone. Nonbiodegradable polymers form another class of osteoconductive grafts. For example, polymethyl methacrylate (PMMA) is a polymer that acts similarly to a bioinert ceramic in that it does not incorporate into newly forming bone, yet it bonds adhesively to the bone surface without interfering with regeneration. Bone preparations such as demineralized bone matrix (DBM) also belong to the weakly osteoinductive/osteoconductive group of bone grafts. These grafts hold tremendous potential because of their osteoinductive capabilities and as such have been used with considerable success in spinal fusion applications.

The chemical composition of a synthetic graft also affects its rate of resorption. For example, tricalcium phosphate (TCP) will be resorbed 10–20 times faster than hydroxyapatite (HA), another calcium phosphate ceramic. Crystalline structure clearly affects the total amount of resorption. Several clinical trials have reported that TCP can be totally resorbed, or converted into hydroxyapatite that may remain in the body for an indefinite period of time (14). In using a hydroxyapatite graft that persists in the host bone, the intrinsic strength of the bone may be compromised at the callus site owing to the weaker synthetic ceramic.

Porosity is another factor to consider when using ceramics. The optimal osteoconductive pore sizes for ceramics appear to be between 150 and 500 μm. Cancellous bone has a complex trabecular pattern in which approximately 20% of the total matrix is bone and the remaining area is marrow space connected through pores. Synthetic ceramics, on the other hand, have various-sized pores but lack pore-to-pore connectivity. Thus, in clinical situations where ceramics are used, the healing osteogenic process must reabsorb the synthetic bone to gain access to the interior pores. An important consideration is that with increased porosity the graft will maintain significantly less compressive strength. The exceptions are ceramics derived from materials such as coral that have a biological network of pore interconnectivity. Factors such as surface area affect the rate of biological degradation, and in general, the larger the surface area, the greater the rate of bioresorption. Dense ceramic blocks with small surface areas biodegrade slowly when compared to porous implants. Thus, the shape and architecture of the ceramic will also have a profound effect on biological resorption rates.

Calcium phosphates ceramics have received attention as osteoconductive bioabsorbable ceramics. Most calcium phosphate ceramics currently under investigation are synthetic and composed primarily of hydroxyapatite, triphasic calcium phosphate, or a combination of the two. A wide difference in the resorption rates and porosity between TCP and hydroxyapatite makes a mixture of the two clinically favorable. Most calcium phosphate ceramics are obtained by sintering calcium phosphate salts at high temperatures to produce a moldable powder that can then be transformed into pellet form by compaction at high pressure. These biomaterials are currently being commercially produced as porous implants, nonporous dense implants, or granular particles with pores. Several injectable calcium phosphates using various crystal types are now available for restoring non-weight-bearing osseous defects. Injectable ceramics have performed reasonably well in a recent clinical trial in metaphyseal fractures (15).

Calcium phosphate bioabsorbable ceramics are brittle and have very little tensile strength; hence use in situations where torsion or shear strength is required is impractical. However, once they have been incorporated and remodeled the mechanical properties of porous ceramics are comparable to those of host cancellous bone. No adverse effects such as inflammation or foreign-body responses to these ceramics have been noted when they are used in a structural block arrangement. Small granules, however, have been shown to elicit a foreign-body giant cell reaction. The lack of complete remodeling can radiographically manifest as a continued presence of the ceramic for a prolonged period of time. Persistent radiographic opacity may cause difficulty in determining the degree of bone ingrowth and incorporation.

Replamineform ceramics are porous hydroxyapatite ceramics derived from the calcium carbonate skeletal structure of sea coral. A hydrothermal exchange method replaces the original calcium carbonate with a calcium phosphate replicate. The pore structure of the coralline calcium phosphate implants is highly organized almost exactly similar to that of human cancellous bone. The genus of the coral used determines the porous size of this graft. The hydroxyapatite ceramic derived from *Gonipora* has large pores measuring 500–600 μm in diameter with interconnections of 220–260 μm, making it similar to human cancellous bone (16). Hydroxyapatite ceramics derived from *Porites* has a smaller pore diameter of 200–2500 μm with parallel channels interconnected by 190-μm fenestrations.

Its microstructure is thus similar to that of interstitial cortical bone. The disadvantage of these ceramics is that as these grafts lack intrinsic strength, they can be used only to fill defects up to 7–8 cm and require some form of internal fixation so the graft does not fail subject to cyclical loading. Another problem with these biological coralline-derived ceramics is their delayed degradation in vivo. Only the surface of the ceramic is resorbed by osteoclasts, thereby leaving the majority of the microstructure intact. This may limit the coralline ceramics to anatomical regions in which bone remodeling is not crucial. In an effort to overcome the slow turnover, a coralline ceramic has been created with surface HA and an interior of calcium carbonate, an easily resorbed material. Boden et al. (17) studied the effectiveness of coralline hydroxyapatite as a bone graft substitute for lumbar spinal fusion when used with bone marrow alone, autogenous bone graft, or a bovine osteoinductive protein extract in an established rabbit model. The rabbits were assigned to one of three groups based on the graft material they received: 3.0 mL of coralline hydroxyapatite (CHA) plus 1.5 mL bone marrow, 3.0 mL CHA plus 500 µg bovine-derived osteoinductive bone protein extract, and 1.5 mL CHA plus 1.5 mL autogenous bone graft on each side. Rabbits were sacrificed at 2, 5, or 10 weeks and the spines were evaluated by radiographs, mechanical testing, and undecalcified histology. Their date indicated that the use of CHA plus bone marrow was not a suitable bone graft substitute in this healing environment. When combined with autogenous bone graft, the CHA acted as a graft extender demonstrating solid fusions in 50% of animals. However, when the CHA was combined with an osteoinductive bone protein extract, fusion rates of 100% were achieved. Hence, it was concluded that CHA served as an excellent carrier for bone proteins in a posterolateral lumbar spine fusion model.

Calcium sulfate ceramics are provided as an implant or are capable of being fabricated as needed. This latter form can incorporate antibiotics during the consolidation stage. The ceramic has weak mechanical properties and resorbs rapidly and acellularly. Bone forms directly adjacent to the resorbing ceramic. Clinically calcium sulfate is an excellent product to fill defects. It has been used successfully to graft defect sites in osteomyelitis as well as provide local antibiotic release.

Bioinert ceramics, as the name suggests, do not react with living tissue and provide the highest mechanical strength of all graft material. They are the most biocompatible of ceramics and are composed of metal oxides, such as alumina (Al_2O_3), zirconia (ZrO_2), and titania (TiO_2) (18). They have been utilized predominantly for long-bone defects because of their compressive strength.

Partially resorbable porous polymers such as polyglycolide (PGA) and poly-L-lactide (PLLA) allow for new bone growth. The development of these polymers is advantageous as they can be shaped into self-reinforcing screws, dowels, rods, and spacers, and have been utilized with some success in large-bone-fracture fixation (19). Polymers may also eventually be important potential carriers for substances such as antibiotics and osteoinduction agents.

IV. DEMINERALIZED BONE MATRIX

Demineralized bone matrix (DBM) is produced from the acid extraction of bone, leaving noncollagenous proteins, bone growth factors, and collagen. DBM is currently prepared by bone banks as pathogen free by virtue of rigorous donor selection and tissue processing. DBM has been utilized to promote bone group regeneration, mainly in well-supported, stable skeletal defects. Demineralized materials have no structural strength, but have enhanced osteoinductive capability afforded by members of the TGF-β superfamily, notably bone morphogenetic proteins (BMPs). The FDA requires sterilization of the DBM as prepared by bone banks and this may in fact decrease some of the viability of the available BMP within the preparation. DBM does afford the potential of enhanced osteoinduction and to date has been used as an adjunctive to more traditional grafting materials.

DBM is currently available as freeze-dried and processed from cortical/cancellous bone in the form of powder, crushed, chips, or as a gel. When successful in achieving union, DBM develops bone of comparable mechanical strength of autograft. However, some commercially available DBM preparations have failed to induce bone in the Urist biological mouse muscle test. DBM is easy to mold intraoperatively; however, it does not provide intrinsic strength.

DBM has been used to augment autogenous bone grafts while repairing cysts, fractures, nonunions, and fusions. Glowacki et al. reported on the clinical applications in craniofacial reconstruction (20–23). Tiedman et al. (24) evaluated the efficacy of DBM used alone and with autogenous bone marrow as graft material in the treatment of a variety of clinical situations such as bone defects and comminuted and nonunited fractures in children. In their series, 30 of 39 patients demonstrated a bony union. These authors concluded that DBM and marrow composite grafts are comparable in efficacy to autogenous iliac crest bone graft alone for use in certain clinical situations. Michelson and Curl (25) compared hindfoot fusions augmented by either iliac crest bone graft or demineralized bone matrix alone. All 29 patients receiving DBM achieved complete fusion, while 13 of 15 patients receiving autologous iliac crest bone graft went on to bony healing. There was no difference in the time required for complete healing, with both groups achieving union in 3–4 months. Killian et al. (26) used DBM to obliterate unicameral bone cysts in 9 of 11 patients, who were cyst free at 2 years' follow-up, clearly showing the effectiveness of using demineralized bone matrix in certain clinical situations.

V. ALLOGRAFTS

The use of allografts to repair skeletal defects is not restricted by harvest availability as autogenous grafting is, nor by donor site morbidity. Current procedures utilize allografts in the form of morselized cancellous and cortical bone chips for the filling of cavitary defects and corticocancellous and cortical struts for structural support.

Infection and allograft fracture are the most common complications, and though stabilization and tissue testing techniques have improved allogenic transplantation greatly, recent studies have found incidence of infection near 10–15% and incidence of fracture between 5 and 15% (27,28). Stringent testing and sterilization of graft tissue prior to use can decrease the incidence of transmissible disease. However, such practices compromise the osteoinductive and osteogenic potential of allogenic grafting significantly. Allograft is harvested, batch-sterilized, and preserved by deep-freezing below −60°C, or freeze-drying. Slow cryopreservation using glycerol or dimethylsulfoxide has been shown to maintain the viability of allogenic osteochondral grafts by preventing water crystallization within cells. Studies demonstrate a wide range of cartilage viability (20–70%) using these techniques, producing controversy as to their true efficacy (29,30). Freeze-drying fully destroys the osteoprogenitor cells and osteo-inductive factors, and alters the biomechanical properties of the graft with losses of hoop and compressive strength upon rehydration. The net result of these procedures produces a bone substitute that can only provide an osteoconductive scaffold, although there is indication that they do provide decreased immunogenicity and antigenicity.

The risk of disease transmission, particularly HIV and hepatitis B and C, is an important issue. The American Association of Tissue Banks (AATB) monitors hospital tissue banks to ensure compliance with a comprehensive sets of standards. Regulations include donor screening, repeated infectious disease testing, sterilization of graft tissue with such substances as ethylene oxide or radiation, long-term tracking of the graft, and inspection of tissue banks. These techniques have significantly lowered the risk of disease transmission.

Incorporation of allograft bone is considerably different than autogenous bone graft. Vascular penetration is more superficial and impeded; indeed, a study demonstrated that allograft revascularization was not as complete at 8 months postsurgery as autogenous graft was at 4 weeks (31). Osteogenesis is initiated by the host immune response as demonstrated by an inflammatory reaction. This results in hyalinization of penetrating and pre-existing blood vessels, prompting necrosis of allograft periosteal cells and osteocytes. It is this necrotic bone that remains after full incorporation of the allograft that is the main reason for the increased incidence of fracture (32,33). This problem is most notable when using massive cortical allografts as supportive struts (33). Fatigue-generated microfractures form at the interface around the necrotic bone near the fracture site, which cannot remodel itself, thus resulting in structural failure (33).

Allografts may also be used for nonstructural purposes such as filling osseous defects after curettage of a benign neoplasm or periarticular bone cyst. In addition, bony cavities at the time of joint arthroplasty revision can be filled with allograft chips. The transient loss of strength, so markedly seen in autogenous cortical grafting, is not demonstrated in this type of allogenic transplantation as revascularization of morselized allograft does not require resorption. Rehydration of these chips produces an open and porous structure, without physical impediment, fully allowing the ingrowth of vasculature.

When needed for structural support a variety of forms of allograft bone are available, including iliac bicortical and tricortical strips, cancellous cortical dowels, fibular shafts and wedges, femoral and tibial cross sections, patellae, and ribs. They can be utilized as an intercalary segment to reconstruct a diaphyseal defect of long bone, and large segments can be modeled to replace acetabular, femoral, and tibial defects during primary and revision arthroplasty. Additionally, structural allografts have been used quite frequently to facilitate in arthodesis about the ankle, hip, and spine. A full array of PLIF and ALIF allografts have been milled for interbody fusion.

Osteochondral allografts replace resected bone and provide a biological bone surface. These grafts are used primarily to treat large or small isolated articular cartilage defects most often about the knee (34,35). Small, cylindrical grafts are harvested arthroscopically and implanted in mosaiclike fashion into the cartilage defect. Since it has become apparent that the life span of conventional joint prostheses is limited, their use has become more prevalent in the past decade.

VI. GROWTH FACTORS

Osteoinduction is mediated by a variety of growth factors within the bone matrix itself that play a critical role in bone healing. These peptides have become an important area of investigation in an effort to enhance fracture healing. Bone healing involves a complex interaction of many local and systemic regulatory factors (36–42). Autocrine and paracrine mechanisms cause undifferentiated mesenchymal cells to migrate, proliferate, and differentiate at the fracture site.

Numerous mediators have been implicated as the predominant growth factors in fracture healing with members of the transforming growth factor betas (TGF-β) superfamily of polypeptide growth factors being the most notable. This group of growth factors appears to regulate the proliferation and expression of differentiated phenotypes for many cell populations, including chondrocyte, osteoblast, and osteoclast precursors. Its members include TGF-β_1–TGF-β_5 and other peptides, including the BMPs, and growth and differentiation factors (GDF). Transforming growth factor-β is present in the graft hematoma after release by the platelet and is synthesized additionally by the mesenchymal cells. Other growth factors present in the developing callus during the fracture healing process include fibroblast growth factor (FGF), platelet-derived growth factor (PDGF), and insulin-like growth factors (IGF) (43–45). FGFs are mitogenic and angiogenic factors that play an essential role in neovascularization and wound healing. PDGFs act as local tissue growth regulators and were initially isolated in blood platelets, hence focusing upon the important role of the clot in fracture healing. IGFs are other examples of matrix-synthesizing growth factors important in bone healing. Readers are directed to a review by Khan et al. for further information regarding these factors (46). This section, however, will be devoted exclusively to the only FDA-approved growth factor for clinical use, the BMPs.

VII. BONE MORPHOGENETIC PROTEINS

Bone morphogenetic proteins are low-molecular-weight glycoproteins that function as morphogens (47,48). The BMPs belong to the TGF-β superfamily and have numerous functions, including extracellular and skeletal organogenesis to bone generation and regeneration. Bone induced by BMP in postfetal life recapitulates the process of embryonic and endochondral ossification. Through recombinant gene technology, BMPs are now available in sufficient amounts for basic research and clinical trials. Recombinant human BMP-2 and -7 (rhBMP-2 and -7) induce structurally sound orthotopic bone in various experimental systems. These BMPs have the capability of healing critical size defects in rodents, dogs, sheep, and primate models when combined with collagen, guanidine hydrochloric-acid-extracted demineralized bone matrix, or biodegradable polymers as carriers (49–54).

Bostrom et al. (55) characterized and localized BMP-2 and BMP-4 in rat fracture callus by implementing immunolocalization techniques.

The authors defined and characterized the physiological presence of BMP in endochondral and membranous fracture healing. During the early stages of fracture healing, only a small number of primitive cells stained positively in the callus. As the process of endochondral ossification proceeded, the presence of BMP-2 and BMP-4 increased significantly, especially within the primitive mesenchymal and chondrocytic cells. Although the cartilage component of the callus matured, there was a concomitant decrease in the number of primitive cells, the intensity of the stain, and the number of the positively staining cells with BMP. As osteoblasts started to lay down woven bone on the chondroid matrix, these osteoblastic cells showed a strong positive staining for BMP. The intensity of the staining decreased, however, as lamellar bone replaced the primitive bone. A similar observation was seen for areas undergoing intramembranous ossification. Initially, within several days after the fracture, periosteal cells and osteoblasts had intense staining for BMP. As woven bone was replaced with lamellar bone, the staining intensity increased. The data from these authors suggested that BMPs were important regulators in osteogenic differentiation during fracture repair. Additional supporting evidence for BMPs' critical role as signaling molecules comes from in vitro studies. Wang et al. (56) showed that BMP-2 causes commitment and differentiation of multipotential stem cell line into osteoblast-like cells.

Native human BMP was used successfully by Johnson et al. (57–59) for the treatment of established nonunions and spinal fusions. In their study of 70 patients union was achieved in over 90% of cases and there were no reports of any adverse events. Animal studies have demonstrated irrefutable proof of the efficacy of these proteins. Kirker-Head et al. (60) evaluated the long-term healing of bone using rhBMP-2 in adult sheep. At 12-month followup, all the defects were intact structurally and were healed rigidly. Woven and lamellar bone bridged the defect site and apparently the normal sequence of ossification, modeling, and remodeling events has occurred. Studies by Cook et al. (61–64) used BMP-7 to heal large segmental defects in rabbits, dogs, and primates. In their latter studies, five of six ulnas and four of five tibias treated with BMP-7 in African green monkeys achieved complete healing in 6–8 weeks with bridging of the defect and new bone formation in 4 weeks. Two unhealed defects had new bone formation. All the tibial defects and all the ulnar defects that had been treated with autogenous bone graft formed fibrous union with little new bone formation. Thus, these studies showed the efficacy of rhBMP in a nonhuman primate.

Perhaps the greatest attention has been directed toward using rhBMPs for spinal fusions. Boden et al. (65,66), Sandhu et al. (67), Schimandle et al. (68,69), and Muschler et al. (70) have developed spine models that can be used to test recombinant factors. Sandhu et al. (67) performed numerous studies using BMP-2 in a canine spine intraspinous process model. They found that the critical element was the dose of BMP and the result was unrelated to whether decortication was performed. The same authors showed that rhBMP-2 with polylactic acid carrier was clearly superior at higher and lower doses ranging from 57 µg and 2.3 mg as compared with autogenous bone graft fusion by 3 months. This study resulted in a 100% clinical fusion rate at 3 months. Fusions resulting from high doses of BMP were mechanically stiffer than fusions that received low-dose BMP in the axial plane. Additionally all fusions that received BMP were stiffer than autograft fusions in all planes. These studies showed the efficacy of higher doses of rhBMP-2 for inducing posteriolateral lumbar fusion in a canine model.

Laursen et al. (71) reported a pilot study performed in five patients with unstable thoracolumbar spine fractures treated with transpedicular rhBMP-7 transplantation, short-segment instrumentation, and posterolateral fusion. Follow-up time was 12–18 months and patients were evaluated clinically, by plain radiographs, and with serial CT scans. In all the five patients there was a lose of correction of anterior and middle-column height and sagittal balance at last follow-up. The authors were forced to discontinue the study in the face of these results and concluded that rhBMP-7 was not capable of inducing an early sufficient structural bone support in the spine. A preliminary trial using the growth factor as an adjunct to iliac crest autograft in lumbar fusion was conducted by Patel et al. (72). Sixteen patients with the diagnosis of spinal stenosis and single-level degenerative spondylolisthesis in the lower lumbar spine (L3–S1) were enrolled in an investigate device exempted (IDE) multicenter trial. The patients were randomized to either a rhBMP-7 group (12 patients) or a control group (four patients). The control group received iliac crest autograft alone while the experimental group received iliac crest autograft plus 3.5 mg of rhBMP-7 in a "putty" carrier per side. Clinical outcomes were measured using the Oswestry score and radiographically by two independent, blinded radiologists.

At 6 months (time point of last report) 9 of 12 (75%) patients receiving autograft with rhBMP-7 were deemed radiologically fused versus two of four (50%) patients in the control group. Clinical success was defined as a minimum 20% improvement in the Oswestry score. With that criterion, at 6 months, 10 of 12 (83%) of rhBMP-7+ autograft-implanted patients were deemed clinical successes compared to two of four (50%) of the control group. The pilot study demonstrated the effectiveness of rhBMP-7 when used in concert with autograft in human posterolateral lumbar fusion.

Recently an FDA-approved IDE multicenter pilot study was performed to report the early results of the first human trial attempting to use rhBMP-2 in interbody fusion cages (73). Fourteen patients with single-level lumbar degenerative disc disease refractory to nonoperative therapy were entered into the prospective randomized trail. The control group received autogenous bone graft inside tapered titanium fusion cages while the investigational group received rhBMP-2 delivered in a collagen sponge inside the fusion cages. Patients were followed at regular intervals with radiographs, sagittally reformatted computerized tomography scans, and Short Form-36 and Oswestry outcome questionnaires. At 3-month followup, 91% (10 of 11) were judged to be fused. At 6 months, 1 year, and 2 years, 100% (11 of 11) of patients were noted to have solid fusion. Of the three control patients, two had solid union and one had an apparent nonunion at 1 year. After 3 months the Oswestry Disability Questionnaire scores of the rhBMP-2 group improved sooner than those of the control group with both groups demonstrating similar improvement at 6 months. This was the first clinical study to clearly demonstrate evidence of osteoinduction by a recombinant growth factor in humans.

In a prospective, randomized controlled clinical trial 450 patients with open tibial fractures were randomized to receive either the standard of care (intramedullary nail fixation and routine soft-tissue management; the control group), the standard of care and an implant containing 0.75 mg/mL of rhBMP-2 (total dose 6 mg), or the standard of care and an implant containing 1.50 mg/mL of rhBMP-2 (total dose 12 mg) (74). The rhBMP-2 implant was placed over the fracture at the time of definitive wound closure and the primary outcome was the proportion of patients requiring secondary intervention because of delayed union or nonunion within 12 months postoperatively. Compared with the control patients, those treated with 1.5 mg/mL of rhBMP-2 also had significantly fewer hardware failures, reduction in the risk of failure, fewer invasive procedures, fewer infections, and faster wound healing. This landmark study once again demonstrated the clinical efficacy of the rhBMP-2 implant for the treatment of human musculoskeletal conditions. Both rhBMP-2 and rhBMP-7 have undergone clinical trails for efficacy in the treatment of long bone fractures. Both are approved for clinical use in Europe. rhBMP-7 (OP-1) is currently available for humanitarian use in the United States (75).

Bone morphogenetic proteins may eventually be used as an alternative to autogenous bone grafts in numerous clinical scenarios including spinal deformity, degeneration, and reconstruction of osseous defects caused by trauma, neoplasia, or infection. In such situations, replacing the need for an additional operative procedure to harvest autogenous bone graft will reduce the morbidity associated with the procedure. Similarly, the availability of such potent osteoinductive factors to produce predictable osseous healing in the future may offer the ability to reduce instrumentation and perhaps lead to more predictable healing. At present the estimated cost of a single BMP application ranges from $3000 to $5000. If data from human trials continue to demonstrate objective clinical benefit from using these recombinant molecules, such expense may be clinically justified. Indeed if the cost-benefit relationship is examined, there may be a potentially significant cost advantage in index surgeries. Predictable healing engendered by these growth factors will not only reduce the need for autogenous graft and the cost associated with its harvest and complications (e.g., operative time, blood loss, etc.) but also reduce the need for revision surgery for any application.

VIII. SUMMARY

Autogenous bone graft is frequently inadequate in size and is associated with undue morbidity. An array of osteoinductive, osteoconductive, and osteoprogenitor alternatives are available. Local requirements and site-specific and host characteristics should be appreciated in chosing the appropriate adjuvant. Biodegradable biosynthetic options now challenge autogenous bone graft as the "gold standard."

Combination products containing osteoprogenitor stem cells, osteoinductive factors, and biodegradable osteoconductive matrices are in clinical use.

REFERENCES

1. Younger EM, Chapman MW. Morbidity at bone graft donor sites. J Orthop Trauma 1989; 3:192–195.
2. Strong DM, Friedlaender GE, Tomford WW, et al. Immunologic responses in human recipients of osseous and osteochondral allografts. Clin Orthop 326: 107–114, 1996.
3. Burwell RG. The function of bone marrow in the incorporation of a bone graft. Clin Orthop 1985; 200:125–141.
4. Salama R, Weissman SL. The clinical use of combined xenografts of bone an autologous red marrow: a preliminary report. J Bone Joint Surg 1978; 60B:111–115.
5. Burwell RG, Friedlaender GE, Mankin HJ. Current perspectives and future directions: the 1983 invitational conference on osteochondral allografts. Clin Orthop 1985; 197:141–157.
6. Werntz JR, Lane JM, Burstein AH, Justin R, Klein R, Tomin E. Qualitative and quantitative analysis of orthotopic bone regeneration by marrow. J Orthop Res 1996; 14(1):85–93.
7. Yamagiwa H, Endo N, Tokunaga K, Hayami T, Hatano H, Takahashi HE. In vivo bone-forming capacity of human bone marrow-derived stromal cells is

stimulated by recombinant human bone morphogenetic protein-2. J Bone Miner Metab 2001; 19(1):20–8.

8. Connolly J, Guse R, Lippiello L, et al. Development of an osteogenic bone marrow preparation. J Bone Joint Surg 71A:684–691, 1989.

9. Connolly JF, Guse R, Tiedeman J, et al. Autologous marrow injection as a substitute for grafting of tibial nonunions. Clin Orthop 266:259–270, 1991.

10. Healy JH, Zimmerman PA, McDonnell JM, Lane JM. Percutaneous bone marrow grafting of delayed union and nonunion in cancer patients. Clin Orthop 1990; 256:280–285.

11. Morrison SJ, Wandycz AM, Akashi K, et al. The aging of hematopoietic stem cells. Net Med 2:1011–1016, 1996.

12. Bruder SP, Fink DJ, Caplan AI. Mesenchymal stem cells in bone development, bone repair, and skeletal regeneration therapy. J Cell Biochem 1994; 56:283–294.

13. Takao Yamamuro. Bone bonding behavior and clinical use of A-W glass-ceramic. In: Urist MR, O'Connor BT, Burwell RG, eds. Bone Grafts, Derivatives and Substitutes. London: Butterworth-Heinemann Ltd, 1994:245–259.

14. Bucholz RW. Nonallograft osteoconductive bone graft substitutes. Clin Orthop 2002; 395:44–52.

15. Kopylov P. Norian SRS versus external fixation in redisplaced distal radial fractures: a randomized study in 40 patients. Acta Orthop Scand 1999; 70:1–5.

16. Bucholz RW. Development and clinical use of coral-derived hydroxyapatite bone graft substitutes. In: Urist MR, O'Connor BT, Burwell RG, eds. Bone Grafts, Derivatives, and Substitutes. London: Butterworth-Heinemann Ltd, 1994:260–270.

17. Boden SD, Martin GJ Jr, Morone M, Ugbo JI, Titus L, Hutton WC. The use of coralline hydroxyapatite with bone marrow, autogenous bone graft, or osteoinductive bone protein extract for posterolateral lumbar spine fusion. Spine 24(4):320–7, 1999.

18. Takao Yamamuro. Bone bonding behavior and clinical use of A-W glass-ceramic. In: Urist MR, O'Connor BT, Burwell RG, eds. Bone Grafts, Derivatives and Substitutes.. London: Butterworth-Heinemann Ltd, 1994:245–259.

19. Partio EK, Tuompo P, Hirvensalo E, Bostman O, Rokkanen P. Totally absorbable fixation in the treatment of fractures of the distal femoral epiphyses. A prospective clinical study. Arch Orthop Trauma Surg 1997; 116:213–216.

20. Glowacki J, Altobelli D, Mulliken JB. Fate of mineralized and demineralized osseous implants in cranial defects. Calcif Tissue Int 1981; 30:71.

21. Glowacki J, Kablan LB, Murray JE et al. Application of the biological principle of induced osteogenesis for craniofacial defects. Lancet 1:959 1981.

22. Glowacki J, Mulliken JB. Demineralized bone implants. Clin Plast Surg 1985; 12:233.

23. Mulliken JB, Glowacki J. Induced osteogenesis for the repair and reconstruction of the craniofacial region. Plast Reconstr Surg 1980; 65:533.

24. Tiedman JJ, Garvin KL, Kile TA, et al. The role of composite, demineralized bone marrow in the treatment of osseous defects. Orthopedics 18:1153–1158, 1995.

25. Michelson JD, Curl LA. Use of demineralized bone matrix in hindfoot arthrodesis. Clin Orthop 1996; 325:203–208.
26. Killian JT, Wilkinson L, White S, et al. Treatment of unicameral bone cyst with demineralized bone matrix. J Pediatr Orthop 18:621–624, 1998.
27. Beresford JN. Osteogenic stem cells and the stromal system of bone and marrow. Clin Orthop 1989; 240:270.
28. Berrey BH, Lord CF, Gebhardt MC, Mankin HJ. Fractures in allografts. Bone Joint Surg Am 1990; 72A:825–833.
29. Ohlendorf C, Tomford W, Mankin HJ. Chondrocyte survival in cryopreserved osteochondral articular cartilage. J Orthop Res 1996; 14:413–416.
30. Tomford W, Springfield DS, Mankin HJ. Fresh and frozen articular cartilage allografts. Orthopedics 1992; 15:1183–1188.
31. Burchardt H. The biology of bone graft repair. Clin Orthop Rel Res 1983; 174:28–42.
32. Ashton BA, Allen TD, Howlett CR, et al. Formation of bone and cartilage by marrow stromal cells in diffusion chambers in vivo. Clin Orthop Rel Res 151:294, 1980.
33. Thompson RC, Pickvance EA, Garry D. Fractures in large-segmented allografts. J Bone Joint Surg 1993; 75A:1663–1673.
34. Bugbee WD, Convery FR. Osteochondral allograft transplantation. Clin Sports Med 1999; 18:67–75.
35. Kish G, Modis L, Hangody L. Osteochondral mosaicplasty for the treatment of focal chondral and osteochondral lesions of the knee and talus in the athlete: rationale, indications, techniques, and results. Clin Sports Med 1999; 18: 45–66.
36. Canalis E, McCarthy T, Centrella M. Growth factors and the regulation of bone remodeling. J Clin Invest 1988; 81:277–281.
37. Celeste AJ, Iannazzi JA, Taylor RC, et al; Identification of transforming growth factor beta family members present in bone-inductive protein purified from bovine bone. Proc Natl Acad Sci USA 87:9843–9847, 1990.
38. Joyce ME, Jingushi S, Bolander ME. Transforming growth factor-beta in the regulation of fracture repair. Orthop Clin North Am 1990; 21:199–209.
39. Joyce ME, Jingushi S, Scully SP, Bolander ME. Role of growth factors in fracture healing. Prog Clin Biol Res 1991; 365:391–416.
40. Nakase T, Nomura S, Yoshikawa H, et al. Transient and localized expression of bone morphogenetic protein 4 messenger RNA during fracture healing. J Bone Min Res 9:651–659, 1994.
41. Simmons DJ. Fracture healing perspectives. Clin Orthop 1985; 200:100–113.
42. Triffitt JT. Initiation and enhancement of bone formation: a review [published erratum appears in Acta Orthop Scand 1988; 59(5):625]. Acta Orthop Scand 58:673–684, 1987.
43. Sandberg MM, Aro HT, Vuorio EI. Gene expression during bone repair. Clin Orthop 1993; 289:292–312.
44. Einhorn TA. Enhancement of fracture healing. Instr Course Lect 1996; 45:401–416.

45. Einhorn TA, Trippel SB. Growth factor treatment of fractures. Instr Course Lect 1997; 46:483–486.
46. Khan SN, Bostrom MP, Lane JM. Bone growth factors. Orthop Clin North Am 2000; 31(3):375–88.
47. Wozney JM, Rosen V. Bone morphogenetic protein and bone morphogenetic protein gene family in bone formation and repair. Clin Orthop 1998; 346: 26–37.
48. Wozney JM, Rosen V, Celeste AJ, et al: Novel regulators of bone formation: molecular clones and activities. Science 242:1528–1534, 1988.
49. Yasko AW, Lane JM, Fellinger EJ, et al: The healing of segmental bone defects, induced by recombinant human bone morphogenetic protein (rhBMP-2): a radiographic, histological, and biomechanical study in rats [published erratum appears in J Bone Joint Surg Am 1992; 74(7):1111]. J Bone Joint Surg Am 74:659–670, 1992.
50. Kirker-Head CA, Gerhart TN, Armstrong R, Schelling SH, Carmel LA. Healing bone using recombinant human bone morphogenetic protein 2 and co-polymer. Clin Orthop 1988; 349:205–217.
51. Heckman JD, Boyan BD, Aufdemorte TB, Abbott JT. The use of bone morphogenetic protein in the treatment of non-union a canine model. J Bone Joint Surg Am 1991; 73:750–764.
52. Cook SD, Dalton JE, Tan EH, Whitecloud TS, III, Rueger DC: In vivo evaluation of recombinant human osteogenic protein (rhOP-1) implants as a bone graft substitute for spinal fusions. Spine 19:1655–1663, 1994.
53. Bostrom M, Lane JM, Tomin E, et al: Use of bone morphogenetic protein-2 in the rabbit ulnar nonunion model. Clin Orthop 327:272–282, 1996.
54. Aspenberg P, Wang E, Thorngren KG. Bone morphogenetic protein induces bone in the squirrel monkey, but bone matrix docs not. Acta Ortho Scand 1992; 63:619–622.
55. Bostrom MP, Lane JM, Berberian WS, et al: Immunolocalization and expression of bone morphogenetic proteins 2 and 4 in fracture healing. J Orthop Res 13:357–367, 1995.
56. Wang EA, Israel DI, Kelly S, Luxenberg DP. Bone morphogenetic protein-2 causes commitment and differentiation in C3H10T1/2 and 3T3 cells. Growth Factors 1993; 9:57–71.
57. Johnson EE, Urist MR, Finerman GA. Bone morphogenetic protein augmentation grafting of resistant femoral nonunions: a preliminary report. Clin Orthop 1988a; 230:257–265.
58. Johnson EE, Urist MR, Finerman GA. Repair of segmental defects of the tibia with cancellous bone grafts augmented with human bone morphogenetic protein: a preliminary report. Clin Orthop 1988b; 236:249–257.
59. Johnson EE, Urist Mr, Finerman GA. Resistant nonunions and partial or complete segmental defects of long bones: treatment with implants of a composite of human bone morphogenetic protein (BMP) and autolyzed, antigen-extracted, allogeneic (AAA) bone. Clin Orthop 1992; 277:229–237.

60. Kirker-Head CA, Gerhart TN, Schelling SH, et al: Long-term healing of bone using recombinant human bone morphogenetic protein 2. Clin Orthop 1995; 318:222–230.

61. Cook SD, Baffes GC, Wolfe MW, Sampath TK, Rueger DC. Recombinant human bone morphogenetic protein-7 induces healing in a canine long-bone segmental defect model. Clin Orthop 1994; 301:302–312.

62. Cook SD, Baffes GC, Wolfe MW, et al: The effect of recombinant human osteogenic protein-1 on healing of large segmental bone defects. J Bone Joint Surg 1994; 76A:827–838.

63. Cook SD, Dalton JE, Tan EH, Whitecloud TS, III, Rueger DC: In vivo evaluation of recombinant human osteogenic protein (rhOP 1) implants as a bone graft substitute for spinal fusions. Spine 1994; 19:1655–1663.

64. Cook SD, Wolfe MW, Salkeld SL, Rueger DC. Effect of recombinant human osteogenic protein-1 on healing of segmental defects in non-human primates. J Bone Joint Surg 1995; 77A:734–750.

65. Boden SD, Schimandle JH, Hutton WC. 1995 Volvo Award in basic sciences. The use of an osteoinductive growth factor for lumbar spinal fusion. Part II. Study of dose, carrier, and species. Spine 1995; 20:2633–2644.

66. Boden SD, Schimandle JH, Hutton WC, Chen MI. 1995 Volvo Award in basic sciences. The use of an osteoinductive growth factor for lumbar spinal fusion. Part I: Biology of spinal fusion. Spine 1995; 20:2626–2632.

67. Sandhu HS, Kanim LE, Kabo JM, et al: Evaluation of rhBMP-2 with an OPLA carrier in a canine posterolateral (transverse process) spinal fusion and model. Spine 20:2669–2682, 995.

68. Schimandle JH, Boden SD. Spine update. The use of animal models to study spinal fusion. Spine 1994; 19:1998–2006.

69. Schimandle JH, Boden SD, Hutton WC. Experimental spinal fusion with recombinant human bone morphogenetic protein-2. Spine 1995; 20:1326–1337.

70. Muschler G, Hyodo A, Manning T, Kambic H, Easley K. Evaluation of human bone morphogenetic protein 2 in a canine spinal fusion model. Clin Orthop 1994; 308:229–240.

71. Laursen M, Hoy K, Hansen ES, Gelineck J, Christensen FB, Bunger CE. Recombinant bone morphogenetic protein-7 as an intracorporal bone growth stimulator in unstable thoracolumbar burst fractures in humans: preliminary results. Eur Spine J 1999; 8(6):485–490.

72. Patel TC, Vaccaro AR, Truumees E, Fischgrund JS, Herkowitz HN, Hillibrand A. A safety and efficacy study of OP-1 (rhBMP-7) as an adjunct to posterolateral lumbar fusion. Presented at the 15th Annual Meeting of the North American Spine Society, New Orleans, LA, 2000.

73. Boden SD, Zdeblick TA, Sandhu HS, Heim SE. The use of rhBMP-2 in interbody fusion cages. Definitive evidence of osteoinduction in humans: a preliminary report. Spine 2000; 25(3):376–381.

74. Govender S, Csimma C, Genant HK, et al. The BMP-2 evaluation in surgery for tibial trauma (BESTT) study group: Recombinant human bone

morphogenetic protein-2 for the treatment of open tibial fractures: a prospective controlled randomized study of four hundred and fift patients. J Bone Joint
Surg Am 84A:2123–2134, 2002.
75.   Friedlaender GE, Perry CR, Cole JD, Cook SD, Cierny G, Muschler GF, Zych
       GA, Calhoun JH, LaForte AJ, Yin S: Osteogenic protein-1 (bone morphoge-
       netic protein-7) in the treatment of tibial nonunions. J Bone Joint Surg Am
       2001; 83-A (suppl 1)(Pt 2):S151–158.

11

Articular Cartilage: Overview

Joseph A. Buckwalter
University of Iowa College of Medicine, Iowa City, Iowa, U.S.A.

I. INTRODUCTION

Synovial joints make possible the movements necessary for essential activities of daily living, work, and recreation. These complex structures, developed and refined by hundreds of millions of years of evolution, form by integration of multiple distinct tissues including joint capsules, ligaments, menisci, subchondral bone, synovium, and articular cartilage into structural and functional units with a wide variety of shapes and sizes. They provide painless stable movement with a level of friction far below that achieved by any prosthetic joint; and, for many people, they perform these functions flawlessly for eight decades or more. The tissue that contributes the most to these latter extraordinary functional capacities is the articular cartilage that forms the bearing surface of every synovial joint (1–3). Although it is at most only a few millimeters thick, it has surprising stiffness to compression, resilience, durability, and exceptional ability to distribute loads (2), thereby minimizing peak stresses on subchondral bone.

Gross inspection of a synovial joint shows that the opposing articular cartilage surfaces are smooth, slick, and firm; and, although they resist indentation by application of pressure from a fingertip they can easily be cut or scratched with a sharp instrument. Light microscopic examination shows

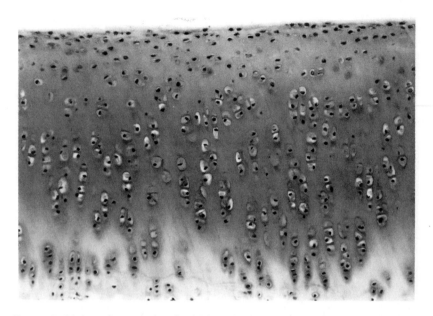

Figure 1 Light micrograph of rabbit articular cartilage showing the homogeneous extracellular matrix containing chondrocytes, but lacking nerves
and blood vessels.

that articular cartilage consists primarily of a homogeneous bland extracellular matrix, with only one type of cell, chondrocytes, scattered throughout
the matrix, and no cell-to-cell connections, blood vessels, lymphatic vessels,
or nerves (Fig. 1). Compared with tissues like muscle or bone, cartilage has
a low level of metabolic activity and appears to be less responsive to changes
in loading or injury. Yet, despite its unimpressive appearance and low level
of metabolic activity and responsiveness, detailed study of the morphology
and biology of adult articular cartilage shows that it has an elaborate highly
ordered structure and that a variety of complex interactions between the
chondrocytes and the matrix maintain the tissue (2,4). The structure, molecular composition, and organization give the tissue the exceptional biomechanical properties that make joint function possible even under the
demanding conditions imposed by strenuous physical activity.

II. STRUCTURE AND COMPOSITION

Unlike most tissues, articular cartilage does not have blood vessels, nerves,
or lymphatics. It consists of a highly organized extracellular matrix with a
sparse population of highly specialized cells (chondrocytes) distributed

throughout the tissue (2). The primary components of the matrix are water, proteoglycans, and collagens, with other proteins and glycoproteins present in lesser amounts.

The structure and composition of the articular cartilage vary throughout its depth, from the articular surface to the subchondral bone. These differences include cell shape and volume, collagen fibril diameter and orientation, proteoglycan concentration, and water content. The cartilage can be divided into four zones: the superficial zone, the middle or transitional zone, the deep zone, and the zone of calcified cartilage. Within each zone, three regions can be identified: the pericellular region, the territorial region, and the interterritorial region.

A. Zones

The superficial zone forms the gliding surface. The chondrocytes in this zone are elongated with the long axis parallel to the surface (Fig. 1). The proteoglycan content in this region is at its lowest and the water content at its highest level. The middle, or transitional, zone contains collagen fibers with a larger diameter and less apparent organization, and the chondrocytes have a more rounded appearance and appear more active. The deep zone contains the highest concentration of proteoglycans and the lowest water content; the collagen fibers have a larger diameter and are organized vertical to the joint surface. The chondrocytes are spherical, often are arranged in a columnar fashion, and appear to be metabolically less active. The deepest layer, known as the zone of calcified cartilage, separates the articular cartilage from the subchondral bone. Cells in this region are small and randomly distributed in a calcified cartilaginous matrix.

B. Regions

In addition to these articular surface-to-bone zonal distinctions, the matrix is divided into pericellular, territorial, and interterritorial regions. These regions differ in proximity to the cells, composition (collagen, proteoglycan, and other matrix components), and collagen fibril diameter and organization. The pericellular matrix is a thin layer adjacent to the cell membrane and completely surrounds the chondrocyte. The territorial matrix surrounds the pericellular matrix, and it is characterized by thin collagen fibrils that, at the boundary of the territorial matrix, appear to form a fibrillar network that is distinct from the surrounding interterritorial matrix. The interterritorial matrix is the largest of the matrix regions and contributes the majority of the biomechanical properties of the articular cartilage. It encompasses all of the matrix between the territorial matrices of the individual cells or clusters of cells and contains large collagen fibers and the majority of the proteoglycans.

C. Chondrocytes

The formation and maintenance of articular cartilage depends on the chondrocytes (2,5,6). They are derived from mesenchymal cells, which differentiate during skeletal morphogenesis and development to assume the appearance and functions of chondrocytes. During skeletal growth, these cells generate the large amount of matrix necessary to form the articular surfaces, and in mature tissue, where they occupy less than 10% of the total tissue volume, they are solely responsible for the maintenance of this matrix. They respond to a variety of stimuli including soluble mediators, such as growth factors, interleukins, and pharmaceutical agents; matrix molecules; mechanical loads; and hydrostatic pressure changes.

D. Extracellular Matrix

Because the chondrocytes of articular cartilage occupy only a small proportion of the total volume of the tissue, its composition is determined primarily by the matrix. Normal cartilage has water contents ranging from 65% to 80% of its total wet weight. The remaining wet weight of the tissue is accounted for principally by two major classes of structural macromolecules, collagens, and proteoglycans. Several other classes of molecules, including lipids, phospholipids, proteins, and glycoproteins, make up the remaining portion of the extracellular matrix.

1. Water

Water is the most abundant component of normal articular cartilage, making up from 65% to 80% of the wet weight of the tissue (7,8). A small percentage of this water is contained in the intracellular space, about 30% is associated with the intrafibrillar space within the collagen, and the remainder is contained in the molecular pore space of the matrix. Inorganic salts, such as sodium, calcium, chloride, and potassium, are dissolved in the tissue water. Water content varies throughout cartilage, decreasing in concentration from approximately 80% at the surface to 65% in the deep zone. Most of the water appears to exist as a gel and much of it may be moved through the extracellular matrix by applying a pressure gradient across the tissue, or by compressing the solid matrix. Frictional resistance against this flow through the matrix is very high, and thus the permeability of the tissue is very low. This frictional resistance to the flow of water and the pressurization of the water within the matrix are the two basic mechanisms from which articular cartilage derives its ability to support very high joint loads. The flow of water through the tissue and across the articular surface also promotes the transport of nutrients and provides a source of lubricant for the joint.

2. Collagens

Collagens are the major structural macromolecules of the matrix (9,10). There are at least 15 distinct collagen types composed of at least 29 genetically distinct polypeptide chains. All members of the collagen family contain a characteristic triple-helical structure that may constitute the majority of the length of the molecule, or may be interrupted by one or more nonhelical domains. Over 50% of the dry weight of articular cartilage consists of collagen. The major cartilage collagen, which represents 90–95% of the total, is known as type II. However, the articular cartilage matrix also contains types IV, V, VI, IX, and XI. Articular cartilage collagens provide the tissue's tensile properties and immobilize the proteoglycans within the matrix. Collagen fibers in cartilage are generally thinner than those seen in tendon or bone, and this may, in part, be a function of their interaction with the relatively large amount of proteoglycan in this tissue.

3. Proteoglycans

Proteoglycans are complex macromolecules that consist of a protein core with covalently bound glycosaminoglycans, unbranched chains of repeating disaccharide units. Articular cartilage contains three major types of glycosaminoglycans: (1) chondroitin sulfate 4- and 6-isomers, (2) keratan sulfate, and (3) dermatan sulfate. Chondroitin sulfates are the most prevalent glycosaminoglycans in cartilage. They account for 55–90% of the total population, depending principally on the age of the subject. Each chain is composed of 25–30 repeating disaccharide units, giving an average chain weight of 15–20 kd. The keratan sulfate constituent of articular cartilage, which resides primarily in the large, aggregating proteoglycan, is not as well defined as the chondroitin sulfates. Keratan sulfate chains from human articular cartilage are shorter than chondroitin sulfate chains, with an average molecular weight of 5–10 kd. Hyaluronate is also a glycosaminoglycan, but, unlike those described above, it is not sulfated and it is not bound to a protein core. In cartilage it is present as unbranched chain.

All the glycosaminoglycan chains found in cartilage have repeating carboxyl (COOH) and/or sulfate (SO_4) groups. In solution, these groups become ionized (COO^- and SO_3^-), and in the physiological environment, they attract positive counterions such as Ca^{2+} and Na^+ to maintain overall electroneutrality. These free-floating ions within the interstitial water give rise to the Donnan osmotic pressure effect. Also, because the proteoglycans are packed to within one fifth of their free-solution volume in the tissue, the fixed-charge groups are spaced 10–15 A° apart, resulting in a strong charge-to-charge repulsive force. The magnitude of this repulsive force also depends on the concentration of the counterions present in the tissue. The Donnan osmotic pressure and the charge-to-charge repulsion are critical in determining the biomechanical properties of articular cartilage.

Eighty to ninety percent of all proteoglycans in cartilage are of the large, aggregating type, called aggrecan. Aggrecan consists of a long, extended protein core with up to 100 chondroitin sulfate and 50 keratan sulfate glycosaminoglycan chains covalently bound to the protein core. In young individuals the concentration of keratan sulfate is relatively low and chondroitin 4 sulfate is the predominant form of chondroitin sulfate. With increasing age, the concentration of keratan sulfate increases and chondroin 6 sulfate becomes the predominant form of chondroitin sulfate. The aggrecan protein core is large and complex, and has several distinct globular and extended domains. One extended domain contains the majority of the keratan sulfate glycosaminoglycan chains, and is adjacent to the longest extended region, which has the chondroitin sulfate chains attached with some interspersed keratan sulfate chains. Small oligosaccharides are also attached along the protein core. At the N-terminal end of the protein core, one of the globular domains (G1) has the specific function of binding to hyaluronan. The functions of the other globular domains of aggrecan are unknown. A separate, smaller molecule called link protein binds to both the G1 domain of aggrecan and the hyaluronan, stabilizing the bond and, thus, forming the aggrecan-hyaluronate-link protein complexes referred to as a proteoglycan aggregates (Fig. 2) (11–13). Aggregation helps stabilize the aggrecan molecules within the matrix, and because each hyaluronate chain is long and unbranched, many aggrecan molecules can bind to a single hyaluronan chain to form a large proteoglycan aggregate (Fig. 2A). Aggregate size varies with age and disease state: with increasing age aggregates decrease in size. Aggregates containing more than 300 aggrecans have been identified in fetal cartilages, but most articular cartilage aggregates are a fraction of this size (13,14).

The other articular cartilage proteoglycans are much smaller than aggrecan and contain different core proteins. These include two small proteoglycans termed biglycan and decorin, both of which have a protein core of approximately 30 kd. Biglycan contains two dermatan sulfate chains, and decorin contains one (15,16). Decorin is located on the surface of collagen fibrils and is thought to be involved with the control of fibrillogenesis and fibril diameter. In addition, type IX collagen usually carries a chondroitin sulfate chain and, thus, is also a proteoglycan. Fibromodulin

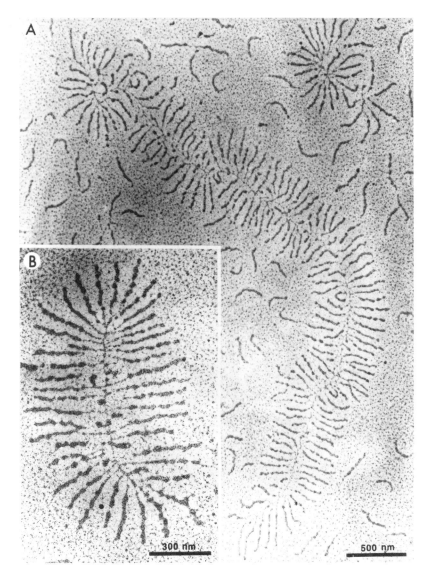

FIGURE 2   Electron micrographs of large (A) and small (B) cartilage proteoglycan aggregates. The aggregates consist of single central hyaluronic acid filament with multiple attached aggrecans projecting from the hyaluronic acid
filament.

(50–65 kd) is another small proteoglycan present in cartilage and contains keratan sulfate. Despite the relatively minor contribution of small proteoglycan molecules to the mass of proteoglycans, there are nearly as many of these small proteoglycan molecules in cartilage as there are aggrecans. Thus, the small proteoglycans are not minor components of the tissue and almost certainly play major, though not yet defined, roles in the tissue.

4. Noncollagenous Proteins and Glycoproteins

A variety of noncollagenous proteins and glycoproteins exist within articular cartilage, but thus far only a few of them have been studied (2,17). In general, they consist primarily of protein and have a few attached monosaccharides and oligosaccharides. At least some of these molecules appear to help organize and maintain the macromolecular structure of the extracellular matrix. Cartilage oligomeric protein (COMP), an acidic protein, is concentrated primarily within the chondrocyte territorial matrix. It appears to be present only within cartilage and have the capacity to bind to chondrocytes. Fibronectin and tenascin, noncollagenous matrix proteins that are found in a variety of tissues, have also been identified within cartilage. Their functions in articular cartilage remain poorly understood, but they may have roles in matrix organization, in cell-matrix interactions, and in the responses of the tissue in inflammatory arthritis and osteoarthritis (18–21).

III. METABOLISM

In adults, chondrocytes derive their nutrition from nutrients in the synovial fluid that necessarily pass through a double diffusion barrier to reach the cell: first the synovium and synovial fluid and then the cartilage matrix. This latter barrier is restrictive not only as to the size of the materials but also to their charge and other features such as molecular configuration. The nature of this system leaves chondrocytes with a low oxygen concentration relative to most other tissues, and therefore they depend primarily on anaerobic metabolism.

   To produce a tissue that can provide normal synovial joint function the chondrocytes must first synthesize appropriate types and amounts of macromolecules and then assemble and organize them into a highly ordered macromolecular framework. Maintenance of the articular surface requires turnover of the matrix macromolecules, that is, continual replacement of degraded matrix components; and probably alteration in the matrix macromolecular framework in response to joint use. To accomplish these activities, the cells must sense changes in the matrix composition due to degradation of macromolecules and in the demands placed on the articular surface, and then respond by synthesizing appropriate types and amounts of macromolecules.

Chondrocytes synthesize and assemble the cartilaginous matrix components and direct their distribution within the tissue. These synthetic and assembly processes are complex, and involve synthesis of proteins, synthesis of glycosaminoglycan chains and their addition to the appropriate protein cores, and secretion of the completed molecules into the extracellular matrix. The final incorporation of these components into the matrix also appears to depend on the chondrocyte. All of these actions take place under avascular and, for the most part, anaerobic conditions, with considerable variation in local pressure and physicochemical states. In addition, the chondrocyte directs internal matrix remodeling by means of an elaborate series of degradative enzymes.

The interdependence of chondrocytes and the matrix makes possible the maintenance of the tissue throughout life. The relationship between the chondrocytes and the matrix does not end when the cells secrete the matrix macromolecules. The matrix protects the chondrocytes from mechanical damage during normal joint use, and it helps maintain their shape and their phenotype. Nutrients, substrates for synthesis of matrix molecules, newly synthesized molecules, degraded matrix molecules, metabolic waste products, and molecules that help regulate cell function, like cytokines and growth factors, all pass through the matrix, and in some instances may be stored in the matrix. The types of molecules that can pass through the matrix and the rate at which they can pass depend on the composition and organization of the matrix—primarily the concentration, composition, and organization of the large proteoglycans.

Throughout life, chondrocytes degrade and synthesize matrix macromolecules. The mechanisms that control the balance between these activities remain poorly understood, but cytokines with catabolic and anabolic effects appear to have important roles (2). Interleukin-1 (IL-1) induces expression of matrix metalloproteases that can degrade the aggrecan and collagen as well as other matrix macromolecules and interferes with synthesis of matrix proteoglycans at the transcriptional level. Insulin-dependent growth factor I (IGF-I), fibroblast growth factor basic (FGFb), and transforming growth factor beta (TGF-β) oppose these catabolic activities by stimulating matrix synthesis and cell proliferation. In response to a variety of stimuli, chondrocytes synthesize and release these cytokines into the matrix where they may bind to receptors on the cell surfaces (stimulating cell activity by either autocrine or paracrine mechanisms) or become trapped within the matrix. The anabolic activities appear in large measure to be responses to matrix structural needs or other stimuli possibly including mechanical loading of the tissue detected by the chondrocytes. In contrast, the degradative response appears to be the result of a complex cascade that includes IL-1, stromelysin, aggrecanase, plasmin, and collagenase being activated or inhibited by factors such as prostaglandins, TGF-β, tumor necrosis factor, tissue inhibitors of metalloproteases (TIMPs 1, 2 and 3), tissue plasminogen activator, plasminogen activator inhibitor, and other molecules.

Because articular cartilage is an aneural tissue, the nerve impulses that regulate many of the body processes cannot provide information to chondrocytes. Cellular and humoral immune responses also are not likely to occur in cartilage, because both monocytes and immunoglobulins tend to be excluded from the tissue by virtue of their size. However, the cells derive considerable information from the mechanical stresses and strains that act on their membranes as a result of physical forces applied to the tissue (22–24) and the matrix acts as a mechanical signal transducer for the chondrocytes. It transmits signals that result from mechanical loading of the articular surface to the chondrocytes and the chondrocytes respond to these signals by altering the structure and density of the matrix, possibly through expression of cytokines that act through autocrine or paracrine mechanisms. How the chondrocytes sense their mechanical environment and convert the information received to changes in gene expression is unknown, although integrins, molecules that span the plasma membrane and are connected to the intracellular cytoplasm, are likely to be involved. The specific mechanisms by which joint loading influences chondrocyte function remain unknown, although various mechanical, physicochemical, and electrical transduction mechanisms have been proposed (22–24). Matrix deformation causes fluid and ion flow, which may facilitate chondrocyte nutrition and chemical transduction signals, and chondrocyte deformation, which may directly control the metabolic activity. Deformation and fluid flow will lead to changes in the local charge density within the matrix, resulting in an electric potential that may serve as an electric transduction mechanism. In vitro studies have shown that loading of the cartilage matrix can cause all of these mechanical, electric, and physicochemical events, but thus far it has not been shown clearly which signals are most important in stimulating the anabolic and catabolic activity of the chondrocytes.

Experimental studies show that joint loading and motion are required to maintain normal adult articular cartilage composition, structure, and mechanical properties (2,25). The type, intensity, and frequency of loadings necessary to maintain normal articular cartilage vary over a broad range. When the intensity or frequency of loading exceeds or falls below these necessary levels, the balance between synthesis and degradation processes will be altered, and changes in the composition and microstructure of cartilage follow. Prolonged reduced joint motion and loading due to rigid immobilization leads to degeneration of the cartilage. These changes result, in part, because normal nutritive transport to cartilage from the synovial fluid by means of diffusion and convection has been diminished. In addition to the alterations in articular cartilage composition, immobilization compromises the mechanical properties of articular cartilage. These biochemical and biomechanical changes are, at least in part, reversible on remobilization of the joint, although the extent of this recovery decreases with increasing periods of joint immobilization and increasing rigidity of the immobilization.

Excessive joint loading, through either excessive use, increased magnitudes of loading, or impact, also may affect articular cartilage. Catabolic effects can be induced by a single-impact or repetitive trauma, and may serve as the initiating factor for progressive degenerative changes. However, regular joint use, including running, has not been shown to cause joint damage in normal joints (26).

IV. BIOMECHANICAL FUNCTION

The articular cartilage of synovial joints is subject to high loads applied statically, cyclically, and repetitively for many decades. Thus, the structural molecules, that is, collagens, proteoglycans, and other molecules, must be organized into a strong, fatigue-resistant, and tough, solid matrix capable of sustaining the high stresses and strains. The solid matrix is porous and permeable, and very soft (27,28). Water resides in the microscopic pores, and application of loads to the tissue makes the water flow through the porous-permeable solid matrix. Thus, articular cartilage is a biphasic material, composed of a solid phase (the matrix macromolecular framework consisting primarily of collagens and proteoglycans) and a fluid phase (matrix water) (27,28). Water flows through the cartilage when a pressure gradient is imposed. However, very high pressures are required to move the water through cartilage. As a result, fluid pressure provides a significant component of total load support, thus minimizing the stress acting on the solid matrix.

The structure and composition of the articular cartilage matrix give it viscoelastic properties; that is, it exhibits time-dependent behavior when subjected to a constant load or constant deformation. When a constant compressive stress is applied to the tissue, its deformation increases with time; and it will deform or creep until an equilibrium value is reached. Similarly, when the tissue is deformed and held at a constant strain, the stress will rise to a peak, followed by a slow stress-relaxation process until an

equilibrium value is reached. Interstitial fluid pressure is generated in cartilage during loading (compression), and it combines with matrix compression in supporting the applied load. However, under constant load, as creep
continues, the load support is gradually transferred from the fluid phase
(as the fluid pressure dissipates) to the solid phase.

V. DEVELOPMENT AND AGING

The articular cartilage of skeletally immature individuals differs from that
found in skeletally mature individuals. On gross inspection, the cartilage
from skeletally immature individuals appears blue-white in color, presumably because of the reflection of the vascular structures in the underlying
immature bone, and is relatively thick. Microscopic examination shows
that the cell density of immature articular cartilage is considerably greater
than that of mature tissue. The structural organization of the immature tissue also differs from that of adult cartilage in that the zonal characteristics
show major variation, particularly in the lower zones. The gliding or tan-
gential layer is evident in immature articular cartilage, although the surface
cells are somewhat larger and less discoid than those seen in adult cartilage.
The midzone is wider and contains a larger number of randomly arranged
cells. In the lower zones, however, the orientation differs markedly; at
about the halfway mark in the distance from the surface to the underlying
bone, the chondrocytes are arranged in irregular columns and, at further
depth, the columniation becomes more evident. With increasing age,
mature cartilage undergoes changes in matrix organization and composition, mechanical properties and cell function that increase the risk of degeneration of the tissue (29–31). Collagen cross-linking increases as the size of
the proteoglycan aggrecans and aggregates decreases. The tensile strength
of the superficial cartilage layer decreases and, perhaps most important,
the ability of the chondrocytes to maintain and restore the tissue declines
(32,33).

VI. MECHANISMS OF ARTICULAR CARTILAGE INJURY

Understanding of the mechanisms of articular surface injuries requires
appreciation of how loads and rate of loading affect articular cartilage.
Slowly applied loads and suddenly applied loads differ considerably in their
effects. Loading of articular surfaces causes movement of fluid within the
articular cartilage matrix that dampens and distributes loads within the cartilage and to the subchondral bone. When this occurs slowly, the fluid movement allows the cartilage to deform and decreases the force applied to the
matrix macromolecular framework. When it occurs too rapidly for fluid

movement through the matrix and deformation of the tissue, as with sudden impact or torsional joint loading of the joint surface, the matrix macromolecular framework sustains a greater share of the force. If this force is great enough, it ruptures the matrix macromolecular framework, damages cells, and exceeds the ability of articular cartilage to prevent subchondral bone damage by dampening and distributing loads.

Acute or repetitive blunt joint trauma can damage articular cartilage and the calcified cartilage zone–subchondral bone region while leaving the articular surface intact (34). The intensity and type of joint loading that can cause chondral and subchondral damage without visible tissue disruption has not been well defined. Physiological levels of joint loading do not appear to cause joint injury, but impact loading above that associated with normal activities, but less than that necessary to produce cartilage disruption, can cause alterations of the cartilage matrix and damage chondrocytes. Loss of proteoglycans or alteration of their organization (in particular, a decrease in proteoglycan aggregation) occurs before other signs of cartilage injury following impact loading. The loss of proteoglycans may be due to either increased degradation of the molecules or decreased synthesis. Significant loss of matrix proteoglycans decreases cartilage stiffness and increases its permeability. These alterations may cause greater loading of the remaining macromolecular framework, including the collagen fibrils, increasing the vulnerability of the tissue to further damage from loading. These injuries may cause other matrix abnormalities besides loss of proteoglycans, such as distortions of the collagen fibril meshwork or disruptions of the collagen fibril proteoglycan relationships and swelling of the matrix, and they may injure chondrocytes.

Disrupting a normal articular surface with a single impact requires substantial force, presumably because of the ability of articular cartilage and subchondral bone to dampen and distribute loads. A transarticular load of 2170 newtons applied to canine patellofemoral joints caused fractures in the zone of calcified cartilage visible by light microscopy and articular cartilage fissures that extended from the articular surface to the transitional or superficial radial zone of the articular cartilage (35). A study of the response of human articular cartilage to blunt trauma showed that articular cartilage could withstand impact loads of up to 25 newtons/mm^2 (25 MPa) without apparent damage. Impact loads exceeding this level caused chondrocyte death and cartilage fissures (36). The authors suggested that reaching a stress level that could cause cartilage damage required a force greater than that necessary to fracture the femur. Another study (37) measured the pressure on human patellofemoral articular cartilage during impact loading and found that impact loads less than the level necessary to fracture bone caused stresses greater than 25 MPa in some regions of the articular surface. With the knee flexed 90 degrees, 50% of the load necessary to cause a bone fracture produced joint pressures greater than 25 MPa for nearly 20% of the patellofemoral joint. At 70% of the bone fracture load, nearly 35% of the contact area of the patellofemoral joint pressures exceeded 25 MPa and at 100% of the bone fracture load, 60% of the patellofemoral joint pressures exceeded 25 MPa. These latter results show that impact loads can disrupt cartilage without fracturing bone.

Repetitive impact loads can split articular cartilage matrix and initiate progressive cartilage degeneration (38–40). Cyclical loading of human cartilage samples in vitro caused surface fibrillation (39), and periodic impact loading of bovine metacarpal phalangeal joints in vitro combined with joint motion caused degeneration of articular cartilage (41). Repeated overuse of rabbit joints in vivo combined with peak overloading caused articular cartilage damage including formation of chondrocyte clusters, fibrillation of the matrix, thickening of subchondral bone, and penetration of subchondral capillaries into the calcified zone of articular cartilage (38). The extent of cartilage damage appeared to increase with longer periods of repetitive overloading, and deterioration of the cartilage continued following cessation of excessive loading. This latter finding suggests that some cartilage damage is not immediately visible.

An investigation of cartilage plugs also showed that repetitive loading disrupted the tissue and that the severity of the damage increased with increasing load and increasing number of loading cycles (42). Two hundred and fifty cycles of a 1000 lb/in². compression load caused surface abrasions. Five hundred cycles produced primary fissures penetrating to calcified cartilage, and 1000 cycles produced secondary fissures extending from the primary fissures. After 8000 cycles the fissures coalesced and undermined cartilage fragments. Higher loads caused similar changes with fewer cycles. The experiments suggested that repetitive loading can propogate vertical cartilage fissures from the joint surface to calcified cartilage and extension of oblique fissures into areas of intact cartilage, extending the damage and creating cartilage flaps and free fragments.

Clinical experience suggests that chondral fractures and osteochondral fractures result from similar impact and twisting joint injuries, but they tend to occur in different age groups, and some individuals may have a greater risk of chondral fractures. Chondral fractures generally occur in skeletally mature people, while osteochondral fractures typically occur in skeletally immature people or young adults. This difference may result from age-related changes in the mechanical properties of the articular surface including the uncalcified cartilage, the calcified cartilage zone, and the subchondral bone. That is, age-related alterations in the articular cartilage matrix decrease the tensile stiffness and strength of the superficial zone;

and the calcified cartilage zone subchondral bone region mineralizes fully following completion of skeletal growth presumably creating a marked difference in mechanical properties between the uncalcified cartilage and the calcified cartilage subchondral bone region. Taken together these changes probably increase the risk of ruptures of the superficial cartilage matrix and of these ruptures extending to the calcified cartilage subchondral bone region. Genetically determined abnormalities of the articular cartilage may also increase the risk of chondral ruptures from a given impact or torsional load, but the relationships between known genetic abnormalities of articular cartilage and cartilage properties have not been well defined.

VII. RESPONSE OF ARTICULAR CARTILAGE TO INJURY

Articular surface injuries can be classified based on the type of tissue damage and the repair response: (1) cartilage matrix and cell injuries, that is, damage to the joint surface that does not cause visible mechanical disruption of the articular surface, (2) chondral fissures, flap tears, or chondral defects, that is, visible mechanical disruption of articular cartilage limited to articular cartilage, and (3) osteochondral injuries, that is, visible mechanical disruption of articular cartilage and bone (4,34,43,44).

A. Matrix and Cell Injuries

Acute or repetitive blunt trauma including excessive impact loading can cause alterations in articular cartilage matrix including a decrease in proteoglycan concentration and possibly disruptions of the collagen fibril framework. The ability of chondrocytes to sense changes in matrix composition and synthesize new molecules makes it possible for them to repair damage to the macromolecular framework (2,45). It is not clear at what point this type of injury becomes irreversible and leads to progressive loss of articular cartilage. Presumably, the chondrocytes can restore the matrix as long as the loss of matrix proteoglycan does not exceed what the cells can rapidly produce, if the fibrillar collagen meshwork remains intact, and if enough chondrocytes remain viable. When these conditions are not met, the cells cannot restore the matrix, the chondrocytes will be exposed to excessive loads, and the tissue will degenerate.

B. Chondral Injuries

Acute or repetitive trauma can cause focal mechanical disruption of articular cartilage including fissures, chondral flaps or tears, and loss of a segment of articular cartilage . The lack of blood vessels and lack of cells that can repair significant tissue defects limit the response of cartilage to injury. Chondrocytes respond to tissue injury by proliferating and increasing the synthesis of matrix macromolecules near the injury, but the newly synthesized matrix and proliferating cells do not fill the tissue defect, and soon after injury the increased proliferative and synthetic activity ceases.

C. Osteochondral Injuries

Unlike injuries limited to cartilage, injuries that extend into subchondral bone cause hemorrhage and fibrin clot formation and activate the inflammatory response. Soon after injury, blood escaping from the damaged bone blood vessels forms a hematoma that temporarily fills the injury site. Fibrin forms within the hematoma and platelets bind to fibrillar collagen. A continuous fibrin clot fills the bone defect and extends for a variable distance into the cartilage defect. Platelets within the clot release vasoactive mediators and growth factors or cytokines (small proteins that influence multiple cell functions including migration, proliferation, differentiation, and matrix synthesis) including TGF-β and platelet-derived growth factor. Bone matrix also contains growth factors including TGF-β, bone morphogenic protein, platelet-derived growth factor, insulin-like growth factor I, insulin-like growth factor II, and possibly others. Release of these growth factors may have an important role in the repair of osteochondral defects. In particular, they probably stimulate vascular invasion and migration of undifferentiated cells into the clot and influence the proliferative and synthetic activities of the cells. Shortly after entering the tissue defect, the undifferentiated mesenchymal cells proliferate and synthesize a new matrix. Within 2 weeks of injury, some mesenchymal cells assume the rounded form of chondrocytes and begin to synthesize a matrix that contains type II collagen and a relatively high concentration of proteoglycans. These cells produce regions of hyaline-like cartilage in the chondral and bone portions of the defect. Six to eight weeks following injury the repair tissue within the chondral region of osteochondral defects contains many chondrocyte-like cells in a matrix consisting of type II collagen, proteoglycans, some type I collagen, and noncollagenous proteins. Unlike the cells in the chondral portion of the defect, the cells in the bony portion of the defect produce immature bone, fibrous tissue, and hyaline-like cartilage.

The chondral repair tissue typically has a composition and structure intermediate between hyaline cartilage and fibrocartilage; and it rarely, if ever, replicates the elaborate structure of normal articular cartilage. Occasionally, the cartilage repair tissue persists unchanged or progressively remodels to form a functional joint surface, but in most large osteochondral injuries the chondral repair tissue begins to show evidence of depletion of matrix proteoglycans, fragmentation and fibrillation, increasing collagen content, and loss of cells with the appearance of chondrocytes within a year or less. The remaining cells often assume the appearance of fibroblasts as the surrounding matrix comes to consist primarily of densely packed collagen fibrils. This fibrous tissue usually fragments and often disintegrates leaving areas of exposed bone. The inferior mechanical properties of chondral repair tissue may be responsible for its frequent deterioration. Even repair tissue that successfully fills osteochondral defects is less stiff and more permeable than normal articular cartilage, and the orientation and organization of the collagen fibrils in even the most hyaline-like cartilage repair tissue does not follow the pattern seen in normal articular cartilage. In addition, the repair tissue cells may fail to establish the normal relationships between matrix macromolecules, in particular, the relationship between cartilage proteoglycans and the collagen fibril network. The decreased stiffness and increased permeability of repair cartilage matrix may increase loading of the macromolecular framework during joint use resulting in progressive structural damage to the matrix collagen and proteoglycans, thereby exposing the repair chondrocytes to excessive loads, further compromising their ability to restore the matrix.

   Clinical experience and experimental studies suggest that the success of chondral repair in osteochondral injuries may depend to some extent on the severity of the injury as measured by the volume of tissue or surface area of cartilage injured and the age of the individual. Smaller osteochondral defects that do not alter joint function heal more predictably than larger defects that may change the loading of the articular surface. Potential age-related differences in healing of chondral and osteochondral injuries have not been thoroughly investigated, but bone heals more rapidly in children than in adults and the articular cartilage chondrocytes in skeletally immature animals show a better proliferative response to injury and synthesize larger proteoglycan molecules than those from mature animals. Furthermore, a growing synovial joint has the potential to remodel the articular surface to decrease the mechanical abnormalities created by a chondral or osteochondral defect.

VIII. SUMMARY

Articular cartilage consists of isolated cells, chondrocytes, embedded in an abundant extracellular matrix consisting of a macromolecular framework filled with water. Chondrocytes form the matrix macromolecular framework from three classes of molecules: collagens, proteoglycans, and noncollagenous proteins. The structural molecules, primarily the collagens and proteoglycans, form a strong, fatigue-resistant, solid matrix capable of sustaining the high stresses and strains developed within the tissue during joint use. This matrix is porous, permeable, soft, and has a water concentration that varies from 65% to 80% or more of the wet weight of the tissue. Compression of cartilage causes the water to flow through the porous-permeable solid matrix and the interaction of the fluid and solid phases of the matrix gives the tissue its biomechanical properties. Throughout life the tissue undergoes continual internal remodeling as the cells replace matrix macromolecules lost through degradation. Loading of the tissue due to joint use creates mechanical, electrical, and physicochemical signals that help direct chondrocyte synthetic and degradative activity. Because it lacks a blood supply and cells capable of producing substantial volumes of new tissue, articular cartilage from skeletally mature individuals has limited capacity for repair following injury or degeneration. For this reason, development of tissue engineering approaches that will make possible replacement of damaged articular surfaces is critical.

REFERENCES

1. Buckwalter JA, Rosenberg LA, Hunziker EB. Articular cartilage: composition, structure, response to injury, and methods of facilitation repair. In: Ewing JW, eds. Articular Cartilage and Knee Joint Function: Basic Science and Arthroscopy. New York: Raven Press, 1990:19–56.
2. Buckwalter JA, Mankin HJ. Articular cartilage I. Tissue design and chondrocyte-matrix interactions. J Bone Joint Surg 1997; 79A(4):600–611.
3. Buckwalter JA, Hunziker EB, Rosenberg LC, Coutts RD, Adams ME, Eyre DR. Articular cartilage: composition and structure. In: Woo SL, Buckwalter JA, eds. Injury and Repair of the Musculoskeletal Soft Tissues. Park Ridge, IL: American Academy of Orthopaedic Surgeons, 1988:405–425.
4. Buckwalter JA, Mow VC, Hunziker EB. Concepts of cartilage repair in osteoarthritis. In: Moskowitz R. et al., eds. Osteoarthritis: Diagnosis and Medical/Surgical Management. Philadelphia: Saunders, 2001: 101–114.
5. Aydelotte MB, Schumacher BL, Kuettner KE. Heterogeneity of articular chondrocytes. In: Kuettner KE. et al., eds. Articular Cartilage and Osteoarthritis. New York: Raven Press, 1992: 237–249.
6. Stockwell RA. Chondrocytes. J Clin Pathol 1978; (suppl):7–13.
7. Mankin HJ. The water of articular cartilage. Simon WHThe Human Joint in Health and Disease. Philadelphia: University of Pennsylvannia Press, 1978:37–42.
8. Mankin HJ, Thrasher AZ. Water content and binding in normal and osteoarthritic human cartilage. J Bone Joint Surg 1975; 57A:76–80.
9. Eyre DR. Collagen structure and function in articular cartilage: metabolic changes in the development of osteoarthritis. In: Kuettner KE, Goldberg VM, eds. Osteoarthritic Disorders. Rosemont, IL: American Academy of Orthopaedic Surgeons1995:219–227.

10. Eyre DR, Wu JJ, and Woods P. Cartilage-specific collagens: structural studies. In: Kuettner KE, et al., eds. Articular Cartilage and Osteoarthritis. New York: Raven Press. 1992:119–131.

11. Buckwalter JA, Rosenberg LC, Tang LH. The effect of link protein on proteoglycan aggregate structure. J Biol Chem 1984; 259(9):5361–5363.

12. Buckwalter JA, Choi H, Tang L, Rosenberg L, Ungar R. The effect of link protein concentration of proteoglycan aggregation. Trans 32nd Meeting Orthop Res Soc 1986; 11:98.

13. Buckwalter JA, Roughley PJ, Rosenberg LC. Age-related changes in cartilage proteoglycans: quantitative electron microscopic studies. Microsc Res Tech 1994; 28:398–408.

14. Buckwalter JA, Rosenberg LC. Electron microscopic studies of cartilage proteoglycans. Elec Microsc Rev 1988; 1:87–112.

15. Rosenberg LC, Structure and function of dermatan sulfate proteoglycans in articular cartilage. In: Kuettner KE, et al., eds. Articular Cartilage and Osteoarthritis. New York: Raven Press, 1992:45–63.

16. Poole AR, Rosenberg LC, Reiner A, Ionescu M, Bogoch E, Roughley PJ. Contents and distribution of the proteoglycans decorin and biglycan in normal and osteoarthritic human articular cartilage. J Orthop Res, 1996; 14:681–689.

17. Heinegard DK, Pimentel ER. Cartilage matrix proteins. In: Kuettner KE, et al., eds. Articular Cartilage and Osteoarthritis. New York: Raven Press. 1992:95–111.

18. Martin JA, Buckwalter JA. Effects of fibronectin on articular cartilage chondrocyte proteoglycan synthesis and response to IGF-I. J Orthop Res 1998; 16:752–757.

19. Chevalier X. Fibronectin, cartilage, and osteoarthritis. Semin Arthritis Rheum 1993; 22:307–318.

20. Gluhak J, Mais A, Mina M. Tenascin-C is associated with early stages of chondrogenesis by chick mandibular ectomesenchymal cells in vivo and in vitro. Dev Dynami 1996; 205(1):24–40.

21. Chevalier X, Groult N, Larget-Piet B, Zardi L, Hornebeck W. Tenascin distribution in articular cartilage from normal subjects and from patients with osteoarthritis and rheumatoid arthritis. Arthritis Rheum 1994; 37:1013–1022.

22. Buschmann MD, Gluzband YA, Grodzinsky AJ, Hunziker EB. Mechanical compression modulates matrix biosynthesis in chondrocyte/agarose culture. J Cell Sci 1995; 108:1497–1508.

23. Gray ML, Pizzanelli AM, Grodzinski AJ, Lee RC. Mechanical and physico-chemical determinants of chondrocyte biosynthesis response. J Orthop Res 1988; 6:788–792.

24. Kim YJ, Sah RL, Grodzinsky AJ, Plaas AH, Sandy JD. Mechanical regulation of cartilage biosynthetic behavior: physical stimuli. Arch Biochem Biophys 1994; 311(1):1–12.

25. Buckwalter JA. Activity vs. rest in the treatment of bone, soft tissue and joint injuries. Iowa Orthop J 1995; 15:29–42.

26. Buckwalter JA, Lane NE. Athletics and osteoarthritis. Am J Sports Med 1997; 25:873–881.

27. Mow VC, Rosenwasser MP. Articular cartilage: Biomechanics. In: Woo SL, Buckwalter JA, eds. Injury and Repair of the Musculoskeletal Soft Tissues. Park Ridge, IL: American Academy of Orthopaedic Surgeons, 1998:427–463.

28. Setton LA, Zhu W, Mow VC. The biphasic poroviscoelastic behavior of articular cartilage: role of the surface zone in governing the compressive behavior. J Biomech 1993; 26:581–592.

29. Buckwalter JA, Woo SL-Y, Goldberg VM, Hadley EC, Booth F, Oegema TR, Eyre DR. Soft tissue aging and musculoskeletal function. J Bone Joint Surg 1993; 75A:1533–1548.

30. Bullough PG, Brauer FU. Age-related changes in articular cartilage. In: Buckwalter JA, Goldberg VM, Woo SL-Y, eds. Soft Tissue Aging: Impact on Musculoskeletal Function and Mobility. Rosemont, IL: American Academy of Orthopaedic Surgeons, 1993:117–135.

31. Roughley PJ. Articular cartilage: matrix changes with aging. In: Buckwalter JA, Goldberg VM, Woo SL-Y, eds. Soft Tissue Aging: Impact on Musculoskeletal Function and Mobility. Rosemont, IL: American Academy of Orthopaedic Surgeons, 1993:151–164.

32. Martin JA, Ellerbroek SM, Buckwalter JA. The age-related decline in chondrocyte response to insulin-like growth factor-I: the role of growth factor binding proteins. J Ortho Res 1997; 15:491–498.

33. Martin JA, Buckwalter JA. Telomere erosion and senescence in human articular cartilage chondrocytes. J Gerontol Biol Sci 2001; 56A:B172–B179.

34. Buckwalter JA. Mechanical injuries of articular cartilage. In: Finerman G, ed. Biology and Biomechanics of the Traumatized Synovial Joint. Park Ridge, IL: American Academy of Orthopaedic Surgeons, 1992:83–96.

35. Thompson RC, Oegema TR, Lewis JL, Wallace L. Osteoarthritic changes after acute transarticular load: an animal model. J Bone Joint Surg 1991; 73A:990–1001.

36. Repo RU, Finlay JB. Survival of articular cartilage after controlled impact. J Bone Joint Surg 1977; 59A:1068–1075.

37. Haut RC. Contact pressures in the patellofemoral joint during impact loading on the human flexed knee. J Orthop Res 1989; 7:272–280.

38. Dekel S, Weissman SL. Joint changes after overuse and peak overloading of rabbit knees in vivo. Acta Orthop Scand 1978; 49:519–528.

39. Weightman B. Tensile fatigue of human articular cartilage. J Biomech 1976; 9:193–200.

40. Weightman BO, Freeman MAR, Swanson SAV. Fatigue of articular cartilage. Nature 1973; 244:303–304.

41. Radin EL, Paul IL. Response of joints to impact loading: in vitro wear. Arthritis Rheum 1971; 14:356–362.

42. Zimmerman NB, Smith DG, Pottenger LA, Cooperman DR. Mechanical disruption of human patellar cartilage by repetitive loading in vitro. Clin Orthop Rel Res 1988; 229:302–307.

43. Buckwalter JA, Rosenberg LC, Coutts R, Hunziker E, Reddi AH, Mow VC. Articular cartilage: injury and repair. In: Woo SL, Buckwalter JA, eds. Injury and Repair of the Musculoskeletal Soft Tissues, 1998:465–482.
44. Buckwalter JA, Mow VC, Ratliff A. Restoration of injured or degenerated articular surfaces. J Am Acad Orthop Surg 1994; 2:192–201.
45. Buckwalter JA, Mankin HJ. Articular cartilage. II. Degeneration and osteoarthrosis, repair, regeneration and transplantation. J Bone Joint Surg 1997; 79A(4):612–632.

12

Cartilage: Current Applications

B. Kinner and M. Spector
Brigham and Women's Hospital, Harvard Medical School, and
VA Boston Healthcare System, Boston, Massachusetts, U.S.A.

I. INTRODUCTION

The term "tissue engineering" has now come to encompass a wide range of treatments involving synthetic and natural materials, cells, tissues, cytokines, and genes. Cell therapies and tissue transplant procedures are thus now often considered under the rubric of tissue engineering. In this respect tissue engineering is not so much a revolution in reconstructive surgery but part of the evolutionary process that this discipline has continuously undergone since its inception over 100 years ago. These myriad aspects of tissue engineering make a complete review of the field, even if focused on only one tissue such as articular cartilage, challenging to prepare.

In recent years several surgical procedures, some involving the transplantation of tissue, have been introduced into the clinic for the treatment of cartilage defects. One procedure involves the implantation of autologous articular chondrocytes that have been isolated from a biopsy and expanded in number in culture. Of the procedures recently implemented in the clinic (and approved for selected clinical applications by the U.S. Food and Drug

Administration), this treatment comes closest to a tissue engineering approach. That is, a procedure that uses exogenous cells for de novo formation of tissue. This chapter addresses this cell-based therapeutic approach and briefly discusses alternative surgical procedures that are also currently being used in the clinic to provide a framework for comparison.

Many investigations are underway to evaluate a host of cell-seeded scaffolds fabricated from synthetic and natural materials. None of these constructs, however, has yet been introduced into the clinic. Several reviews have been published that deal with these approaches (1). In this chapter selected examples of cell-seeded constructs undergoing investigation are discussed.

It is important to point out that no "tissue engineering" procedure, or any other treatment, has yet been successful in truly regenerating articular cartilage. This is concerning as it has been known for many years that the long-term function of articular cartilage is exquisitely related to its composition and architecture, and to the associated mechanical properties, as discussed in the previous chapter. A promising observation, however, has been that under certain circumstances—sometimes those occurring in an untreated cartilage defect—regeneration of articular cartilage can take place, albeit it only in a region of the lesion (Fig. 1). This indicates that articular cartilage regeneration is a possibility. The challenge, then, is to identify the elements of the regeneration process that need to be supplied to a particular defect: cells, matrix, cytokines individually, or some combination.

It is also important to recognise that despite the absence of articular cartilage regeneration, many patients report a dramatic relief of pain as a result of certain treatments. This has raised fundamental questions about the criteria for success that should be adopted in the evaluation of new procedures. For example, a clinically meaningful outcome might be one that provides pain relief for 5 years, and this may be achieved through the formation of a tissue that falls short of replicating the composition and structure of articular cartilage. Thus, is it more appropriate to use histological or clinical criteria for success of a new tissue engineering procedure? The problem with using the clinical endpoint is that patients may report a relief of symptoms for a few years only to experience subsequently a precipitous decline in their condition. There is no reason to expect that there would be a gradual decline in patient function that would signal potential problems and thus allow for adjustments to be made in the procedure or for it to be abandoned before it is applied to large numbers of patients. Fundamental questions thus remain as to how to gauge the success of a new cartilage repair procedure.

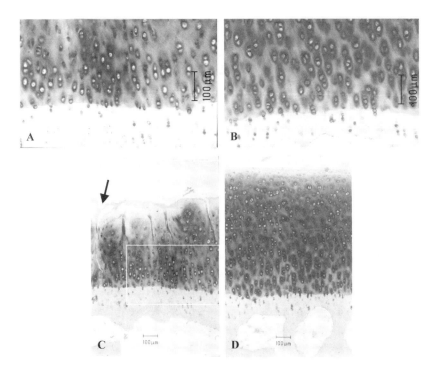

Figure 1 (A) Histological micrograph of an untreated chondral defect, 6 months postoperative. The region shown is that outlined in (C). Hematoxylin and eosin stain. (B) Histological micrograph showing normal canine articular cartilage. Hematoxylin and eosin stain. (C) Micrograph of an untreated chondral defect, 6 months postoperative. The arrow shows the interface between the reparative tissue on the right and the adjacent articular cartilage on the left. The white box shows the area presented at higher magnification in (A). Hematoxylin and eosin stain. (D) Histology of normal canine articular cartilage. Hematoxylin and eosin stain.

A. Limitations to Healing of Articular Cartilage

"Cartilage once destroyed never heals" (2,3). This 200-year-old observation stands as a challenge to tissue engineering approaches to the biological repair of injured and diseased articular cartilage. As with other tissues, cartilage depends on fibrin clot formation and the subsequent migration of progenitor cells into the repair site. The chondroprogenitor cells are derived from adjacent cartilage, underlying marrow, or synovium. Owing to the rather unique anatomical and physiological characteristics of cartilage, as discussed in the previous chapter, e.g., avascularity, low mitotic activity of chondrocytes, and the chondrocytic release of degrading enzymes, this reparative process will not be initiated if the defect does not penetrate the subchondral bone. This, then, is the basis of Hunter's observation that cartilage defects do not heal.

Even if a defect in the articular surface of a joint extends into the subchondral bone, patients are more likely to develop fibrocartilage of questionable functional value instead of hyaline cartilage (4). Thus while healing ensues, the result is "repair" with a scar-like tissue instead of "regeneration" of articular cartilage. One solution to this problem in the past has been osteotomy to unload the affected area and then prosthetic replacement of the joint, if the damage ultimately led to complete joint destruction. Although total joint replacement has been successful in the elderly patient, there is still a high enough incidence of failure due to mechanical and biological problems in the active individual that joint arthroplasty is not a satisfying solution for the younger patient. The potential risks of surgery and the higher likelihood of prosthetic loosening have led to a more conservative attitude toward joint replacement in younger individuals.

B.   Tissue Engineering and Regenerative Medicine

The term "tissue engineering" was initially introduced to describe the technology for producing tissue in vitro (5). More recently the term "regenerative medicine" has been used to describe the development of technology and surgical procedures for the regeneration of tissue in vivo. There are advantages and disadvantages to both strategies. One advantage of the synthesis of tissue in vitro is the ready ability to examine the tissue as it forms, and to make nondestructive measurements to establish its characteristics prior to implantation. However, a disadvantage, particularly in the production of musculoskeletal tissue that must play a load-bearing role, is the absence of a physiological mechanical environment during the formation of the tissue in vitro. It is now well established that mechanical force serves as a critical regulator of cell function, and can profoundly influence the architecture of tissue as it is forming. Because the mechanical environment extant during the formation of most musculoskeletal tissues in vivo is not well understood, it is not yet possible to recreate such an environment in vitro during the engineering of most tissues. Another disadvantage of the formation of musculoskeletal tissue outside of the body is the necessary integration into the host tissue after implantation. This integration requires the engineered tissue to be mechanically coupled to the surrounding structures. Union of the implanted tissue with the host organ requires degradation and new tissue formation at the interfaces of the implant with the host tissues. That remodeling of the implanted tissue is essential for its functional incorporation.

The current strategy most often used for the treatment of cartilage defects is to facilitate tissue formation in vivo, under the influence of the physiological mechanical environment. However, one disadvantage of this approach is that the regenerating tissue may be dislodged or degraded by the mechanical forces normally acting at the site before it is fully formed and incorporated. This underscores the importance of postoperative rehabilitation protocols.

C. Alternative Cartilage Repair Procedures

Myriad surgical procedures have been implemented for the treatment of defects in the articulating surfaces of joints. These methods are directed toward accessing the subchondral vascularity and marrow by either abrasion of the calcified cartilage and subchondral bone plate using powered burrs (6–8), drilling of the subchondral bone (9), spongialization (10), or microfracturing (11,12). These procedures are usually combined with debridement of loose cartilage particles and lavage of the joint. The fibrocartilage-like reparative tissue that results from these techniques lacks the composition, structure, and mechanical properties of normal cartilage and the long-term clinical outcomes are unpredictable (13). Patients treated with these techniques often experience short-term pain relief but develop progressive symptoms when the reparative tissue breaks down (8).

Other surgical procedures have been developed to deliver autologous chondrogenic cells to the cartilage defect in the form of precursor cells derived from the periosteum (14) or the perichondrium (15), with the expectation that the cells will eventually undergo terminal differentiation to chondrocytes. While these procedures have been used in selected clinics for many years, there is not yet widespread implementation. In the case of the grafting of periosteum, there have not yet been sufficient studies demonstrating reproducibility of the procedure and in the case of perichondrium there appears to be a disturbing incidence of ossification of the implanted defect site.

Recently an alternative surgical approach has been to transplant autologous osteochondral plugs from a minimally loaded region of the joint to the site of the lesion (16). While the short-term results have not revealed donor site morbidity, this issue demands further follow-up, particularly before the procedure is employed in patients with an otherwise healthy joint.

II. CELL THERAPIES

Of the tissue engineering triad—exogenous cells, matrix, and soluble regulators—it has been the cells that have first made it to the clinic. The principal cell of interest for such therapies has understandably been the chondrocyte derived from articular cartilage. The technology that has enabled such endeavors has been cell culture methodology that facilitates expansion of the number of cells in vitro under conditions that allow the cells to retain, or at least to recover, their phenotypic traits. However, questions about the long-term function of tissue formed by these cells, difficulties in harvesting donor tissue, concern about donor site morbidity and the slow growth of the cells in culture have directed attention to other cell types that might be used instead of articular chondrocytes.

A comprehensive understanding of the results of cell-based therapies for cartilage repair is important because lessons can be learned that apply to tissue engineering strategies employing cell-seeded matrices.

A. Autologous Chondrocyte Implantation (ACI)

The rationale for using articular chondrocytes for a cell-based therapy is that they already possess the desired phenotype (1). Chondrocytes comprise the single cellular component of adult hyaline cartilage and are considered to be terminally differentiated, thus being highly specialized. Their main function is to maintain the cartilage matrix, synthesizing: types II, IX, and XI collagen; the large aggregating proteoglycan, aggrecan; the smaller proteoglycans biglycan and decorin; and several specific and nonspecific matrix proteins that are expressed at defined stages during growth and development. Freshly isolated articular chondrocytes continue to exhibit their specific phenotype for at least several days to weeks in culture. This makes them a suitable cell type for a cell-based treatment of chondral defects.

1. Cell Biological Issues

Articular chondrocytes do not readily proliferate in vitro. Cells from a younger population (e.g., third and fourth decades of life) have been found to undergo 0.3 doublings per day, using a standardized and validated approach for culturing cells for later implantation (17). Even lower cellular proliferation rates are obtained when cells are harvested from older patients or from arthritic cartilage (18). This requires that cells be subcultured (passaged) in monolayer culture to obtain the necessary number of cells for implantation. However, the longer chondrocytes are deprived of their native three-dimensional environment, their phenotype switches to a more fibroblastic cell form, expressing types I and III collagen instead of cartilage-specific type II collagen (19–21).

The process of "dedifferentiation" is dependent upon specific culture conditions. Expression of fibroblast-like proteins and morphology can by promoted by seeding at low density and treatment with certain cytokines (19). On the other hand, "redifferentiation," or re-expression of cartilage-specific behavior, can be accomplished:

1. using selected culture systems, including spinner-flasks (22) and dishes coated with materials that prevent cell adherence—agar-ose or collagen gels (23);
2. seeding in high-density micromass cultures (24,25);
3. using hypoxic culture conditions (26); and
4. by embedding the cells in solid matrices that do not allow adhe-rence—agarose (27), collagen, or alginate gels (28–30).

The chondrocytic phenotype can also be maintained when the cells are seeded in certain sponge-like scaffolds used for tissue engineering (31,32). Additionally, different cytokines have influence on the degree of expression of cartilage specific molecules. Members of the TGF-β superfamily can trigger the expression of the chondrocytic phenotype (33). Staurosporine, a protein kinase C inhibitor (25,26,34), insulin-like growth factor (IGF) with or without addition of insulin (35–37), hepatocyte growth factor (HGF), and fibroblast growth factor (FGF) (32,38) have been shown to increase the expression of cartilage-specific matrix products.

Other studies propose that chondrocytes, even if dedifferentiated after an extended time in monolayer culture, re-express their chondrocytic phenotype if implanted into a cartilage defect in vivo. The release of growth and differentiation factors from the adjacent host tissue (39) may be the driving biological cue for this re-expression. However, more recent studies suggest that this re-expression of the hyaline cartilage phenotype does not occur (31).

Other recent studies have demonstrated that as articular chondro-cytes are expanded in monolayer culture a greater percentage of cells express the gene that encodes for a contractile muscle actin, α-smooth muscle actin (SMA). These studies have also demonstrated that SMA-expressing cells in articular cartilage are capable of contracting a colla-gen-glycosaminoglycan analog of extracellular matrix in vitro (40,41). Moreover, cells with a higher passage number express higher levels of SMA and display higher levels of contractility (41). This work raises the question of the role that SMA expression may play once the cells are injected into the cartilage defect.

2. Autologous Chondrocyte Implantation in Animal Models

Animal investigation of articular chondrocytes (viz., allogeneic cells), expanded in vitro, for cartilage repair dates back more than 20 years (42). An experiment evaluating the possibilities of autologous chondrocyte implantation (ACI) was first reported in 1987. In a study in rabbits Grande et al. (43) showed that defects that had received transplants had a significant amount of cartilage reconstituted 82%, compared to ungrafted controls 18%. Brittberg, et al. (44) later obtained similar results treating 51 New Zealand white rabbits. ACI significantly increased the amount of newly formed repair tissue up to 52 weeks in contrast to the lack of intrinsic repair with periosteal grafts alone. However, these authors also noted that repair tissue was incompletely bonded to the adjacent cartilage.

Subsequently, Breinan et al. (45,46) repeated these experiments in a canine model (Fig. 2). They found significantly more hyaline cartilage in the ACI-treated group after 3 and 6 months (Fig. 3) compared to the untreated control. At 6 months there was a promising amount of defect filling with articular cartilage-like tissue (Fig. 3). However, by 1 year there were no significant differences among the treated and control (periosteum alone and nontreated defects) groups. By 18 months neither a complete filling nor the restoration of the architecture was found (45). Moreover, cartilage surrounding the defect showed degenerative changes, some of which were related to suturing of the periosteal flap.

The varying results of ACI from different animal studies may have been due in part to differences in the animal models. Dogs have a thin subchondral bone plate that can easily be damaged. As a consequence, mesenchymal stem cells can gain access to the defect and mix with the implanted chondrocytes. Related work showed a significant correlation between the degree to which the calcified cartilage layer and subchondral bone were disturbed and the amount of defect filling (47). The amount of reparative tissue was inversely proportional to the remaining intact calcified cartilage. Comparing microfracture treatment with ACI showed that defect filling was more completely achieved using microfracture technique, whereas the defect was more likely to be filled with hyaline cartilage after ACI. This work suggests the importance of an intact calcified cartilage layer for obtaining repair tissue composed mainly of articular cartilage (47).

Additionally, the observation that some spontaneous regeneration can occur in a canine model (48) raised the question of the degree to which such regeneration can occur in humans. In a surgically created chondral defect (to the tidemark) in adult mongrel dogs, 40% of the untreated defect

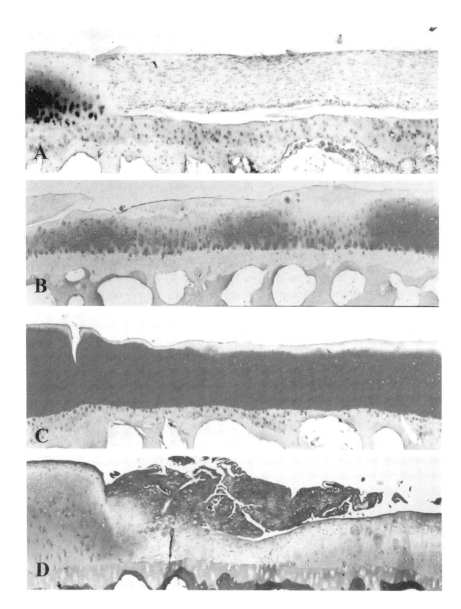

FIGURE 2 Micrographs showing the histology of ACI-treated canine chondral defects (to the tidemark) defects 1.5 (A), 3 (B), 6 (C), and 12 (D) months postoperative. (A) Hematoxylin and eosin stain. (B–D) Safranin O stain.

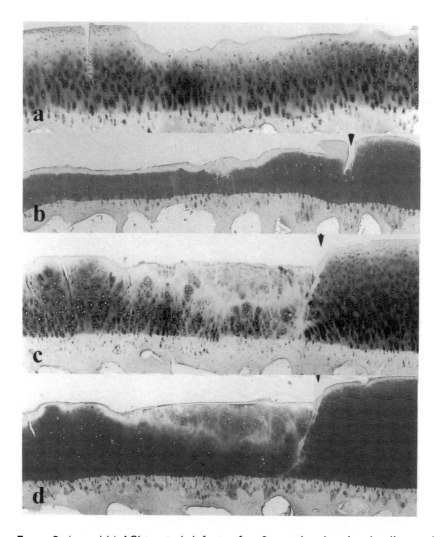

Figure 3 (a and b) ACl-treated defects after 6 months showing hyaline and articular cartilage extending over much of the lesion but with an irregular surface comprising fibrocartilage and fibrous tissue. The regenerated cartilage is well integrated with the calcified cartilage and along one half of the height of the adjacent articular cartilage. (c and d) Serial sections of a 6-month untreated defect with articular cartilage extending along the base of the lesion. (a and c) Hematoxylin and eosin. (b and d) Safranin O. (a) 60×. (b) 50×. (c and d) 50×.

was filled with reparative tissue, 19% of which was found to be hyaline cartilage (48). Therefore, investigations of new modalities treating lesions in articular cartilage have to consider, through careful design of controls, the potential for spontaneous regeneration (48).

3. Procedures for Procuring and Isolating Chondrocytes

While there appear to be general similarities in the procedures used by various commercial and academic laboratories for the isolation and expansion of articular chondrocytes for ACI, there may be important differences. One such difference is the use of the patient's own serum for culturing the cells, as described in the original method by Brittberg et al. (49). One commercial enterprise, Genzyme Biosurgery, uses approved and validated fetal bovine serum, instead of the patient's serum, in the culture media. Another potentially important difference is that Genzyme needs to freeze and store the isolated cells to allow for verification of adequate insurance coverage prior to the implantation procedure. A recent study has indicated that this freeze-thaw cycle may adversely affect the outcome of the procedure. Perka et al. (50) demonstrated that cryopreserved chondrocytes seeded into polymer scaffolds yielded an 85% repair of an osteochondral defect in rabbits, whereas 100% of the defects treated with noncryopreserved cells were filled. Additional work is necessary to more fully explore the effects of certain handling and culture procedures on the performance of monolayer-expanded chondrocytes in ACI.

Since first published in 1994, techniques of cell isolation, expansion in culture and implantation have remained essentially the same. Cartilage (150–300 mg) is harvested arthroscopically from a minimally load-bearing area of the upper aspect of the medial condyle of the affected knee. The biopsy is then transported to a laboratory facility using transport media. Chondrocytes are isolated using standard techniques. After a certain period of cell expansion [11–21 days (18), depending on the growth kinetics] a certain number of cells (e.g., minimally 12×10^6 for Genzyme's Carticel procedure) are provided in a serum-free and gentamycin-free transport medium.

4. Surgical Procedure for ACI in the Knee Joint

With a medial or lateral parapatellar incision, the defect is exposed and debrided. It is generally desirable to maintain the integrity of the tidemark to avoid infiltration of undifferentiated mesenchymal cells from the marrow and blood, which could contribute to the formation of fibrocartilagenous repair tissue (51). However, this is not always possible. A periosteal flap is harvested from the anterior aspect of the proximal tibia or femur, formed to the shape of the lesion, and sutured to the rim of the defect. More recently, an off-the-shelf collagen membrane (Geistlich Biomaterials, Wolhusen, Switzerland) is being used in place of the periosteal flap (not yet FDA approved for use in the United States). The border of periosteal (or collagen) cover is then sealed using fibrin glue. The chondrocyte suspension is subsequently injected under the periosteal flap or collagen membrane. Postoperative rehabilitation protocols generally involve continuous passive motion and limited weight bearing for an extended time. Cooperation of the patient in this respect is essential for a favorable outcome, hence, difficult to control. This difficulty in controlling the postoperative rehabilitation contributes to the challenge in evaluating outcome data.

5. Initial Clinical Study

On the basis of promising animal studies (rabbit) ACI was introduced into the clinic. Brittberg et al. (49) were the first to publish their results on 23 patients treated in Sweden for symptomatic cartilage defects. Thirteen patients had femoral condylar defects, ranging in size from 1.6 to 6.5 cm^2, due to trauma or osteochondritis dissecans. Seven patients had patellar defects. Ten patients had previously been treated with shaving and debridement of unstable cartilage. The results were very promising for the condylar defects. Patients were followed for 16–66 months (mean, 39 months). Initially, the transplants eliminated knee locking and reduced pain and swelling in all patients. After 3 months, arthroscopy showed that the transplants were level with the surrounding tissue and spongy when probed, with visible borders. A second arthroscopic examination showed that in many instances the transplants had the same macroscopic appearance as they had earlier but were firmer when probed and similar in appearance to the surrounding cartilage. Two years after transplantation, 14 of the 16 patients with femoral condylar transplants had good-to-excellent results. Two patients required a second operation because of severe central wear in the transplants, with locking and pain. A mean of 36 months after transplantation, the results were excellent or good in two of the seven patients with patellar transplants, fair in three, and poor in two; two patients required a second operation because of severe chondromalacia. Biopsies showed that 11 of the 15 femoral transplants and one of the seven patellar transplants had the appearance of "hyaline-like" cartilage. These results and the fact that a commercial service for culturing autologous chondrocytes was established led to a dramatic increase in the use of this cell-based therapy for cartilage repair.

6. Clinical Results

Follow-up investigations of the two largest patient groups have been reported: patients treated in Sweden predominantly by L. Peterson,

M.D., and M. Brittberg, M.D., and the Genzyme Cartilage Repair Registry. Peterson et al. (18) reported their 2–9-year results including clinical, arthroscopic, and histological evaluations of 101 patients. In this retrospective study ACI yielded good results in 92% for isolated femoral lesions, 67% for multiple lesions, 89% for osteochondritits dissecans, and 65% for patella defects after an average follow-up of 4.2 years. Arthroscopic follow-up in 65 of 93 patients showed slow maturing of the tissue during the first year, but repair tissue at the subsequent follow-ups was as firm as the adjacent tissue. Histopathological analysis in 21 patients revealed a homogeneous matrix with low cellularity considered to be "hyaline-like" in 17 patients, whereas four patients showed fibrous repair tissue. Immunohistochemistry for collagen type II was positive in all of the patients with "hyaline-like" repair tissue, and negative in the fibrous repair tissue. Adverse events were reported in 51% of the patients, including seven graft failures (7%) and 10 adhesions that needed arthroscopic intervention. Graft hypertrophy, attributed to the periosteal flap, was seen in 26 patients.

One of the Genzyme Biosurgery Patient Registry Reports that included 5-year patient outcome data for individuals treated outside of Sweden showed that there was progressive improvement in the overall condition of the patients and in symptomatology from 24 to 60 months. Improvement compared to baseline was 79% (i.e., percentage of patients improved) for all treated locations as rated by the clinician. However, there was a difference among the treatment sites, with ACT being most successful where the lesion treated was on the lateral femoral condyle (100% improvement) and less successful if the defect was in the trochlea (50%). Adverse events were reported in 7% of the patients (n=4834, at the time of the report). These included adhesions or fibroarthrosis and hypertrophic changes. The cumulative incidence of treatment failure was estimated to be 3% at 60 months. Six percent of the patients reported an additional knee operation following ACT.

7. Federal Regulations

Since the clinical introduction of the procedure much attention has been paid to the standardization and validation of the cell culture procedures. In August 1997 the U.S. Food and Drug Administration granted accelerated approval for Genzyme's Carticel procedure for the repair of symptomatic, cartilaginous defects of the femoral condyle, including both first- and second-line repairs. As a condition of this approval, Genzyme agreed to conduct two studies, including a multicenter, randomized controlled trial in 300 patients comparing Carticel to other primary repair techniques, to confirm the benefits of Carticel in this setting.

However, to date Genzyme has not been able to enroll an adequate number of patients in either of the planned studies. As a result Genzyme changed the product labeling, narrowing the indications for Carticel to second-line therapy for the repair of cartilage defects of the femoral condyle.

8. Quality Control

Significant challenges exist in assuring a safe and reproducible product for ACI. Genzyme Biosurgery established a quality assurance program based on U.S. FDA Good Manufacturing Practice regulations, which was reviewed recently (17). Process variables have to be controlled rigorously and implantation delayed for sterility and endotoxin testing. Moreover, assessment of cell viability and growth kinetics is a crucial part of nonconformance reporting.

According to Genzyme data, 1.64% of the cartilage biopsies received were contaminated. Contamination was recorded only for 0.03% during processing and in 0.16% at release. Endotoxin content ranged between less than 0.15 to 0.5 EU/mL (allowable limit 82.5 EU/mL), and cell viability was $90.9 \pm 4.06\%$ at release. Measurement of growth kinetics revealed 0.311 doublings per day. Out of 1377 cartilage biopsies, 86 nonconformances were identified related to biopsy quality; only 12 were related to cell processing.

9. Risks

The risks associated with the currently used cell-based products are unknown, but might include the following: (1) adverse effects of the harvest procedure to procure the articular cartilage tissue for cell isolation, (2) effects of the arthrotomy currently required for the open implantation of the cells, (3) degeneration of the adjacent articular cartilage related to the damage due to suturing, (4) flap detachment, and (5) malignant transformation of cells in culture.

Fortunately, while there is a finite possibility (albeit small) for malignant or dysplastic transformation of cells during their in vitro expansion, no such occurrence has been reported. In addition, implantation of normal autologous chondrocytes could potentially stimulate growth of malignant cells in the area of the implant, although there have been no reported incidents in humans.

Another issue in employing autologous articular chondrocytes relates to donor site morbidity. To obtain autologous chondrocytes, healthy cartilage must be harvested from uninvolved regions of the joint. Although it has been assumed that there are no major problems associated with the harvest of cartilage, evidence is scarce. There are no published clinical studies focusing on the harvest site. Harvesting cartilage for ACI makes a second operation necessary with all theoretical possibilities of complication (e.g., infection). Moreover, harvesting cartilage might initiate additional damage to the joint. A recent study in a canine animal model (52) could show that the harvest of articular cartilage introduces distinct changes of selected mechanical properties of the cartilage distant from the harvest site. The articular cartilage in the harvested joint displayed a three fold increase of dynamic stiffness and steaming potential. These changes were consisted with hypertrophic changes that may precede degeneration. Clearly, additional studies are necessary to investigate the consequences of harvest of articular cartilage for the isolation of chondrocytes for cell-based therapies.

B. Allogeneic Chondrocytes

Transplantation of allogeneic osteochondral grafts has been used clinically for many years (53–55), and several investigations have focused on studying tissue engineering using allogeneic cells or cell-based tissue engineered constructs (56,57). It has been proposed (58) that allogeneic chondrocytes from amputated limbs or joint arthoplasties might play a major role in the future. However, this approach is less attractive for cell therapy because issues related to immune response and transmission of disease have to be taken into account.

C. Adult Mesenchymal Stem Cells

The difficulty in obtaining chondrocytes and maintaining differentiated cell cultures has led to research on other cell types for cell-based therapies for cartilage repair. Several studies have shown that autologous bone-marrow-derived progenitor cells and periosteum-derived cells are able to exhibit a chondrocytic phenotype in vivo (59) and in vitro under certain conditions (60).

Friedenstein et al. (61,62) were the first to describe the adherence of bone-marrow-derived stromal cells to tissue culture plastic. Using this phenotypic characteristic they were able to easily separate mesenchymal from hematopoietic progenitor cells. Subsequently Haynesworth et al. (63), Bruder et al. (64), and Johnstone and Yoo (65) developed a culture system that facilitated the chondrogenic differentiation of bone-marrow-derived mesenchymal progenitor cells. Cells obtained in bone marrow aspirates were first isolated by monolayer culture and then transferred into conical tubes and allowed to form three-dimensional aggregates in a chemically defined medium that included dexamethasone and/or TGB-β1. The chondrogenic differentiation of cells within the aggregate was evidenced by

the appearance of toluidine blue metachromasia and the immunohistochemical detection of type II collagen (60). Chondrogenic differentiation in this
environment seemed to recapitulate embryonic chondrogenesis.

Other approaches describe the isolation of progenitor cells, viz.,
cells capable of differentiation along multilineage pathways, from trabecular bone explants (66), skeletal muscle (67), and fat tissue (68). Culturing these cells at high density or under hypoxic conditions (micromass
cultures) promoted differentiation toward a chondrocytic phenotype,
viz., the expression of chondrogenic genes (24,65,69). This process may
be facilitated by addition of selected cytokines including TGF-β1 or β3
and BMP-2, and perhaps by merely adding dexamethasone to the culture
medium (65). The principal advantages associated with the use of these
cells over autologous articular chondrocytes for cartilage repair procedures are their ready availability and minimal donor site morbidity.

Moreover, with the development of gene transfer techniques, stem
cells have become the target of in vitro and in vivo gene therapy—involving
direct injection of viral and nonviral vectors carrying transgenes. Other in
vitro data suggest that the chondrogenic potential of these cells is maintained with virally mediated ex vivo gene transfer (70,71).

Several animal studies have demonstrated the promise of human
mesenchymal stem cells (hMSC) for cartilage repair (72,73). Some reports
have even suggested a lower chondrogenic activity of articular chondrocytes compared to MSC isolated from the same animal (goat model) (74).
Recent investigations carried out by Osiris Therapeutics indicated that
MSC, delivered by direct injection to the osteoarthritic joint, may bind to
the surface of fibrillated host tissue and potentially alter the progression of
the disease (72). Murphy et al. (73) could show that injection of MSC into
destabilized, osteoarthritic joints of 24 goats resulted in marked regeneration of the medial meniscus, which had been previously excised. The newly
formed tissue had a hyaline appearance with focal areas rich in type II
collagen similar to developing meniscus. In parallel with this tissue regeneration there was a marked chondroprotective effect.

While the reports implementing hMSC for the treatment of musculoskeletal defects are promising, no clinical trials have yet been published.
Osiris Therapeutics has begun a Phase 1 safety trial with autologous hMSC
delivered on a hydroxyapatite matrix in alveolar ridge regeneration prior
to dental implantation.

D. Embryonic Stem Cells

Recently embryonic stem cells have also attracted interest for cell therapy
and transplantation. The feasibility of isolating and culture-expanding

embryonic stem cells as well as their differentiation into bone and cartilage has been shown (75). Transplantation of mouse embryonic stem cells has been used to repair the ventricular myocardium of mdx dystrophic mice (76,77). However, legal and ethical issues have restricted widespread embryonic stem cell research and cell therapy approaches for human subjects.

E. Fibroblasts

Recently a model has been described for the conversion (transdifferentiation) of human dermal fibroblasts to chondrocyte-like cells in vitro (26). Human neonatal foreskin fibroblasts were seeded in two-dimensional, high-density micromass cultures in the presence of staurosporine and lactic acid to induce functional hypoxia. Cells were also seeded into three-dimensional polymer scaffolds. Northern analysis revealed aggrecan core protein expression in lactate-treated micromass cultures, and type I collagen gene expression was virtually abolished in all cultures supplemented with staurosporine. Moreover, the cells in these cultures displayed a rounded, cobblestone-shaped morphology typical of differentiated chondrocytes and were organized into nodules that stained positive with alcian blue. When seeded on polyglycolide/poly-L-lactide scaffolds, a chondrocyte-like morphology was observed in cultures treated with lactate and staurosporine in contrast to the flattened sheets of fibroblast-like cells seen in untreated controls. This approach holds promise for the use of readily accessible nonchondrocytic autologous cells for cartilage repair procedures.

Many issues remain related to this approach; however, the debate about whether this effect is due to transdifferentiation of already terminally differentiated fibroblasts or due to the presence of mesenchymal progenitor cells in neonatal foreskin dermis appears central.

III. USE OF MATRICES ALONE

Several animal studies have investigated the implantation of porous, absorbable scaffolds alone in cartilage defects. However, none of these materials has yet been investigated in a clinical trial. Most studies have evaluated the reparative process in osteochondral defects implanted with these scaffold materials. Implantation of such a matrix into a chondral defect (i.e., a defect that does not initially penetrate the subchondral bone plate) was found to have little effect in facilitating the reparative process (78). Recent work has shown that even small penetrations through the subchondral bone, such as those produced by "microfracture," can increase the amount of reparative tissue formed in the implanted scaffold (79). In one canine model the benefit of the matrix implanted alone in a microfracture-treated defect was to significantly increase the amount of tissue filling the defect. However, the composition of the reparative tissue was principally fibrocartilage (79). The initial function of the scaffold appeared to be to stabilize the fibrin clot that formed as a result of the bleeding from the subchondral bone. Clinical studies will now be required to determine the extent to which implantation of a porous scaffold into a microfracture-treated site will improve the clinical outcome.

IV. CELL-SEEDED MATRICES

Because phenotypic changes of chondrocytes in monolayer culture have been shown to occur, interest has focused on three-dimensional systems in which to culture and deliver the cells to the defect. These systems can act as templates for growth and hence contribute to phenotypic stability of the chondrocytes. The matrix, or scaffold, can play several roles in the process of tissue engineering. These roles include:

1. structural support for the defect site,
2. barrier to the ingrowth of undesirable cell and tissue types,
3. scaffold for cell migration and proliferation, and
4. carrier or reservoir of cells or regulators (e.g., growth factors).

A variety of scaffolds have shown promise thus far (1).

Bell (80) described the ideal scaffold for tissue engineering as one that provides a transitional framework whereby the cells populating it create a replacement tissue as the scaffolding material disappears. Ideally this scaffold should be degraded at the same speed that the cells produce their own framework. Other studies have demonstrated that matrix composition affects cell viability, cell attachment, morphology, and synthesis of matrix components. As an example, chondrocytes seeded into agarose proliferated and synthesized matrix molecules over a period of weeks (81), whereas cellulose matrix was found to be toxic. Grande et al. (82) found that chondrocytes seeded onto type I collagen matrices were more strongly attached, more spherical in shape, and produced more type II collagen and higher levels of proteoglycan than chondrocytes seeded onto polyglycolide or Vicryl (polylactide-polyglycolide copolymer) matrices.

Although type I collagen matrices have been extensively studied, recently it was shown that a type II collagen matrix supported a more chondrocytic morphology and biosynthetic activity (31,83). In addition to chemical composition, matrix geometry can influence the performance of the implant. Collagen can be employed as gel (58) or as a sponge with varying degrees of porosity and a range of pore diameters (31,82,84).

Not only is there a lack of clinical data on matrix applications for cartilage repair, there are also only a few preclinical studies in larger animals. Most of the animal work has been done in rabbits and has shown comparatively uniform good results (58,60,85–89).

Few studies have systematically compared different cell-seeded matrices in a large animal model. One such study conducted in dogs (78) demonstrated no notable differences in the makeup of the reparative tissue after 15 weeks in defects treated with chondrocyte-seeded type I and type II collagen scaffolds. Of importance was that a subsequent study that cultured the chondrocyte-seeded type II collagen matrix in vitro for 4 weeks prior to implantation (90) reported a greater amount of tissue filling the defect and more hyaline cartilage that in defects in which the cell-seeded construct was implanted 24 h after being seeded with cells (79). Moreover, the construct cultured for 4 weeks also yielded a greater percentage of reparative tissue in the treated defect, while having the same amount of hyaline cartilage, than previously found with ACI employed in the same animal model (46). These results demonstrate the potential advantage of growing monolayer-expanded chondrocytes in a biomaterial scaffold in vitro prior to implantation compared to ACI.

V. CURRENT CLINICAL IMPLEMENTATION OF SURGICAL PROCEDURES FOR ARTICULAR CARTILAGE REPAIR

It is instructive to place the aforementioned tissue engineering strategies in the context of other currently used clinical cartilage repair procedures.

A. Microfracture

The fact that cartilage has some limited healing potential has led to methods of improving the healing processes by increasing the number of progenitor cells able to form a cartilage-like matrix in the defect, by creating access to the underlying bone marrow. Specially designed awls have been used to make multiple perforations, or "microfractures," through the subchondral bone plate. The perforations are made as close together as necessary, but not so close that one breaks into another. Consequently, the microfracture holes are approximately 3–4 mm apart (or 3–4 holes/cm^2). Importantly, the integrity of the subchondral bone plate is maintained, at least intraoperatively. The released marrow elements form a "superclot," which provides an enriched environment for tissue regeneration. Follow-up with long-term results of more than 8 years have been encouraging (12). Because this procedure is technically the easiest one, and the least expensive, it is also the most widely utilized. There have been no long-term or controlled studies published using this procedure.

B. Autologous Periosteal Grafting

The use of autologous periosteum alone (14,91,92) has also been investigated for cartilage repair. Animal studies by several groups showed that neochondrogenesis of hyaline cartilage is also possible with this approach (93–95). Periosteal transplantation was initially described by Rubak (96). He used a periosteal flap to treat cartilage defects in rabbits. The results revealed that the defects were repaired and filled after 4 weeks with a hyaline-like cartilage whereas the empty control defect showed fibrocartilage-like repair tissue. The first trial in humans was published 3 years later by Niedermann et al. (97). They reported successful results in all of their four initially treated patients. Hoikka et al.(98) treated 13 patients, of whom eight had a good result, four a fair outcome, and one a poor result. O'Dirscoll contributed in the following years valuable basic science data (14,91,99–101). It was found that orientation of the periosteal flap (cambium layer facing up), postoperative factors such as the use of continuous passive motion (102), and the age (91) and skeletal maturity of the experimental animal were of importance when dealing with periosteal transplants. O'Driscoll (14) himself treated approximately 40 patients, 20 of whom had defects in the knee and were followed up by the author. Twelve individuals had a good outcome, four had poor results, and four patients had inadequate length of follow-up.

O'Driscoll also contributed useful technical detail on harvesting the periosteal flap. In an animal model he showed that training the surgeon leads to a significant increase of the chondrogenic potential of the harvested periosteum (91,92).

Collectively the results using this approach are promising, but as with the other techniques, there are no controlled studies that would allow for comparison with other methods.

C. Autologous Perichondrial Grafting

Autologous perichondrium has also been employed for cartilage repair (15,103–105). Perichondrium, taken from the cartilaginous covering of the rib, has been placed into the chondral defect of the affected joint. The first clinical study of this approach was performed by Homminga et al. (15). Twenty-five patients with 30 symptomatic chondral lesions received autologous perichondrial grafts taken from the costal arch and fixed to the subchondral bone with human fibrin glue. The majority of the lesions were graded Outerbridge grade III/IV and half were located on the medial femoral condyle. The opposing articulating surface had no greater than Outerbridge II changes. Preparation of the defect used techniques very similar to those employed for ACI. Postoperative, continuous passive motion was started 2 weeks after surgery and non-weight-bearing was continued for 3 months. All patients were examined arthroscopically at an average of 10 months after implantation. Of the 30 grafted defects 27 had completely filled with tissue resembling cartilage. In two cases the defect was unchanged, and one patella graft was covered with white tissue with a fibrillated surface. Three biopsies were taken at 1 year, two of which showed disruption of the cartilage-bone junction. Histologically, the regenerated cells appeared to be chondrocytes. Clinically at 1 year the mean clinical improvement was 80%, as rated by the Hospital for Special Surgery grading scheme; 18 of the 25 patients were completely symptom-free. These results remained stable even after 23.5 months, but at 5 years 20 of the 27 grafts were associated with pain and degeneration.

A total of 88 patients were treated between 1986 and 1992 in another series (106). After a mean follow-up of 4 years only 38% showed a good, 8% a fair, but 55% a poor result. Graft failure ranged between 33 and 62%, according to the location of the defect. Only a small, carefully selected group of patients (isolated defects) showed good results in 91% of the tissue.

Animal experiments subsequently demonstrated an increased calcification of the basal layer of the repair tissue (105) and this was confirmed clinically. Twenty-five of 47 patients showed calcification of the graft, so the authors used indomethacin to prevent this from occurring (106).

One of the main shortcomings of perichondrial grafting is the limited availability of large grafts. Graft size is limited to the rib size, so that several rib perichondrial grafts have to be harvested to fill a large defect. Additionally endochondral ossification and delamination of the cartilage from the subchondral bone plate are potentially significant limitations to the long-term efficacy of this repair.

D. Osteochondral Transplantation

Osteochondral transplantation has been used clinically for more than 25 years. Large osteochondral allografts have been used in orthopedic tumor surgery and in a smaller amount for repairing degenerative defects (54),(107). However, this method has never been widely accepted.

The reports presented by Matsusue et al. (16) and Bobic (108) using autografts, however, renewed interest in this method. Matsusue was the first to harvest and implant osteochondral autografts from a patient with a cartilage defect after rupture of the anterior cruciate ligament. Later Bobic (108) reported the treatment of 12 patients with multiple osteochondral transplants (5–10 mm in width and 10–15 mm in length). As with the ACI method, the osteochondral plug was harvested from a non-weight-bearing area of the knee joint and was implanted into the drilled defect using press-fit technique. Using this approach Bobic was able to treat defects up to 4 cm^2.

Since 1992 Hangody et al. (109) treated a total of 227 patients with full-thickness lesions resulting from chondropathy, traumatic chondral defects, and osteochondritis dissecans; the procedure was evaluated in 57 patients who had >3 years of follow-up. Magnetic resonance imaging, computed tomography arthrographies, ultrasound, and arthroscopy were used to evaluate the technique. Using the modified Hospital for Special Surgery knee scoring system, 91% of the patients achieved a good or excellent result. Graft matching and contouring to the recipient articular surface was reported to be challenging. The availability of donor sites was also a limiting factor. Furthermore, the fibrocartilaginous interface between the donor and recipient site may contribute to breakdown in the long run.

As with ACI, the early results have been promising (108–111). However, no long-term patient outcomes or data of controlled clinical studies are available using this method and there is limited knowledge about integration and survival of the chondral graft, to judge the procedure. Application of this method for larger defects, requiring the harvest of several plugs, may compromise the integrity of the harvest site. This is also of particular interest if the cartilage cannot be taken from the involved joint. For example, to treat a cartilage defect in the ankle, osteochondral plugs usually have to be harvested from the knee joint (112).

E. Composition of Reparative Tissue from Symptomatic Patients

Sufficient data are not yet available to allow a correlation to be drawn between clinical (viz., pain relief) and histological outcomes of cartilage repair procedures. Such a correlation would be valuable for the evaluation of new tissue engineering procedures studied in animal models. An understanding of the type of reparative tissues recovered from symptomatic patients can begin to add to this database.

A recent study (113) compared the histological outcomes of different cartilage repair procedures that failed to relieve patient symptoms. The reparative tissue was retrieved during revision surgery from full-thickness chondral defects in 18 patients in whom abrasion arthroplasty ($n = 12$), grafting of perichondrial flaps ($n = 4$), and periosteal patching augmented by autologous chondrocyte implantation in cell suspension ($n = 6$) failed to provide lasting relief of symptoms. The Histological and immunohisto-chemical investigations showed fibrous, spongiform tissue comprising type I collagen in 22% ± 9% (mean ± standard error of the mean) of the cross-sectional area, and degenerating hyaline tissue (30% ± 10%) and fibrocartilage (28% ± 7%) with positive type II collagen staining. Three of four specimens obtained after implantation of perichondrium failed as a result of bone formation that was found in 19% + 6% of the cross-sectional area, including areas staining positive for type X collagen, as an indicator for hypertrophic chondrocytes. Revision after autologous chondrocyte implantation was associated with partial displacement of the periosteal graft from the defect site because of insufficient ongrowth or early suture failure. When the graft edge displaced, repair tissue was fibrous (55%±11%), whereas graft tissue attached to subchondral bone displayed hyaline tissue (to 6%) and fibrocartilage (to 12%).

F. Summary

Competing and alternative techniques like osteochondral autograft trans-fer (16,114), mosaicplasty (109), or osteochondral paste have to be consid-ered or included into a therapeutic algorithm (115) when considering tissue engineering strategies for treating cartilage defects. Moreover, correction of predisposing anatomical factors such as malalignment of the knee or maltracking of the patella have been shown to be necessary for a good clinical outcome (116). Of importance also is the etiology of the defect, whether traumatic or degenerative in nature. Many studies of cartilage repair fail to distinguish adequately between lesions resulting from disease and those resulting from acute injury. Methods for the effec-tive treatment of these lesions may be different.

Considering that clinical trials employ "pain" as the major outcome parameter, meaningful outcome instruments (e.g., the SF-36 question-naire) are necessary to account for the overall physical and mental health of the patient. In addition, the patient's clinical and functional goals must be considered.

A number of fundamental questions will have to be answered as more and more procedures are introduced into the clinic for treatment of carti-lage problems: For how long does a particular biological cartilage repair procedure have to provide pain relief—for 3, 5, or 10 years? Which risks are we willing to take to achieve a particular clinical outcome (e.g., donor site morbidity)? What are the financial costs we are willing to accept for a certain level of functional performance?

VI. FUTURE DEVELOPMENTS

Current investigations are addressing the following issues:

1. refinement of surgical procedure (viz., arthroscopic delivery of cells and cell-seeded matrices and suturing of the covering flap),
2. alternative cell sources,
3. optimization of culture conditions with respect to enhancing cell growth and maintenance of chondrocyte phenotype,
4. engineered scaffolds for cell delivery, and
5. genetic modification of cells.

As outlined above, different cell types are under investigation. To date the committed chondrocytes are the most investigated cell type for cartilage repair, although they do undergo phenotypic changes in monolayer culture. However, a final judgment is impossible, because of lack of information. Further studies have to show clearly the advantages and disadvantages of each cell type. Moreover, culture conditions have a profound effect on cell growth kinetics, phenotypic stability, and matrix production, but the optimal conditions have yet to be defined. The use of selected growth factors is under intensive investigation (35,36,38,117,118). Culture of cells under hydrodynamic pressure (119), continuous medium perfusion (120), or using microgravity in bioreactors (121–127) has also been implemented and shown promise.

A. Genetically Modified Cells

In recent years interest in combining tissue engineering and gene therapy approaches has been growing. Principal applications of genetically augmented engineered tissues of the musculoskeletal system have been reviewed recently (128). A target gene, encoding a specific protein molecule, can be introduced into the cell using different vectors. There are several advantages to delivering genes, rather than the gene products, to patients, including the ability to achieve high concentrations of the gene products locally in a sustained manner for extended times. Such capabilities are likely to be especially valuable in orthopedic tissue engineering and tissue repair, where it may be necessary to expose discrete populations of cells to various growth factors in precise anatomical locations for lengths of time that go beyond conventional means of delivery (129). Also, endogenously synthesized proteins might have greater biological activities than exogenously administered recombinant proteins (130).

Cell therapies and tissue engineering provide the ideal partner for ex vivo gene therapy since in vivo gene transfer in humans is constrained by safety concerns and the lack of suitable vectors (129). Ex vivo gene transfer is safer because vectors are not introduced directly into the patient, and genetically modified cells can be screened extensively before they are implanted. Moreover, gene delivery to chondrocytes may require ex vivo techniques, because the dense cartilaginous matrix is likely to restrict access of vectors to the cells by in vivo delivery. Different feasibility studies delivering marker genes like the lacZ marker gene—encoding for the enzyme β-galactosidase—to different musculoskeletal tissues have been carried out (131–135). Genetically modified mesenchymal stem cells may also prove to be useful agents of tissue repair in orthopedics (128). Moreover, recent studies could show an increased matrix synthesis after adenoviral transfer of TGF-β1 gene to canine and human meniscal cells (135) and disc cells (136). However, as for the application of the growth factor alone, the exact combination of cell types and genes to be delivered as well as the timing of the gene expression are unknown. (See earlier chapter for complete review of genetic engineering.)

B. Effects of Mechanical Loading on Chondrocyte-Seeded Constructs

It has long been appreciated that mechanical forces can affect cell functions. For example, it is well known that chondrocytes in intact articular cartilage and in agarose and alginate gels can respond to dynamic mechanical stimulation by up-regulating collagen and proteoglycan synthesis (137,138). However, it has been only recently that studies have investigated how serially passaged cells (e.g., chondrocytes) seeded into porous scaffolds, designed for tissue engineering, respond to mechanical loading (139). Future studies will be needed to better determine how mechanical loading protocols in vitro can be used to prepare cell-seeded matrices for tissue engineering and regenerative medicine. (See earlier chapter for additional aspects of bioreactors as strategies in tissue engineering.)

VII. CONCLUSIONS

In recent years biological (including tissue engineering) therapies of cartilage defects have progressed significantly and are becoming important modalities of treatment in orthopedic surgery. However, for all these therapies long-term outcome is unknown, and there is a lack of controlled studies comparing the different treatment options. Prospective studies are needed to better understand which of the different options will be the most suitable for specific indications.

We have to answer several questions in the near future: Do we need to deliver cells to the defect or might it be suitable to recruit enough endogenous cells, locally, capable of migration, proliferation, differentiation, and biosynthesis (perhaps with a method similar to microfracture)? Using in vitro tissue engineering methods, how much preformed matrix (in vitro tissue engineering) do we need in our construct to obtain a mechanically stable implant that will eventually integrate into the surrounding healthy articular cartilage? Is it better to have a defect fully filled with fibrocartilage or partly filled with hyaline cartilage; what will be the long-term result of these two repair tissues? And finally, is the regeneration of true (normal) articular cartilage necessary to achieve a satisfactory clinical result; no study has yet shown that the regeneration of normal articular cartilage is possible?

Tissue engineering holds the promise of providing effective, long-term solutions to the cartilage problems affecting a large segment of the population. While more work will be required to achieve this goal, during the course of future studies it is likely that much will be learned about cartilage biology that will inform still newer approaches for the treatment of joint problems.

REFERENCES

1. Lee CR, Spector M. Status of articular cartilage tissue engineering. Curr Opin Orthop 1998; 9:88–93.
2. Hunter W. Of the structure and diseases of articulating cartilages. Philosoph Trans 1743; 470:514–521.
3. Paget J. Healing of injuries in various tissues. Lect Surg Pathol (Lond) 1853; 1:262.
4. Wirth CJ, Rudert M. Techniques of cartilage growth enhancement: a review of the literature. Arthroscopy 1996; 12:300–308.
5. Langer R, Vacanti JP. Tissue engineering. Science 1993; 260:920–926.
6. Friedmann MJ, Berasi DO, Fox JM, Pizzo WD, Snyder SJ, Ferkel RD. Preliminary results with abrasion arthroplasty in the osteoarthritic knee. Clin Orthop 1984; 182:200–205.
7. Ewing JW. Arthroscopic treatment of degenerative meniscal lesion and early degenerative arthritis of the knee. In: Ewing JW, ed. Articular Cartilage and Knee Joint Function: Basic Science and Arthroscopy. New York: Raven Press, 1990:137–145.
8. Johnson LL. Arthroscopic abrasion arthroplasty historical and pathologic perspective: present status. Arthroscopy 1986; 2:54–69.
9. Pridie K. A method of resurfacing osteoarthritic knee joints. J Bone Joint Surg 1959; 41-B:618–619.
10. Ficat RP, Ficat C, Gedeon PK, Toussaint JF. Spongialization: a new treatment for diseased patella. Clin Orthop 1984; 182:200–205.

11. Frisbie DD, Trotter GW, Powers BE, et al. Arthroscopic subchondral bone plate microfracture technique augments healing of large chondral defects in the radial carpal bone and medial femoral condyle of horses. Vet Surg 1999; 28:242–255.

12. Rodrigo JJ, Steadman JR, Silliman JF, Fulstone HA. Improvement of full-thickness chondral defect healing in the human knee after debridement and microfracture using continuous passive motion. Am J Knee Surg 1994; 7:109–116.

13. Johnson LL. Characteristics of the immediate postarthroscopic blood clot formation in the knee joint. Arthroscop J Arthroscop Rel Surg 1991; 7:14–23.

14. O'Driscoll SW. Articular cartilage regeneration using periosteum. Clin Orthop 1999; 367 Suppl:S186–203.

15. Homminga GN, Bulstra S, Bouwmeester PSM, Van Der Linden AJ. Perichondral grafting for cartilage lesions of the knee. J Bone Joint Surg 1990; 72-B:1003–1007.

16. Matsusue Y, Yamamuro T, Hama H. Arthroscopic multiple osteochondral transplantation to the chondral defect in the knee associated with anterior cruciate ligament disruption. Arthroscopy 1993; 9:318–321.

17. Mayhew TA, Williams GR, Senica MA, Kuniholm G, Du Moulin GC. Validation of a quality assurance program for autologous cultured chondrocyte implantation. Tiss Eng 1998; 4:325–334.

18. Peterson L, Minas T, Brittberg M, Nilsson A, Sjogren-Jansson E, Lindahl A. Two- to 9-year outcome after autologous chondrocyte transplantation of the knee. Clin Orthop 2000; 374:212–234.

19. Goldring MB, Birkhead J, Sandell LJ, Kimura T, Krane SM. Interleukin 1 suppresses expression of cartilage-specific types II and IX collagens and increases types I and III collagens in human chondrocytes. J Clin Invest 1988; 82:2026–2037.

20. Goldring MB, Sandell LJ, Stephenson ML, Krane SM. Immune interferon suppresses levels of procollagen mRNA and type II collagen synthesis in cultured human articular and costal chondrocytes. J Biol Chem 1986; 261:9049–9055.

21. Saadeh PB, Brent B, Mehrara BJ, et al. Human cartilage engineering: chondrocyte extraction, proliferation, and characterization for construct development. Ann Plast Surg 1999; 42:509–513.

22. Norby DP, Malemud CJ, Sokoloff L. Differences in the collagen types synthesized by lapine articular chondrocytes in spinner and monolayer culture. Arth Rheum 1977; 20:709–716.

23. Watt FM, Dudhia J. Prolonged expression of differentiated phenotype by chondrocytes cultured at low density on a composite substrate of collagen and agarose that restricts cell spreading. Differentiation 1988; 38:140–147.

24. Denker AE, Nicoll SB, Tuan RS. Formation of cartilage-like spheroids by micromass cultures of murine C3H10T1/2 cells upon treatment with transforming growth factor-beta 1. Differentiation 1995; 59:25–34.

25. Kulyk WM, Reichert C. Staurosporine, a protein kinase inhibitor, stimulates cartilage differentiation by embryonic facial mesenchyme. J Craniofac Genet Dev Biol 1992; 12:90–97.

26. Nicoll SB. Induction of a chondrocyte-like phenotype in human dermal fibroblasts: application to cartilage tissue engineering. Trans Soc Biomat 1998; 24th Annual Meeting p.236.

27. Benya PO, Schaffer JD. Dedifferentiated chondrocytes re-express the differentiated collagen phenotype when cultured in agarose gels. Cell 1982; 30:215–224.

28. Guo JF, Jourdian GW, MacCallum DK. Culture and growth characteristics of chondrocytes encapsulated in alginate beads. Connect Tiss Res 1989; 19:277–297.

29. Hauselmann HJ, Fernandes RJ, Mok SS, et al. Phenotypic stability of bovine articular chondrocytes after long-term culture in alginate beads. J Cell Sci 1994; 107:17–27.

30. Häuselmann HJ, Masuda K, Hunziker EB, et al. Adult human chondrocytes cultured in alginate form a matrix similar to native human articular cartilage. Am J Physiol 1996; 271:C742–C752.

31. Nehrer S, Breinan HA, Ramappa A, et al. Matrix collagen type and pore size influence behaviour of seeded canine chondrocytes. Biomaterials 1997; 18:769–776.

32. Martin I, Vunjak-Novakovic G, Yang J, Langer R, Freed LE. Mammalian chondrocytes expanded in the presence of fibroblast growth factor 2 maintain the ability to differentiate and regenerate three-dimensional cartilaginous tissue. Exp Cell Res 1999; 253:681–688.

33. Frenkel SR, Saadeh PB, Mehrara BJ, et al. Transforming growth factor beta superfamily members: role in cartilage modeling. Plast Reconstr Surg 2000; 105:980–990.

34. Kulyk WM, Franklin JL, Hoffman LM. Sox9 expression during chondrogenesis in micromass cultures of embryonic limb mesenchyme. Exp Cell Res 2000; 255:327–332.

35. Chopra R, Anastassiades T. Specificity and synergism of polypeptide growth factors in stimulating the synthesis of proteoglycans and a novel high molecular weight anionic glycoprotein by articular chondrocyte cultures. J Rheum 1998; 25:1578–1584.

36. Dunham BP, Koch RJ. Basic fibroblast growth factor and insulin-like growth factor I support the growth of human septal chondrocytes in a serum-free environment. Arch Otolaryngol Head Neck Surg 1998; 124: 1325–1330.

37. Goto K, Yamazaki M, Tagawa M, et al. Involvement of insulin-like growth factor I in development of ossification of the posterior longitudinal ligament of the spine. Calcif. Tissue Int 1998; 62:158–165.

38. Fujisato T, Sajiki T, Liu Q, Ikada Y. Effect of basic fibroblast growth factor-on cartilage regeneration in chondrocyte-seeded collagen sponge scaffold. Biomaterials 1996; 17:155–162.

39. Shortkroff S, Barone L, Hsu H-P, et al. Healing of chondral and osteo-chondral defects in a canine model: the role of cultured autologous chondro-cytes in regeneration of articular cartilage. Biomaterials 1996; 17:147–154.
40. Lee CR, Breinan HA, Nehrer S, Spector M. Articular cartilage chondrocytes in type I and type II collagen-GAG matrices exhibit contractile behavior in vitro. Tiss Eng 2000; 6:555–565.
41. Kinner B, Spector M. Smooth muscle actin expression by human articular chondrocytes and their contraction of a collagen-glycosaminoglycan matrix in vitro. J Orthop Res 2001; 19:233–241.
42. Green WT. Articular cartilage repair behavior of rabbit chondrocytes during tissue culture and subsequent allografting. Clin Orthop 1977; 124: 237–250.
43. Grande DA, Singh IJ, Pugh J. Healing of experimentally produced lesions in articular cartilage following chondrocyte transplantation. Anat Rec 1987; 218:142–148.
44. Brittberg M, Nilsson A, Lindahl A, Ohlsson C, Peterson L. Rabbit articular cartilage defects treated with autologous cultured chondrocytes. Clin Orthop 1996; 326:270–283.
45. Breinan HA, Minas T, Hsu H-P, Nehrer S, Sledge CB, Spector M. Effect of cultured autologous chondrocytes on repair of chondral defects in a canine model. J Bone Joint Surg 1997; 79-A:1439–1451.
46. Breinan HA, Minas T, Hsu H-P, Nehrer S, Shortkroff S, Spector M. Auto-logous chondrocyte implantation in a canine model: change in composition of reparative tissue with time. J Orthop Res 2001; 19:482–492.
47. Breinan HA, Hsu H-P, Spector M. Chondral defects in animal models: effects of selected repair procedures in canines. Clin Orthop 2001; 391S: 219–230.
48. Wang Q, Breinan HA, Hsu HP, Spector M. Healing of defects in canine articular cartilage: Distribution of nonvascular alpha-smooth muscle actin-containing cells. Wound Repair Regen 2000; 8:145–158.
49. Brittberg M, Lindahl A, Nilsson A, Ohlsson C, Isaksson O, Peterson L. Treatment of deep cartilage defects in the knee with autologous chondrocyte transplantation. N Engl J Med 1994; 331:889–894.
50. Perka C, Sittinger M, Schultz O, Spitzer R-S, Schlenzka D, Burmester GR. Tissue engineered cartilage repair using cryopreserved and noncryopre-served chondrocytes. Clin Orthop 2000; 378:245–254.
51. Brittberg M. Autologous chondrocyte transplantation. Clin Orthop 1999; 367S:147–155.
52. Lee CR, Grodzinsky AJ, Hsu H-P, Martin SD, Spector M. Effects of harvest and selected cartilage repair procedures on the physical and biochemical properties of articular cartilage in the canine knee. J Orthop Res 2000; 18:790–799.
53. Ghazavi MT, Pritzker KP, Davis AM, Gross AE. Fresh osteochondral allo-grafts for post-traumatic osteochondral defects of the knee. J Bone Joint Surg 1997; 79-B:1008–1013.

54. Gross AE, Silverstein EA, Falk J, Falk R, Langer F. The allotransplantation of partial joints in the treatment of osteoarthritis of the knee. Clin Orthop 1975; 108:7–14.

55. McDermott AG, Langer F, Pritzker KP, Gross AE. Fresh small-fragment osteochondral allografts: long-term follow-up study on first 100 cases. Clin Orthop 1985; 197:96–102.

56. Rahfoth B, Weisser J, Sternkopp F, Aigner T, Von der Mark K, Brauer R. Transplantation of allograft chondrocytes embedded in agarose gel into cartilage defects of rabbits. Osteoarthr Cart 1998; 6:50–65.

57. Wakitani S, Goto T, Young RG, Mansour JM, Goldberg VM, Caplan AI. Repair of large full-thickness articular cartilage defects with allograft articular chondrocytes embedded in a collagen gel. Tiss Eng 1998; 4:429–444.

58. Kawamura S, Wakitani S, Kimura T, et al. Articular cartilage repair. rabbit experiment with a collagen gel-biomatrix and chondrocytes cultured in it. Acta Orthop Scand 1998; 69:56–62.

59. Wakitani S, Goto T, Pineda SJ, et al. Mesenchymal cell-based repair of large, full-thickness defects of articular cartilage. J Bone Joint Surg 1994; 76-A:579–592.

60. Johnstone B, Hering TM, Caplan AI, Goldberg VM, Yoo JU. In vitro chondrogenesis of bone marrow-derived mesenchymal progenitor cells. Exp Cell Res 1998; 238:265–272.

61. Friedenstein AJ, Gorskaja JF, Kulagina NN. Fibroblast precursors in normal and irradiated mouse hematopoietic organs. Exp Hematol 1976; 4:267–274.

62. Friedenstein AJ, Chailakhyan RK, Gerasimov UV. Bone marrow osteogenic stem cells: in vitro cultivation and transplantation in diffusion chambers. Cell Tissue Kinet 1987; 20:263–272.

63. Haynesworth SE, Goshima J, Goldberg VM, Caplan AI. Characterization of cells with osteogenic potential from human marrow. Bone 1992; 13:81–88.

64. Bruder SP, Fink DJ, Caplan AI. Mesenchymal stem cells in bone development, bone repair, and skeletal regeneration therapy. J Cell Biochem 1994; 56:283–294.

65. Johnstone B, Yoo JU. Autologous mesenchymal progenitor cells in articular cartilage repair. Clin Orthop 1999; 367 (suppl):S156–162.

66. Noth U, Osyczka A, Tuli R, Danielson KG, Tuan RS. Multipotential mesenchymal cell cultures derived from human trabecul bone, 47th Annual Meeting, Orthopaedic Research Society, February 25–28, 2001, San Francisco, 2001.

67. Bosch P, Musgrave DS, Lee JY, et al. Osteoprogenitor cells within skeletal muscle. J Orthop Res 2000; 18:933–944.

68. Zuk PA, Zhu M, Mizuno H, et al. Multilineage cells from human adipose tissue: implications for cell- based therapies. Tiss Eng 2001; 7:211–228.

69. Dennis JE, Merriam A, Awadallah A, Yoo JU, Johnstone B, Caplan A. A quadripotential mesenchymal progenitor cell isolated from the marrow of an adult mouse. J Biomed Mater Res 1999; 14:700–709.

70. Yoo JU, Mandell I, Angele P, Johnstone B. Chondrogenitor cells and gene therapy. Clin Orthop 2000; 379 (suppl):S164–170.

71. Evans CH, Ghivizzani SC, Smith P, Shuler FD, Mi Z, Robbins PD. Using gene therapy to protect and restore cartilage. Clin Orthop 2000; 379 (suppl):S214–219.

72. Murphy M, Kavalkovich K, Barry F. Distribution of injected mesenchymal stem cells in the osteoarthritic knee., 47th Annual Meeting, Orthopaedic Research Society, San Francisco, 2001.

73. Murphy M, Kavalkovich K, Fink D, Hunziker E, Barry F. Injected mesenchymal stem cells stimulate meniscal repair and protection of articular cartilage, 47th Annual Meeting, Orthopaedic Research Society, San Francisco, 2001.

74. Kavalokovich K, Murphy M, Barry F. Chondrogenic activity of mesenchymal stem cellls compared to articular chondrocytes, 47th Annual Meeting, orthopaedic Research Society, San Francisco, 2001.

75. Thomson JA, Itskovitz-Eldor J, Shapiro SS, et al. Embryonic stem cell lines derived from human blastocysts. Science 1998; 282:1145–1147.

76. Klug MG, Soonpaa MH, Koh GY, Field LJ. Genetically selected cardiomyocytes from differentiating embronic stem cells form stable intracardiac grafts. J Clin Invest 1996; 98:216–224.

77. Klug MG, Soonpaa MH, Field LJ. DNA synthesis and multinucleation in embryonic stem cell-derived cardiomyocytes. Am J Physiol 1995; 269: H1913–1921.

78. Nehrer S, Breinan HA, Ramappa A, et al. Chondrocyte-seeded collagen matrices implanted in a chondral defect in a canine model. Biomaterials 1998; 19:2313–2328.

79. Breinan HA, Martin SD, Hsu H-P, Spector M. Healing of canine articular cartilage defects treated with microfracture, a type II collagen matrix, or cultured autologous chondrocytes. J Orthop Res 2000; 18:781–789.

80. Bell E. Strategy for the selection of scaffolds for tissue engineering. Tiss Eng 1995; 1:163–179.

81. Cook JL, Kreeger JM, Payne JT, Tomlinson JL. Three-dimensional culture of canine articular chondrocytes on multiple transplantable substrates. Am J Vet Res 1997; 58:419–424.

82. Grande DA, Halberstadt C, Naughton G, Schwartz R, Manji R. Evaluation of matrix scaffolds for tissue engineering of articular cartilage grafts. J Biomed Mater Res 1997; 34:211–220.

83. Nehrer S, Breinan HA, Ramappa A, et al. Autologous chondrocyte-seeded type I and II collagen matrices implanted in a chondral defect in a canine model, Orthop Res Soc, New Orleans, LA, 1998.

84. Frenkel SR, Toolan B, Menche D, Pitman MI, Pachence JM. Chondrocyte transplantation using a collagen bilayer matrix for cartilage repair. J Bone Joint Surg 1998; 79-B:831–836.

85. Grande DA, Pitman MI, Peterson L, Menche D, Klein M. The repair of experimentally produced defects in rabbit articular cartilage by autologous chondrocyte transplantation. J Orthop Res 1989; 7:208–218.

86. Ponticiello MS, Schinagl RM, Kadiyala S, Barry FP. Gelatin-based resorbable sponge as a carrier matrix for human mesenchymal stem cells in cartilage regeneration therapy. J Biomed Mater Res 2000; 52:246–255.

87. Dounchis JS, Bae WC, Chen AC, Sah RL, Coutts RD, Amiel D. Cartilage repair with autogenic perichondrium cell and polylactic acid grafts [In Process Citation]. Clin Orthop 2000; 377:248–264.

88. von Schroeder HP, Kwan M, Amiel D, Coutts RD. The use of polylactic acid matrix and periosteal grafts for the reconstruction of rabbit knee articular defects. J Biomed Mater Res 1991; 25:329–339.

89. van Susante JL, Buma P, Homminga GN, van den Berg WB, Veth RP. Chondrocyte-seeded hydroxyapatite for repair of large articular cartilage defects: a pilot study in the goat. Biomaterials 1998; 19:2367–2374.

90. Lee CR, Grodzinsky AJ, Hsu H-P, Spector M. Effects of a cultured autologous chondrocyte-seeded type II collagen scaffold on the healing of a chondral defect in a canine model. J Orthop Res, 2003; 21:272–281.

91. O'Driscoll SW, Saris DB, Ito Y, Fitzimmons JS. The chondrogenic potential of periosteum decreases with age. J Orthop Res 2001; 19:95–103.

92. O'Driscoll SW, Fitzsimmons JS. The importance of procedure specific training in harvesting periosteum for chondrogenesis. Clin Orthop 2000; 380:269–278.

93. O'Driscoll SW, Salter RB. The induction of neochondrogenesis in free intra-articular periosteal antografts under the influence of continuous passive motion: an experimental study in the rabbit. J Bone Joint Surg 1984; 66A:1284–1257.

94. Carranza-Bencano A, Garcia-Paino L, Armas Padron JR, Cayuela Dominguez A. Neochondrogenesis in repair of full-thickness articular cartilage defects using free autogenous periosteal grafts in the rabbit. A follow-up in six months. Osteoarth Cartilage 2000; 8:351–358.

95. Zarnett R, Salter RB. Periosteal neochondrogenesis for biologically resurfacing joints: its cellular origin. Can J Surg 1989; 32:171–174.

96. Rubak JM. Reconstruction of articular cartilage defects with free periosteal grafts: an experimental study. Acta Orthop Scand 1982; 53:175–180.

97. Niedermann B, Boe S, Lauritzen J, Rubak JM. Glued periosteal grafts in the knee. Acta Orthop Scand 1985; 56:457–460.

98. Hoikka VE, Jaroma HJ, Ritsila VA. Reconstruction of the patellar articulation with periosteal grafts. 4- year follow-up of 13 cases. Acta Orthop Scand 1990; 61:36–39.

99. O'Driscoll SW, Salter RB. The induction of neochondrogenesis in free intra-articular periosteal autografts under the influence of continuous passive mation. An investigation in the rabbit. J Bone Joint Surg 1994; 66-B:1248–1257.

100. Ito Y, Sanyal A, Fitzsimmons JS, Mello MA, O'Driscoll SW. Histomorphological and proliferative characterization of developing periosteal neochondrocytes in vitro. J Orthop Res 2001; 19:405–413.

101. Ito Y, Fitzsimmons JS, Sanyal A, Mello MA, Mukherjee N, O'Driscoll SW. Localization of chondrocyte precursors in periosteum. Osteoarth Cartilage 2001; 9:215–223.

102. O'Driscoll SW, Keeley FW, Salter RB. The chondrogenic potential of free autogenous periosteal grafts for biological resurfacing of major full-thickness defects in joint surfaces under the influence of continuous passive motion: an experimental study in the rabbit. J Bone Joint Surg 1986; 68A:1017–1035.

103. Homminga GN, van der Linden TJ, Terwindt-Rouwenhorst EA, Drukker J. Repair of articular defects by perichondrial grafts: experiments in the rabbit. Acta Orthop Scand 1989; 60:326–329.

104. Homminga GN, Linden van der AJ, Terwindt-Rouwenhorst WAW, Drukker J. Repair of articular cartilage defects by perichondrial grafts. Experiments in the rabbit. Acta Orthop Scand 1989; 60.326–329.

105. Homminga GN, Bulstra SK, Kuijer R, van der Linden AJ. Repair of sheep articular cartilage defects with a rabbit costal perichondrial graft. Acta Orthop Scand 1991; 62:415–418.

106. Bouwmeester SJM, Beckers JMH, Kuijer R, van der Linden AJ, Bulstra SK. Long-term results of rib perichondrial grafts for repair of cartilage defects in the human knee. Int Orthop 1997:313–317.

107. Gross AE, Beaver RJ, Mohammed MN. Fresh small fragment osteochondral allografts used for post traumatic defects in the knee joint. In: Fineramann GAM, FR Noyes, eds. Biology and Biomechanics of the Traumatized Synovial Joint: The Knee as a Model. Rosemount, IL: American Academy of Orthopaedic Surgeons, 1992:123–141.

108. Bobic V. Arthroscopic osteochondral autograft transplantation in anterior cruciate ligament reconstruction: a preliminary clinical study. Knee Surg Sports Traumatol Arthrosc 1996; 3:262–264.

109. Hangody L, Kish G, Karpati Z, Udvarhelyi I, Szigeti I, Bely M. Mosaicplasty for the treatment of articular cartilage defects: application in clinical practice. Orthopedics 1998; 21:1–6.

110. Hangody L, Kish G, Karpati Z, Szerb I, Udvarhelyi I. Arthroscopic autogenous osteochondral mosaicplasty for the treatment of femoral condylar defects. Knee Surg Sports Traumatol Athrosc 1997; 5:262–267.

111. Hangody L, Karpati Z, Szigeti I, Sukosd L. Clinical experience with the Mosaic Technique. Rev Osteol 1996; 4:32–36.

112. Hangody L, Kish G, Karpati Z, Szerb I, Eberhardt R. Treatment of osteochondritis dissecans of the talus: use of the mosaicplasty technique—a preliminary report. Foot Ankle 1997; 18:628–634.

113. Nehrer S, Spector M, Minas T. Histologic analysis of tissue after failed cartilage repair procedures. Clin Orthop 1999; 365:149–162.

114. Bobic V. [Autologous osteo-chondral grafts in the management of articular cartilage lesions]. Orthopade 1999; 28:19–25.

115. Minas T. The role of cartilage repair techniques, including chondrocyte transplantation, in focal chondral knee damage. Instr Course Lect 1999; 48:629–643.

116. Minas T, Nehrer S. Current concepts in the treatment of articular cartilage defects. Orthopedics 1997; 20:525–538.

117. van Susante JL, Buma P, van Beuningen HM, van den Berg WB, Veth RP. Responsiveness of bovine chondrocytes to growth factors in medium with different serum concentrations. J Orthop Res 2000; 18:68–77.

118. de Haart M, Marijnissen WJ, van Osch GJ, Verhaar JA. Optimization of chondrocyte expansion in culture: effect of TGF beta-2, bFGF and L-ascorbic acid on bovine articular chondrocytes. Acta Orthop Scand 1999; 70:55–61.

119. Klein-Nulend J, Veldhuijzen JP, van de Stadt RJ, van Kampen GP, Kuijer R, Burger EH. Influence of intermittent compressive force on proteoglycan content in calcifying growth plate cartilage in vitro. J Biol Chem 1987; 262: 15490–15495.

120. Sittinger M, Schultz O, Keyszer G, Minuth WW, Burmester GR. Artificial tissues in perfusion culture. Int J Artif Organs 1997; 20:57–62.

121. Freed LE, Vunjak-Novakovic G, Langer R. Cultivation of cell-polymer cartilage implants in bioreactors. J Cell Biochem 1993; 51:257–264.

122. Freed LE, Langer R, Martin I, Pellis NR, Vunjak-Novakovic G. Tissue engineering of cartilage in space. Proc Natl Acad Sci USA 1997; 94:13885–13890.

123. Freed LE, Vunjak-Novakovic G. Microgravity tissue engineering. In Vitro Cell. Dev Biol Anim 1997; 33:281–285.

124. Freed LE, A.P. H, Martin I, Barry JR, Langer R, G. V-N. Chondrogenesis in a cell-polymer-bioreactor system. Exp Cell Res 1998; 240:58–65.

125. Baker TL, Goodwin TJ. Three-dimensional culture of bovine chondrocytes in rotating-wall vessels. In Vitro Cell. Dev Biol Anim 1997; 33:358–365.

126. Martin I, Obradovic B, Treppo S, et al. Modulation of the mechanical properties of tissue engineered cartilage. Biorheology 2000; 37:141–147.

127. Vunjak-Novakovic G, Martin I, Obradovic B, et al. Bioreactor cultivation conditions modulate the composition and mechanical properties of tissue-engineered cartilage. J Orthop Res 1999; 17:130–138.

128. Evans CH, Robbins PD. Genetically augmented tissue engineering of the musculoskeletal system. Clin Orthop Rel Res 1999:S1–S8.

129. Kang R, Ghivizzani SC, Muzzonigro TS, Herndon JH, Robbins PD, Evans CH. Orthopaedic applications of gene therapy: from concept to clinic. Clin Orthop 2000; 375:324–337.

130. Sandhu JS, Gorczynski RM, Waddell J, et al. Effect of interleukin-6 secreted by engineered human stromal cells on osteoclasts in human bone. Bone 1999; 24:217–227.

131. Kang R, Marui T, Ghivizzani SC, et al. Ex vivo gene transfer to chondrocytes in full-thickness articular cartilage defects: a feasibility study. Osteoarth Cart 1997; 5:139–143.

132. Gerich TG, Fu FH, Robbins PD, Evans CH. Prospects for gene therapy in sports medicine. Knee Surg Sports Traumatol Arthrosc 1996; 4:180–187.

133. Lou J, Tu Y, Ludwig FJ, Zhang J, Manske PR. Effect of bone morphogenetic protein-12 gene transfer on mesenchymal progenitor cells. Clin Orthop 1999; 369:333–339.

134. Nakamura N, Timmermann SA, Hart DA, et al. A comparison of in vivo gene delivery methods for antisense therapy in ligament healing. Gene Ther 1998; 5:1455–1461.
135. Goto H, Onodera T, Hirano H, Shimamura T. Hyaluronic acid suppresses the reduction of alpha2(VI) collagen gene expression caused by interleukin-1beta in cultured rabbit articular chondrocytes. Tohoku J Exp Med 1999; 187:1–13.
136. Nishida K, Kang JD, Gilbertson LG, et al. Modulation of the biologic activity of the rabbit intervertebral disc by gene therapy: an in vivo study of adeno-virus-mediated transfer of the human transforming growth factor beta 1 encoding gene. Spine 1999; 24.2419–2425.
137. Sah RL-Y, Kim Y-J, Doong J-YH, Grodzinsky AJ, Plaas AHK, Sandy JD. Biosynthetic response of cartilage explants to dynamic compression. J Orthop Res 1989; 7:619–636.
138. Buschmann M, Gluzband Y, Grodzinsky A, Hunziker E. Mechanical compression modulates matrix biosynthesis in chondrocyte/agarose culture. J Cell Sci 1995; 108:1497–1508.
139. Lee CR, Grodzinsky AJ, Spector M. . Effects of short term dynamic loading on adult canine chondrocytes seeded into porous collagen-glycosamino-glycan scaffolds. Trans Orthop Res Soc., San Francisco, 2001.

13

Tissue Engineering of Meniscus

Brian Johnstone, Jung Yoo, and Victor Goldberg
Case Western Reserve University, Cleveland, Ohio, U.S.A.

Peter Angele
University of Regensburg, Regensburg, Germany

I. INTRODUCTION

The meniscus has several important functions in the knee joint. In addition to its obvious load-bearing and shock absorption functions, the meniscus provides stability to the joint (1). The finding of nerve endings in the anterior and posterior horns of the menisci led to the suggestion that they also have a proprioceptive function (2,3). It has also been hypothesized that they may be involved in joint cartilage lubrication (4). Given the important functional roles of the meniscus, the ability to repair the damaged meniscus is an obvious clinical goal. The reparative properties of the meniscus are region-dependent, so various treatment strategies have been devised. In this chapter, we will describe the tissue engineering strategies that have been used to attempt repair and regeneration of various meniscal lesions. Meniscus tissue engineering research can be categorized as either augmentation of tear repair or larger block tissue replacement.

II. REGIONAL VARIATION OF MENISCUS STRUCTURE

Morphologically, the menisci are semilunar structures in the knee joint that overlay the tibial articular cartilage. They are attached peripherally to the joint capsule and their anterior and posterior horns are attached to the capsule, ligaments, and the tibial plateau in the intercondylar fossae. The menisci are wedge-shaped in cross section, with inside borders that taper to a free edge. Biochemically, the meniscus is composed mainly of collagen (70% of the dry weight), with 90% of this being type I collagen fibers. The remaining extracellular matrix consists of the other typical components of connective tissues, namely minor collagens, large and small proteoglycans, and noncollagenous proteins. There is some detectable type II collagen, so the meniscus is defined as a fibrocartilage. Ultrastructurally, there are three distinguishable collagenous matrix organizations. The superficial collagen fibers are small and woven into a mesh. There is a subjacent layer of thicker, but irregularly arranged, fibers. The inner region (the bulk of the meniscus) is composed of thick fiber bundles that are chiefly arranged circumferentially, but there are also radial fibers that appear to provide structural rigidity. This description of the meniscus is relatively consistent for larger animals and humans. In some animals, including the rabbit, the meniscus contains more type II collagen, concentrated in the inner zone, but varying in extent from posterior to anterior horns. This probably reflects the different mechanical forces that are present in rabbit knee joints.

Menisci are relatively avascular structures. Blood vessels penetrate only approximately the outer third of the medial meniscus and slightly less of the lateral meniscus (5). The peripheral zone of the meniscus is thus often referred to as the red-red zone. The middle third is termed the red-white zone, since there may be some blood vessel penetration. The inner third is denoted the white-white zone. This blood vessel distribution is important since it correlates with the regional differences in healing capability. Currently, injuries in the red-white zone are seen as clinically the most challenging, since their healing capability is difficult to judge and resection involves a significant portion of the meniscus.

III. HEALING PROPERTIES OF THE MENISCUS

A typical wound healing response occurs if there is injury in the outer vascular red-red zone of the meniscus (5). Initially, there is the creation of a fibrin clot. This is replaced by fibrovascular scar that will completely fill defects in the region and be eventually remodeled to normal meniscal tissue. In contrast, injuries in the avascular white-white zone do not heal. Because of this, surgeons have developed clinical indications for which types of meniscal injuries to attempt to repair with the techniques currently available. The current treatment of meniscal injury at or near the meniscal-synovial junction is surgical repair by direct approximation of the meniscus to surrounding tissue. These types of injuries are commonly associated with a tibial plateau fracture and resection of the meniscus is not recommended. The opposite end of the spectrum is the medial (inner) meniscal tear. These tears are treated by simple resection of the torn portions.

The current debate surrounding the most efficacious treatment of meniscal injuries concerns mid substance tears. These lesions are too large to resect without some alteration of meniscal function and the loss of joint stability, and conversely, they are too difficult to preserve because of poor healing potential. Surgeons must assess the relative vascularity of the torn portion of the meniscus to determine whether there is enough healing capacity of the lesion. If the vascularity appears poor by direct visualization (white-zone lesion), then resection is performed. Even if the tear is present in the vascular region, age and activity level of the patient may play an important role in the decision-making process. In general, those who are young and physically active are recommended to have a repair rather than a resection. In those patients with a completely detached large midsubstance meniscal lesion, the only option is a surgical resection of the detached piece. These patients and those who have had previous complete resection of the meniscus may be a candidate for meniscal replacement surgery. In the following sections, we will describe how tissue engineering has been applied to the area of meniscal repair and regeneration, noting the different strategies needed for the diverse types of injury.

IV. TISSUE ENGINEERING FOR MENISCAL TEARS

The clinical treatment of meniscal tears varies depending on the zone and extent of injury, but suturing of the tear is commonly done. Since this does not work well in the avascular zone, researchers have tried to enhance the healing response with a variety of additions to the wound site. How many of these alternative treatments can be really defined as tissue engineering is debatable, but most consist of inserting some kind of matrix into the repair site. The matrices may be modified with the inclusion of cells or growth factors. In 1988, Arnoczky et al. (6) placed autogenous fibrin clot into full-thickness lesions in the avascular portion of canine menisci. The model used 2-mm-diameter punch biopsy holes, and thus was not a model of a typical meniscal tear, but the fibrin clot was seen to provoke a healing response. Fibrin clot then began to be used clinically as an adjunct to meniscal tear repair with reported enhancement of reparative response and clincial outcome (7–9). The fibrin clot contains not only cells that may assist in the reparative process, but also growth factors that may stimulate both host and clot-introduced cells. However, the sucess of fibrin clot as an implant in healing meniscal tears appears zone-dependent (10) and long-term clinical outcome studies are still awaited. In one randomized prospective clinical study of 40 patients, intrameniscal fibrin clot addition provided a poorer clinical outcome at early follow-up than partial meniscectomy (11).

Since its introduction, researchers have attempted to enhance the fibrin clot's efficacy by considering the clot as a scaffold for delivery of growth factors or cells. Port et al. (12) added autogenous marrow-derived cells to an autologous fibrin clot in a goat model of a full-thickness lesion in the avascular zone. The addition did not alter the poor outcome of the repair found with fibrin alone. The extent to which the marrow cell population that was used contained at least a subpopulation of mesenchymal progenitor cells known to be in marrow (13–15) was not tested, so it is difficult to draw conclusions regarding the use of such cells for meniscal tears from this study. Commercially available fibrin, devoid of cells or intrinsic growth factors, has been used as a sealant for meniscal tears, and apparently enhanced the biomechanical properties of experimental meniscal tears in a rabbit model (16). In a small study, addition of endothelial growth factor to a commercial fibrin sealant was attempted with some implied success (17). Addition of marrow-derived cells to fibrin, presumably including mesenchymal progenitor cells, has also been tested and appeared to enhance healing in a full-thickness defect. In summary, data concerning the use of fibrin sealant for meniscal tear repair is not extensive, and the studies with additional components such as growth factors or cells are not rigorous. Thus, at this time, it is difficult to evaluate the efficacy of fibrin for meniscal tear repair.

Alternative surgical techniques have been created for treating meniscal tears, such as trephination (18–21) or insertion of a vascularized synovial flap into the tear (22), but few tissue engineering alternatives to fibrin-based additions have been attempted. Klompmaker et al. (23–25) did a series of in vivo animal studies with a porous polyurethane scaffold implanted into a wedge-shaped defect extending form the periphery through a longitudinal lesion. It was hypothesized that such an implant would promote both vascular and mesenchymal cell ingrowth from the periphery into the surgically created tear site. The approach taken by this group is interesting because they attempted to build on the idea of regeneration from the periphery, rather than treating the isolated tear or replacing inner meniscus as far out as the tear. The potential risk with such an approach is that a large portion of apparently intact tissue must be removed, so failure of the implant could lead to complete meniscus breakdown. The results indicated that fibrocartilage, rather than the typical fibrous tissue, was found in the repair site. The group has since modified the implant in an attempt to decrease the problems associated with toxic breakdown products of the polyurethane (26). The use of polymeric scaffolds has been extended by several groups, but has been used for the creation of larger meniscal implants, for meniscal replacement rather than tear repair.

V. TISSUE ENGINEERING FOR MENISCAL TISSUE REPLACEMENT

Currently, few options are available to the surgeon for replacement of either portions or the whole meniscus. Total allograft replacement of the meniscus is being done, but it is difficult to assess the success of the studies done to date (for recent review see Ref. (27)). Concerns about immunogenicity, long-term viability, and shrinkage have limited the use of these implants. As alternatives to allograft, researchers have experimented with other tissues as autograft meniscus replacements. Animal model studies with tendon and fat pad indicated that these tissues might provide some cartilage protection initially, but do not remodel appropriately to produce functional meniscal tissue (28,29). Tissues with obvious mesenchymal progenitor cell populations, such as periosteum and perichondrium, have also been tried. Walsh et al. (30) created a partial defect in the rabbit medial meniscus and implanted a periosteal autograft. The autograft underwent

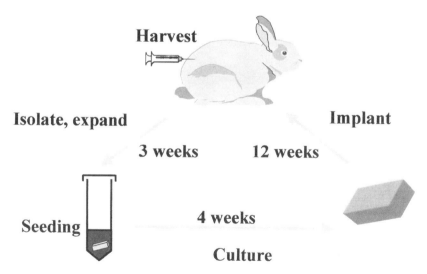

FIGURE 1 Scheme for tissue engineering of cartilage implants for partial meniscal replacement.

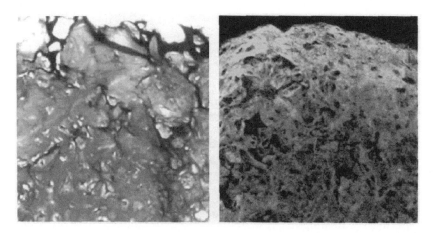

FIGURE 2 Sections of tissue-engineered cartilage stained (A) with toluidine blue and (B) immunohistochemically for type II collagen. The tissue was created from mesenchymal progenitor cells seeded into a composite bio-degradable matrix. (Reproduced with permission from Ref. 45.)

endochondral ossification in the center with a hyaline cartilage cap accelerating degenerative changes in those joints when compared with natural repair controls. This compares with results obtained by Bruns et al. (31), who noted areas of calcification in the center of perichondrial tissue used as a meniscal implant. The results illustrate the point that simply placing cells/tissues with differentiation potential into the appropriate biochemical and biochemical milieu, the joint space in this case, is not sufficient to produce the appropriate differentiation and tissue formation. There are several possible reasons for this. Since the initial biomechanical parameters of the implanted tissues were inferior, the cells may have received different signals to those required for appropriate differentiation and creation of a meniscal matrix. It may also be true that the differentiation potential of the cells used was restricted, or that the vascularity of the tissue, and perhaps its potential to be further vascularized inappropriately, contributed to the improper differentiation.

FIGURE 3 Meniscus repair in New Zealand White rabbits. Gross morphology of defects in the pars intermedia of the medial meniscus after 12 weeks. (A) Empty defect. (B) Empty scaffold implant. (C) Tissue-engineered cell-composite scaffold implant. Box indicates defect area. Note the extensive regenerated tissue in (C).

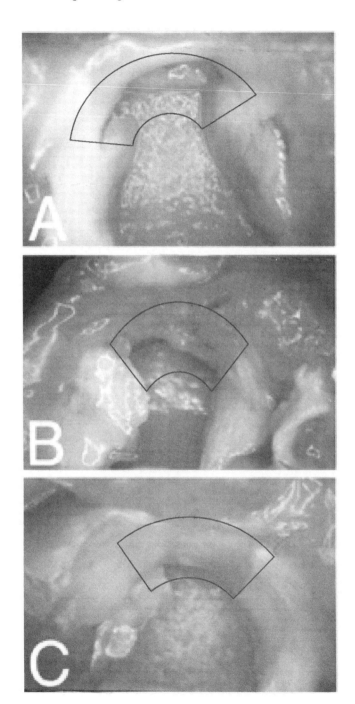

As alternatives to autograft tissue implants, there have been several studies of polymeric scaffolds and various composite matrices as meniscal tissue replacements. An early preliminary report concerning the use of a Teflon net indicated that there may be potential benefit from the use of such matrices (32), although no further reports concerning that matrix have appeared. Wood et al. (33) fabricated a polyester-carbon fiber meniscus prosthesis consisting of concentrically stacked hoops of carbon fibers with a woven polyester fiber sheath. Unfortunately, the implant fragmented in some knees and did little to promote regeneration. Sommerlath and Gillquist (34–36) investigated the utility of a Dacron meniscus prosthesis in rabbits. They found some ingrowth of tissue into the implant and some initial cartilage-protecting effect, but this effect did not continue long-term.

Biodegradable scaffolds have also been investigated and there is ongoing work with several types, including copolymeric constructs of polyglycolic and polylactic acid (37). More extensive work has been done with a collagen-based meniscal implant (38–42). The implant is actually a copolymeric scaffold, consisting of bovine Achilles tendon collagen cross-linked with glycosaminoglycans (40). The animal studies used the implant as a replacement for 80% of the meniscus, leaving a peripheral ring for attachment. Fibrocartilage formation occurred in the implants and meniscal regeneration was evident at 1 year. Only limited clinical experience has been reported and long-term survival is not yet known, but the implant may have some clinical utility for large meniscus defects. A comprehensive multicenter trial is ongoing. Recently, another collagenous biomaterial derived from porcine small intestine submucosa has been studied as a meniscal block replacement (43,44). In two small studies in dogs and rabbits, the submucosa derivative was sutured into meniscal defects. The preliminary results indicated tissue ingrowth and retention of the grafts. These studies show the potential of tissue engineering for meniscal repair, but it is unclear whether scaffold alone is sufficient for meniscal replacement.

A more complicated approach involves the use of cell-scaffold combinations. In the study of Walsh et al. (30), in which periosteum was used as a replacement tissue, alternatives including a type I collagen sponge, or the same sponge loaded with autologous, bone-marrow-derived mesenchymal stem cells, were also used. The collagen sponge functioned as a scaffold that resulted in more abundant fibrous repair tissue, but with marrow-derived mesenchymal stem cells added, fibrocartilage was detected in some specimens. Taking this idea a step further, Angele et al. used tissue engineering methods to create cartilage in vitro with these cells (45) prior to implantation into large meniscal defects (46). A complete resection of the pars intermedia of the medical meniscus was performed in New Zealand White rabbits and the defect was repaired with a composite scaffold containing cartilage (Fig. 1). To create the implant, autologous bone-marrow-derived mesenchymal progenitor cells were seeded into a biodegradable composite matrix of hyaluronan and gelatin and cultured in a chondrogenic medium for 14 days prior to implantation (Fig. 2). Empty defects had only a muted healing response, with fibrous tissue appearing only at the meniscal edges (Fig. 3). Some fibrocartilage formed in some of the composite scaffolds implanted without cell seeding, but the outcome was not significantly different form that of the empty controls. In contrast, cell-loaded, precultured implants integrated well with the surrounding host tissue and 8 of 11 defects contained meniscus-like fibrocartilage, compared with 2 of 11 controls. The mean cross-sectional width of the cellular implants was significantly wider than that of the controls. However, the cartilage protection was minimal and degeneration was seen. The study did demonstrate the feasibility of creating a large tissue-engineered cartilage implant and the use of such an implant for the repair of a significant meniscal defect. The potential drawback to this type of therapy is that the procedure is time and labor-intensive (Fig. 1). For this reason, alternatives such as growth factor–scaffold combinations or gene transfer may prove more useful. There is work indicating the effects of growth factors on meniscal cells (47–50), and some preliminary work with gene therapy techniques (51,52), but no full in vivo studies where these were used for large meniscal defects, either alone or with scaffolds. Undoubtedly, this is an area where meniscal repair experimentation will be expanded in the future. At present it is unclear which tissue engineering techniques will ultimately succeed in producing functional meniscus tissue, but this is a worthy goal given the present lack of choices for the patient with meniscal injuries.

REFERENCES

1. DeHaven KE, Arnoczky SP. Meniscus repair: basic science, indications for repair, and open repair. Instr Course Lect 1994; 43:65–76.
2. O'Connor BL, McConnaughey JS. The structure and innervation of cat knee menisci, and their relation to a "sensory hypothesis" of meniscal function. Am J Anat 1978; 153:431–442.
3. Wilson AS, Legg PG, McNeur JC. Studies on the innervation of the medical meniscus in the human knee joint. Anat Rec 1969; 165:485–491.
4. Arnoczky SP, Adams ME, DeHaven K, Eyre D. V.C.M. Meniscus. In: SL-Y Woo, J Buckwalter, eds. Injury and Repair of the Musculoskeletal Soft Tissues. Park Ridge, IL: American Academy of Orthopaedic Surgeons, 1988.
5. Arnoczky SP, Warren RF. The microvasculature of the meniscus and its response to injury: an experimental study in the dog. Am J Sports Med 1983; 11:131–141.

6. Arnoczky SP, Warren RF, Spivak JM. Meniscal repair using an exogenous fibrin clot. An experimental study in dogs. J Bone Joint Surg Am 1988; 70:1209–1217.
7. Henning CE, Lynch MA, Yearout KM, Vequist SW, Stallbaumer RJ, Decker KA. Arthroscopic meniscal repair using an exogenous fibrin clot. Clin Orthop 1990:64–72.
8. Cannon WD Jr, Morgan CD. Meniscal repair: arthroscopic repair techniques. Instr Course Lect 1994; 43:77–96.
9. van Trommel MF, Simonian PT, Potter HG, Wickiewicz TL. Arthroscopic meniscal repair with fibrin clot of complete radial tears of the lateral meniscus in the avascular zone. Arthroscopy 1998; 14:360–365.
10. McAndrews PT, Arnoczky SP. Meniscal repair enhancement techniques. Clin Sports Med 1996; 15:499–510.
11. Biedert RM. Treatment of intrasubstance meniscal lesions: a randomized prospective study of four different methods. Knee Surg Sports Traumatol Arthrosc 2000; 8:104–108.
12. Port J, Jackson DW, Lee TQ, Simon TM. Meniscal repair supplemented with exogenous fibrin clot and autogenous cultured marrow cells in the goat model. Am J Sports Med 1996; 24:547–555.
13. Friedenstein AJ. Precursor cells of mechanocytes. Int Rev Cytol 1976; 47:327–355.
14. Owen M. The origin of bone cells in the postnatal organism. Arthritis Rheum 1980; 23:1073–1080.
15. Caplan AI. The mesengenic process. Clin Plast Surg 1994; 21:429–435.
16. Roeddecker K, Muennich U, Nagelschmidt M. Meniscal healing: a biomechanical study. J Surg Res 1994; 56:20–27.
17. Hashimoto J, Kurosaka M, Yoshiya S, Hirohata K. Meniscal repair using fibrin sealant and endothelial cell growth factor: an experimental study in dogs. Am J Sports Med 1992; 20:537–541.
18. Zhang ZN, Tu KT, Xu YK, Zhang WM, Liu ZT, Ou SH. Treatment of longitudinal injuries in avascular area of meniscus in dogs by trephination. Arthroscopy 1988; 4:151–159.
19. Fox JM, Rintz KG, Ferkel RD. Trephination of incomplete meniscal tears. Arthroscopy 1993; 9:451–455.
20. Zhang Z, Arnold JA, Williams T, McCann B. Repairs by trephination and suturing of longitudinal injuries in the avascular area of the meniscus in goats. Am J Sports Med 1995; 23:35–41.
21. Shelbourne KD, Rask BP. The sequelae of salvaged nondegenerative peripheral vertical medial meniscus tears with anterior cruciate ligament reconstruction. Arthroscopy 2001; 17:270–274.
22. Gershuni DH, Skyhar MJ, Danzig LA, Camp J, Hargens AR, Akeson WH. Experimental models to promote healing of tears in the avascular segment of canine knee menisci. J Bone Joint Surg Am 1989; 71:1363–1370.
23. Klompmaker J, Jansen HW, Veth RP, Nielsen HK, de Groot JH, Pennings AJ. Porous implants for knee joint meniscus reconstruction: a preliminary study

on the role of pore sizes in ingrowth and differentiation of fibrocartilage. Clin Mater 1993; 14:1–11.

24. Klompmaker J, Jansen HW, Veth RP, et al. Meniscal repair by fibrocartilage? An experimental study in the dog. J Orthop Res 1992; 10:359–370.

25. Klompmaker J, Jansen HW, Veth RP, de Groot JH, Nijenhuis AJ, Pennings AJ. Porous polymer implant for repair if meniscal lesions: a preliminary study in dogs. Biomaterials 1991; 12:810–816.

26. de Groot JH, de Vrijer R, Pennings AJ, Klompmaker J, Veth RP, Jansen HW. Use of porous polyurethanes for meniscal reconstruction and meniscal prostheses. Biomaterials 1996; 17:163–173.

27. Rodeo SA. Meniscal allografts—where do we stand? Am J Sports Med 2001; 29:246–261.

28. Kohn D, Wirth CJ, Reiss G, et al. Medical meniscus replacement by a tendon autograft. Experiments in sheep. J Bone Joint Surg Br 1992; 74:910–917.

29. Kohn D, Rudert M, Wirth CJ, Plitz W, Reiss G, Maschek H. Medical meniscus replacement by a fat pad autograft: an experimental study in sheep. Int Orthop 1997; 21:232–238.

30. Walsh CJ, Goodman D, Caplan AI, Goldberg VM. Meniscus regeneration in a rabbit partial meniscectomy model. Tissue Eng 1999; 5:327–337.

31. Bruns J, Kahrs J, Kampen J, Behrens P, Plitz W. Autologous perichondral tissue for meniscal replacement. J Bone Joint Surg Br 1998; 80:918–923.

32. Toyonaga T, Uezaki N, Chikama H. Substitute meniscus of Teflon-net for the knee joint of dogs. Clin Orthop 1983:291–297.

33. Wood DJ, Minns RJ, Strover A. Replacement of the rabbit medical meniscus with a polyester-carbon fibre bioprosthesis. Biomaterials 1990; 11:13–16.

34. Sommerlath K, Gillquist J. The effects of an artificial meniscus substitute in a knee joint with a resected anterior cruciate ligament: an experimental study in rabbits. Clin Orthop 1993:276–284.

35. Sommerlath KG, Gillquist J. The effect of anterior cruciate ligament resection and immediate or delayed implantation of a meniscus prosthesis on knee joint biomechanics and cartilage: an experimental study in rabbits. Clin Orthop 1993:267–275.

36. Sommerlath K, Gillquist J. The effect of a meniscal prosthesis on knee biomechanics and cartilage: an experimental study in rabbits. Am J Sports Med 1992; 20:73–81.

37. Ibarra C, Koski JA, Warren RF. Tissue engineering meniscus: cells and matrix. Orthop Clin North Am 2000; 31:411–418.

38. Stone KR, Steadman JR, Rodkey WG, Li ST. Regeneration of meniscal cartilage with use of a collagen scaffold: analysis of preliminary data. J Bone Joint Surg Am 1997; 79:1770–1777.

39. Stone KR, Rodkey WG, Webber RJ, McKinney L, Steadman JR. Future directions: collagen-based prostheses for meniscal regeneration. Clin Orthop 1990:129–135.

40. Stone KR, Roadkey WG, Webber R, McKinney L, Steadman JR. Meniscal regeneration with copolymeric collagen scaffolds: in vitro and in vivo studies

evaluated clinically, histologically, and biochemically. Am J Sports Med 1992; 20:104–111.

41. Rodkey WG, Steadman JR, Li ST. A clinical study of collagen meniscus implants to restore the injured meniscus. Clin Orthop 1999:S281–292.

42. Rodkey WG. Basic biology of the meniscus and response to injury. Instr Course Lect 2000; 49:189–193.

43. Cook JL, Tomlinson JL, Kreeger JM, Cook CR. Induction of meniscal regeneration in dogs using a novel biomaterial. Am J Sports Med 1999; 27:658–665.

44. Gastel JA, Muirhead WR, Lifrak JT, Fadale PD, Hulstyn MJ, Labrador DP. Meniscal tissue regeneration using a collagenous biomaterial derived from porcine small intestine submucosa. Arthroscopy 2001; 17:151–159.

45. Angele P, Kujat R, Nerlich M, Yoo J, Goldberg V, Johnstone B. Engineering of osteochondral tissue with bone marrow mesenchymal progenitor cells in a derivatized hyaluronan-gelatin composite sponge. Tissue Eng 1999; 5:545–554.

46. Angele P, Johnstone B, Kujat R, Nerlich M, Goldberg V, Yoo J. Meniscus repair with mesenchymal progenitor cells in a biodegradable composite matrix. Trans Orthop Res Soc 2000; 25:605.

47. Collier S, Ghosh P. Effects of transforming growth factor beta on proteoglycan synthesis by cell and explant cultures derived from the knee joint meniscus. Osteoarthritis Cartilage 1995; 3:127–138.

48. Spindler KP, Mayes CE, Miller RR, Imro AK, Davidson JM. Regional mitogenic response of the meniscus to platelet-derived growth factor (PDGF-AB). J Orthop Res 1995; 13:201–207.

49. Bhargava MM, Attia ET, Murrell GA, Dolan MM, Warren RF, Hannafin JA. The effect of cytokines on the proliferation and migration of bovine meniscal cells. Am J Sports Med 1999; 27:636–643.

50. Tanaka T, Fujii K, Kumagae Y. Comparison of biochemical characteristics of cultured fibrochondrocytes isolated from the inner and outer regions of human meniscus. Knee Surg Sports Traumatol Arthrosc 1999; 7:75–80.

51. Goto H, Shuler FD, Lamsam C, et al. Transfer of lacZ marker gene to the meniscus. J Bone Joint Surg Am 1999; 81:918–925.

52. Nakata K, Shino K, Hamada M, et al. Human meniscus cell: characterization of the primary culture and use for tissue engineering. Clin Orthop 2001; S208–218.

14

Tissue Engineering of Intervertebral Disc

Jung Yoo and Brian Johnstone
Research Institute of University Hospitals and
Case Western Reserve University, Cleveland, Ohio, U.S.A.

I. INTRODUCTION

Degeneration of the intervertebral disc is one of the greatest health problems of the modern industrial age. It is one of the few health problems that result in disability for both the young adult population and the elderly. Despite the fact that this condition causes the loss of billions of dollars from the economy, it is poorly studied. Furthermore, the treatments advanced to date, none being particularly successful, have not focused on the regeneration of new and healthy intervertebral discs.

At present, the most common surgical treatments of this condition consist of either anterior spinal fusion, which eliminates the painful intervertebral disc altogether (replacing the disc with bone), or posterior fusion, which never addresses the diseased disc directly but rather attempts to bypass its function. The creation of new bone during spinal fusion can be viewed as the earliest used of tissue engineering. Tremendous progress has been made in this area, including the introduction of bone-conducting agents and, recently, powerful growth factors, which can induce progenitor cell differentiation into bone cells and the creation of bone de novo. Although spinal fusion can be an effective treatment, the greater load and stresses placed on adjacent discs can result in their premature degeneration (1).

The intervertebral disc has a number of important functions in the spine. It allows multidirectional motion but also provides stability. In addition, it has load-bearing and shock absorption functions. Although joint arthroplasty has been very successful in the treatment of peripheral joints such as hips or knees, the development of artificial intervertebral discs has not been successful and remains at an experimental level. Artificial discs made with similar materials to those used for artificial peripheral joints may provide stability and motion, but have not produced the shock absorption properties of the natural disc. Thus, if disc replacement is to be successful, it requires not only new designs but also new materials as well. Given the important functional roles of the intervertebral disc, the regeneration and repair of degenerated discs are obvious clinical goals. However, the challenges involved in the creation of artificial discs are enormous.

Tissue engineering of the intervertebral disc is complex because disc degeneration involves different regions of the intervertebral disc that have different properties. Although much attention has been given to alterations in the nucleus pulposus being the main facet of intervertebral disc degeneration, the process involves all the components of the disc/vertebral body complex including annulus fibrosus, cartilaginous endplate, and subchondral bone as well as the nucleus pulposus. Therefore, it may be overly simplistic to imagine that regeneration of a single component such as the nucleus pulposus can solve the entire problem of disc degeneration. At same time, it may not be possible to facilitate regeneration of all components of the degenerated intervertebral disc with the technology currently available for tissue engineering. In this chapter, we will describe the pathological anatomy of the degenerated intervertebral disc and possible tissue engineering strategies that may be useful in repair and regeneration of these components.

II. DISC DEGENERATION

A. Nucleus Pulposus

One of the most important physical properties of a normal intervertebral disc is thought to be the hydrophilic nature of the nucleus pulposus. This is due to the presence of highly negatively charged glycosaminoglycan-rich proteoglycans. The resulting mucopolysaccharide gel formed from the mixture of water and proteoglycan enables isotrophic loading of the nucleus pulposus. The earliest recognizable magnetic resonance imaging (MRI) of disc degeneration is the early loss of water from that structure. This is due to loss of proteoglycans from the disc. Proteoglycans are lost with both aging and degeneration, making it is more difficult to distinguish those changes that are due to degeneration, but MRI can show interpretable differences.

Histologically, as the degeneration proceeds, the nucleus loses its gel-like appearance. The border between the nucleus and annulus becomes less distinguishable as the nucleus becomes more fibrous. This fibrous matrix is mainly collagen. The major fibrillar collagen of the healthy nucleus pulposus is type II collagen. However, both with aging and with degeneration, there is a significant increase in type I collagen. There is also a noted increase in type III collagen, both the nucleus pulposus and annulus fibrosus, with degeneration (2,3). In addition to these synthetic changes, there are increases in degradative events. With aging, there is an accumulation of proteoglycan breakdown products and the percentage of denatured type II collagen increases (2,3), but it is unclear what contribution these make to the initiation of disc degeneration. Increased matrix degradation during disc degeneration is observed in the nucleus pulposus and clearly, the loss of nucleus pulposus matrix will alter the ability of the disc to respond appropriately to mechanical loads. However, the sequence of biochemical events in the nucleus pulposus that are involved in the initiation of disc degeneration is presently unclear.

B. Annulus Fibrosus

The annulus fibrosus is mainly collagen fibers arranged in a highly organized lamellar structure. With degeneration and age, separation of fibers can occur and a cyst-like cavity forms. It is thought that this can develop into an annular tear (4). These defects in the annulus most frequently involve the posterolateral region where the number of collagen fibers is greatly reduced (6,7) and these changes have been described in patients as young as 14 years old (8). These posterolateral tears frequently occur without breaching the annulus completely. However, isolated lateral or anterior annular rupture in the absence of posterior annular involvement is not observed.

With the development of cysts and annular tears, the radial tensile properties of the annulus fibrosus are reduced. Degenerated discs have been shown to have approximately 30% decrease in yield and ultimate strength compared with normal discs (5). The motions are increased by the presence of tears in the annulus fibrosus when torque is applied to the motion segment. Tears of the annulus fibrosus have a greater effect on axial rotation than on flexion, extension, or lateral bending (9). This abnormal motion not only affects the intervertebral disc but can lead to increased contact forces on the facet joint leading to facet arthritis.

The intervertebral disc is the largest avascular and aneural structure in the body. However, with degeneration, blood vessel invasion has been noted (12). In the healthy disc, only the outer third of the annulus fibrosus is innervated. However, nerve ingrowth into the degenerate disc has been described (10). Extension of nerves into the inner third of the annulus fibrosus and even into the nucleus pulposus was documented in the discs of individuals with chronic low back pain. The presence of substance P in these nerve fibres suggests that they may play an important role in pain production (10). Strategies for regenerating intervertebral discs may have to consider the prevention of ingrowth of both blood vessels and nerves. This may be a particular problem for strategies involving growth factors that stimulate endochondral ossification, since the presence of blood vessels could lead to ossification of the disc.

C. Endplates

Although solute transport can occur through either the endplate or the annulus fibrosus, most of the nutritional supply to the nucleus pulposus comes through the endplates (11,12). Therefore, subtle changes in the endplate may interfere with the overall health of the disc. The proteoglycans within the endplate regulate solute transport into and out of the disc. Thus, a healthy cartilage endplate may prevent fragments of osmotically active proteoglycans from leaving the disc. Conversely, the transport of the nutritionally important small solutes is increased when the endplates are healthier and a greater proteoglycan concentration is present (13).

Fissures and breaches in the endplate increase with age and degeneration (14). With aging, there is also an increased calcification of the cartilaginous endplate, which may decrease solute transport and lead to disc degeneration. It is likely that pathological sclerosis of the trabecular bone found adjacent to the degenerated discs significantly interferes with the nutritional pathway of the disc as well (15). Therefore, it is imperative that any strategies of regeneration or repair must take into consideration all the unique components of the intervertebral disc and the vertebral body if it is to be successful.

III. HEALING PROPERTIES OF THE INTERVERTEBRAL DISC

A. Nucleus Pulposus

Degenerated nucleus pulposus may have a limited ability to regenerate. Clinically, there has never been a report of any injured or degenerated intervertebral disc wholly reconstituting itself. It is unlikely that any significant regeneration can take place once symptomatic degeneration is present. In animal models where nucleus pulposus matrix depletion has been initiated by chymopapain injection (19), there is partial reconstitution of the matrix. However, these experiments are done in animals with healthy discs where the cells of nucleus pulposus retain sufficient ability to restore the depleted matrix over time. This may be due to the presence of notochordal cells in the nucleus pulposus of these animals, unlike the situation in human discs, in which notochordal cells are lost by puberty (21)

B. Annulus Fibrosus

A typical wound healing requires formation of fibrin clot and then replacement of this clot by cells brought into the site of injury. In the meniscus, another fibrocartilage of the body, peripheral tears of the meniscus can repair by the porgenitor cells brought to the site of injury by the new blood vessels. However, the fibrocartilaginous annulus fibrosus is avascular, with cells encased in an expansive extracellular matrix and thus not easily mobilized to effect repair of the injured region. Fibrovascular scar formation has been noted within the annulus fibrosus but formation of the scar may actually be detrimental to the function of this normally avascular structure.

C. Endplate

The cartilaginous endplates of the intervertebral disc are hyaline cartilage with no perichomdrium since they are directly connected to vertebral bone on one side and annulus fibrosus and nucleus pulposus on the other side. Thus, it is unlikely that they have much regenerative potential. There is no literature describing any form of healing in the endplate's structure, but this area has not received much scrutiny.

IV. TISSUE ENGINEERING FOR DEGENERATED INTERVERTEBRAL DISC

At present, there is no treatment designed to regenerate or repair an entire intervertebral disc using tissue engineering strategies. Total allograft replacement of the intervertebral disc has been proposed (17), but unless the concerns of immunogenicity and long-term viability are addressed, this implant will have no use in the treatment of disc degeneration. It is unlikely that cells within such a large allograft can survive the reimplantation process, as suggested by animal studies indicating the allograft disc would undergo rapid degeneration (23).

The complicated structural arrangement of the intervertebral disc makes tissue engineering of an entire disc a very difficult task at this time. Therefore, strategies of repair and regeneration have focused on individual components of the intervertebral disc. However, it should be noted that scientific work focused on the regeneration or repair of any component of the disc has been little compared with the work done on regeneration of articular or meniscal cartilage.

Tissue engineering strategies including growth factors, cells, and scaffolds have all been employed for regeneration or repair of degenerated nucleus pulposus in the few studies that have been done. Early studies in vitro indicated that cells isolated from both normal and degenerated nucleus pulposus responded to TGF-β1 by increasing proteoglycan production (24,25). Thus, growth factor introduction into the disc may be of use for regeneration, since the earliest changes seen in disc degeneration are generally loss of proteoglycan and subsequent loss of water from the nucleus pulposus. Replenishment of proteoglycan may re-establish the normal viscoelastic properties of the nucleus pulposus. A problem with this approach is the possible need for a more sustained concentration of any bioactive factor introduced. To this end, Kang and co-workers have attempted to use gene transfer techniques (26). They noted a sustained expression of the lacZ reporter gene after injection of adenoviral vector containing the lacZ gene into healthy rabbit discs (18) and then increased proteoglycan production from cells of discs injected with TGF-β1 transgene in the same vector (27). It should be noted that the various growth factor strategies all assume that there is a sufficient number of healthy cells in the nucleus pulposus that can respond to exogenously introduced growth factors. Depending on the extent of degeneration, this may not be true.

This is the basis of nucleus pulposus regeneration that involves introduction of healthy cell into the nucleus pulposus. In a series of reports, Mochida et al. transplanted nucleus pulposus cells in animal models of disc degeneration (29,31). In studies in rat tail and rabbit discs, they transplanted nucleus pulposus tissue and reported a delay in the destruction of disc architecture and greater elaboration of type II collagen as assessed immunohistochemically (29). However, when isolated cells (presumably mostly notochordal cells) were used, the results were less impressive (31), indicating the possibility that the main effect is due to the reintroduction of extracellular matrix that augments the structure of the disc. This idea is the basis for the other attempts at tissue engineering within the nucleus pulposus—the use of artificial matrices to provide structure in a degenerating disc.

Although the cells of nucleus pulposus have been grown in a variety of matrices in vitro (22,23) and in vivo in nude mice subcutaneously (34), there is no in vivo animal or clinical study that has introduced both cell and matrix into the nucleus pulposus. However, various matrices support nucleus cells in culture, including matrices of hyaluronan and fibrin (23). In vitro, the most commonly used matrix has been alginate, which appears to facilitate maintenance of nucleus cell phenotype (22). However, Kusior et al. noted that polyglyolic acid polymer scaffolds facilitated more nucleus pulposus matrix elaboration than alginate in vivo, in implants placed sub-cutaneously in nude mice (34).

Growth factor, cell-based, or implant strategies may facilitate nucleus pulposus regeneration, but the assumption is that the rest of the intervertebral disc is healthy. Therefore, the most effective use of these techniques may be in the treatment of those discs that demonstrate early loss of matrix from the nucleus pulposus, as detectable by T2-weighted MRI images. However, once the collapse of the disc and degenerative changes in the annulus fibrosus and endplates are present, it is unclear that the greater production of the matrix macromolecules in the nucleus pulposus will restore the disc to normal state.

V. TISSUE ENGINEERING FOR DEGENERATED OR INJURED ANNULUS FIBROSUS

At this time, no one has proposed a replacement of an entire degenerated annulus fibrosus with a tissue-engineered implant. The forces that are borne by the intervertebral disc are large and the hoop stresses placed on the annulus fibrosus under pressure make production of a suitable implant an extremely difficult task. It is unlikely that a large matrix alone or a cell-matrix implant made using current technology would be sufficient to withstand such stress without significant deformation while regeneration takes place.

At present, the only clinically useful tissue engineering strategy for annulus fibrosus repair may be to facilitate repair of surgically created annular defects. Such defects are always created after the resection of posterior annulus following the surgical discectomy of a herniated disc. These annular defects may reconstitute or heal inadequately, leading to a recurrent disc herniation through the same defect (24). There can be replacement of the annular defect with scar, but frequently the scar does not provide enough of a structural barrier to prevent recurrent disc hernia-tion. This is one of the most frequent complications following surgical discectomy with the rate of recurrent disc herniation reported to be as high as 7.3% (25). Frequently, recurrent disc herniation is an early phenomenon after surgery but can also occur decades later.

The strategy to regenerate a surgically removed portion of the annulus fibrosus could employ all the currently available techniques of cartilaginous tissue regeneration. These include implantation of a suitable matrix than can facilitate local cellular response or implantation of cell/matrix composite to form a new fibrocartilaginous tissue. However, at this time, there are no reports of such a strategy being used for annular regeneration. Therefore, the discussion of possible strategies must be based on what has been learned from the repair and regeneration of the other cartilaginous tissues.

One possible matrix to be used is fibrin. During spine surgery, fibrin is frequently used to prevent cerebrospinal fluid leak after accidental surgical durotomy. No adverse reaction to fibrin has been reported. Arnoczky et al. (37) reported use of autogenous fibrin clot in the repair of a meniscal defect in a dog model. The punch model used is actually unlike a typical meniscal tear, but much like an annular defect. They found improved repair when fibrin clot was introduced into the defect, suggesting possible utility of such material in annular repair. Other matrices with possible utility include both natural and man-made scaffolds. These matrices have been used to facilitate repair and regeneration of fibrocartilaginous meniscus and they may be useful in the regeneration of annulus fibrosus, which is also a fibrocartilaginous tissue. These scaffolds include man-made scaffolds, such as polyglycolic and polylactic acid (34,38), and scaffolds made of natural polymers, such as bovine tendon collagen cross-linked with glycosaminoglycans (39),(40). Animal and clinical studies with implants that faciliate more complete repair of the annular defect are needed. At this time, no biocompatible and bioregenerative scaffold technology exists that can facilitate whole annulus fibrosus production in vivo or in vitro.

VI. SUMMARY

There has been little progress in the field of intervertebral disc tissue engineering. Despite the potentially enormous market for appropriately designed strategies, the area suffers from a lack of scientific interest. The reasons for this include the difficulty of working with the very acellular, avascular tissues that make up the disc-vertebrae complex and the lack of understanding of either normal disc cell biology or the etiology of degeneration. There is also a lack of good animal models of disc degeneration. In addition, any regenerative or repair strategy in the spine must contend with the large and varied biomechanical forces that are constantly placed on the disc. Regenerative tissue engineering of the intervertebral disc is an immense challenge.

REFERENCES

1. Hilibrand AS, Carlson GD, Palumbo MA, Jones PK, Bohlman HH. Radiculo-pathy and myelopathy at segments adjacent to the site of a previous anterior cervical arthrodesis. J Bone Joint-Surg Am 1999; 81(4):519–528.
2. Roberts S, Menage J, Duance V, Wotton SF. Type III collagen in the inter-vertebral disc. Histochem J 1991; 23:503–508.
3. Adam M, Deyl Z. Degenerated annulus fibrosus of the intervertebral disc contains collagen type II. Ann Rheum Dis 1984; 43:258–263.
4. Johnstone B, Bayliss MT. The large proteoglycans of the human intervertebral disc: changes in their biosynthesis and structure with age, topography, and pathology. Spine 1995; 20(6):674–678.
5. Antoniou J, Steffen T, Nelson F, Winterbottom N, Hollander AP, Poole RA, Aebi M, Alini M. The human lumbar intervertebral disc: evidence for changes in the biosynthesis and denaturation of the extracellular matrix with growth, maturation, ageing and degeneration. J Clin Invest 1996; 98(4):996–1003.
6. Motoe T. Studies on the topographic architecture of the annulus fibrosus in developmental and degenerative processes in the lumbar intervertebral disc in man. Nippon Seikeigeka Gakkai Zasshi 1986; 60(5):495–509.
7. Richie JH, Farhni WH. Age changes in lumbar intervertebral discs. Can J Surg 1970; 13:65.
8. Osti OL, Vernon-Roberts B, Moore R, Fraser RD. Annular tears and disc degeneration in the lumbar spine: a post-mortem study of 135 discs. J Bone Joint Surg Br 1992; 74(5):678–682.
9. Hirsh C, Schajowicz F. Studies of structural changes in the lumbar annulus fibrosus. Acta Orthop Scand 1952; 22:184.
10. Fujita Y, Duncan NA, Lotz JC. Radial tensile properties of the lumbar annulus fibrosus are site and degeneration dependent. J Orthop Res 1997; 15(6):814–819.
11. Haughton VM, Schmidt TA, Keele K, An HS, Lim TH. Flexibility of lumbar spinal motion segments correlated to type of tears in the annulus fibrosus. J Neurosurg 2000; 92(1 Suppl):81–86.
12. Kauppila LI. J Bone Joint Surg Am 1995; 77(1):26–31.
13. Freemont AJ, Peacock TE, Goupille P, Hoyland JA, O'Brien J, Jayson MI. Nerve ingrowth into diseased intervertebral disc in chronic back pain. Lancet 1997; 350:178–181.
14. Holm S, Maroudas A, Urban JP, Selstam G, Nachemson A. Nutrition of the intervertebral disc: solute transport and metabolism. Connect Tissue Res 1981; 8(2):101–119.
15. Ogab K, Whiteside LA. Nutritional pathways of the intervertebral disc. Spine 1981; 6:211–216.
16. Roberts S, Urban JP, Evans H, Eisenstein SM. Transport properties of the human cartilage endplate in relation to its composition and calcification. Spine 1996; 21(4):415–420.

17. Yasuma T, Suzuki F, Koh S, Yamauchi Y. Pathological changes in the carti-laginous plates in relation to intervertebral disc lesions. Acta Pathol Jpn 1988; 38(6):735–750.

18. Roberts S, McCall IW, Menage J, Haddaway MJ, Eisenstein SM. Does the thickness of the vertebral subchondral bone reflect the composition of the intervertebral disc?. Eur Spine J 1997; 6(6):385–389.

19. Fraser RD. Chemonucleolysis. In: Jayson MIV, ed. The Lumbar Spine and Back Pain. Churchill Livingstone: 1992.

20. Melrose J, Taylor TK, Ghosh P, Holbert C, Macpherson C, Bellenger CR. Intervertebral disc reconstitution after chemonucleolysis with chymopapain is dependent on dosage. Spine 1996; 21(1):9–17.

21. Meachim G, Cornah MS. Fine structure of juvenile human nucleus pulposus. J Anat 1970; 107(2):337–350.

22. Matsuzaki H, Wakabayashi K, Ishihara K, Ishikawa H, Ohkawa A. Allo-grafting intervertebral discs in dogs: a possible clinical application. Spine 1996; 21(2):178–183.

23. Frick SL, Hanley EN, Meyer RA, Ramp WK, Chapman TM. Lumbar inter-vertebral disc transfer: a canine study. Spine 1994; 19:1826–1835.

24. Thompson JP, Oegema TR, Bradford DS. Stimulation of mature canine intervertebral disc by growth factors. Spine 1991; 16:253–260.

25. Yoo JU, Song KJ, Malemud CM. TGF-B1 stimulation of proteoglycan and protein synthesis in cells derived from human cervical intervertebral disc. Orthop Trans 1996; 20:198.

26. Cassinelli EH, Hall RA, Kang JD. Biochemistry of intervertebral disc degeneration and the potential for gene therapy applications. Spine 2001; 1:205–214.

27. Nishida K, Kang JD, Suh JK, Robbins PD, Evans CH, Gilbertson LG. Ade-novirus-mediated gene transfer to nucleus pulposus cells: implications for the treatment of intervertebral disc degeneration. Spine 1998; 23(22):2437–2442.

28. Nishida K, Kang JD, Gilbertson LG, Moon SH, Suh JK, Vogt MT, Robbins PD, Evans CH. Modulation of the biologic activity of the rabbit intervertebral disc by gene therapy: an in vivo study of adenovirus-mediated transfer of the human transforming growth factor betal enconding gene. Spine 1999; 24:2419–2425.

29. Nishimura K, Mochida J. Percutaneous reinsertion of the nucleus pulposus. Spine 1998; 14:1531–1539.

30. Okuma M, Mochida J, Nishimura K, Sakabe K, Seiki K. Reinsertion of stimulated nucleus pulposus cells retards intervertebral disc degeneration: an in vitro and in vivo experimental study. J Orthop Res 2000; 18(6):988–997.

31. Nomura T, Mochida J, Okuma M, Nishimura K, Sakabe K. Nucleus pulposus allograft retards intervertebral disc degeneration. Clin Orthop Rel Res 2001; 389:94–101.

32. Masuda K, Miyabayashi T, Meachum SH, Eurell TE. Proliferation of canine intervertebral disk chondrocytes in three-dimensional alginate microsphere culture. J Vet Med Sci 2002; 64(1):79–82.

33. Stern S, Lindenhayn K, Schultz O, Perka C. Cultivation of porcine cells from the nucleus pulposus in a fibrin/hyaluronic acid matrix. Acta Orthop Scand 2000; 71(5):496–502.

34. Kusior LJ, Vacanti CA, Bayley JC et al. Tissue engineering of nucleus pulposus in nude mice. Trans Orthop Res Soc 1999 24:807.

35. Ahlgren BD, Lui W, Herkowitz HN, Panjabi MM, Guiboux JP. Effect of anular repair on the healing strength of the intervertebral disc: a sheep model. Spine 2000; 25(17):2165–2170.

36. Loupasis GA, Stamos K, Katonis PG, Sapkas G, Korres DS, Hartofilakidis G. Seven-to-20-year outcome of lumbar discectomy. Spine 1999; 24(22): 2313–2317.

37. Arnoczky SP, Warren RF, Spivak JM. Meniscal repair using an exogenous fibrin clot. An experimental study in dogs. J Bone Joint Surg Am 1988; 70:1209–1217.

38. Ibarra C, Koski JA, Warren RF. Tissue engineering meniscus: cells and matrix. Orthop Clin North Am 2000; 31:411–418.

39. Stone KR, Rodkey WG, Webber R, McKinney L, Steadman JR. Meniscal regeneration with copolymeric collagen scaffolds: in vitro and in vivo studies evaluated clinically, histologically, and biochemically. Am J Sports Med 1992; 20:104–111.

40. Angele P, Johnstone B, Nerlich M, Goldberg VM, Yoo J. Meniscus repair with mesenchymal proge-nitor cells in a biodegradable composite matrix. Trans Orthop Res Soc 2000.

15

Clinical Applications of Orthopedic Tissue Engineering: Ligaments and Tendons

Lee D. Kaplan
University of Wisconsin School of Medicine
Madison, Wisconsin, U.S.A.

Freddie Fu
University of Pittsburgh School of Medicine
Pittsburgh, Pennsylvania, U.S.A.

I. INTRODUCTION

The biological and biomechanical properties of ligaments and tendons influence the treatment of patients both in their acute care and after reconstructive surgery. The tissue properties of these structures and the characteristic phases of the healing process are currently used to treat soft-tissue sports medicine injuries. Technical advances made through less invasive surgery and early emphasis on load and motion in the postoperative period have led to better clinical outcomes. These results, however, are still inferior to the native ligaments and tendons.

The healing of ligaments and tendons is regulated by a highly orchestrated sequence of events. Understanding this sequence of events, the delivery of growth factors and cells to the site of healing tissue is crucial to future developments directed toward enhancing clinical outcomes. Tissue engineering of ligaments and tendons incorporates cell therapy, gene therapy, and biological scaffolding.

The clinical understanding of ligament and tendon tissue engineering begins with an understanding of the array of injuries we treat as orthopedic surgeons. Athletic injuries commonly involve ligaments and tendons. Common shoulder injuries involve the biceps tendon and the rotator cuff tendon. Throwing athletes may injure the medial collateral ligament of the elbow. The ligamentous structures of the knee are commonly injured in sports, including the medical collateral ligament, the lateral collateral ligament, and the anterior and posterior cruciate ligaments.

Ligament healing is divided into a four-phase process (1). The first phase is the hemorrhagic phase, which results in formation of a clot. Cytokines within the clot influence the beginning of the inflammatory cascade. Various inflammatory cells, including polymorphonuclear leukocytes, migrate into the injured area and release growth factors. These growth factors are the regulatory instruments of the healing process. Platelets release platelet-derived growth factor (PDGF), transforming growth factor-beta (TGF-β), and epidermal growth factor (EDG) (2). Macrophages produce cytokines that are involved in the neovascularization process. Macrophages produce basic fibroblast growth factor (bFGF), TGF-β, and PDGF (3).

The second phase, the proliferative phase, involves migration of stem cells to the wound sites. The clot is becoming a vascular granulation tissue. Fibroblasts produce matrix proteins during this phase. Fibroblasts, influenced by growth factors, produce collagen types I, III, and V. Angiogenesis is occurring with the diffusion of adjacent capillary networks (4).

The third phase, the early remodeling phase, occurs at 6 weeks after insult. Collagen becomes denser and there is a decrease in the cellularity and vascularity of the scar. The collagen becomes more organized and aligned with the axis of the alignment (3). The fourth phase, later remodeling, may extend over a several-year period while the strength and ligament stiffness increase. The healing process is an integrated network of biomechanical and biochemical signaling, which leads cells to be at the site of healing and primed to perform their individual purpose. Tissue engineering involves enhancing this process.

Intra-articular ligaments such as the anterior cruciate ligament (ACL) are unable to have a functional recovery, as opposed to extra-articular ligaments such as the medical collateral ligament (MCL), which have this potential. There are a number of anatomical and histological reasons for this difference in healing potential. The posttraumatic or postoperative knee usually has some degree of hematoma formation. A tissue envelope or synovial sheath must be present for the hematoma to have the ability to organize into a fibrinogen mesh that will allow for the influx of reparative cells. These cells produce cytokines growth factors, which will attract fibroblasts and stem cells to facilitate repair (5). Different healing capabilities distinguish the MCL of the knee and the ACL. The MCL has the potential to heal and the standard of clinical care is to treat MCL injuries conservatively without surgical intervention. The ACL does not have the same capacity for spontaneous healing. The ACL is composed of collagen bundles. It lies within a synovial sheath surrounded by synovial fluid (3). Therefore, clot formation is very poor at the site of ACL tears. The MCL is extraarticular, so the synovial fluid does not have a negative effect on its healing. The resulting ACL instability risks damage to the menisci and future articular cartilage injury.

The resident fibroblasts within these two ligaments differ, which also influences the healing potential of the ligaments. The fibroblasts of the MCL have cytoplasmic processes that are in contact with collagen fibrils. The ACL fibroblasts do not contain these projections (6). The fibroblasts of the MCL are able to fill cell-free areas more expeditiously than ACL fibroblasts (7). The fibroblasts also differ in their response to growth factors (8). MCL fibroblasts produced twice the amount of matrix when exposed to the same amount of TGF-β1 growth factor when compared to ACL fibroblasts.

Nitric oxide has been shown to inhibit collagen and proteoglycan synthesis. The ACL produces a large amount of nitric oxide in response to the interleukins (IL-1) and inflammatory mediators. This inhibits healing capacity. The medial collateral ligament, which has good healing potential, does not produce significant amounts of nitric oxide (9). These differences in healing potential must be taken in consideration when designing tissue engineering treatment strategies.

II. CLINICAL ISSUES

Reconstruction techniques used in the knee illustrate the advances and future hurdles encountered with ligament and tendon tissue engineering. Approximately 50,000 ACL reconstructions are done in the United States annually (5). Surgical reconstruction of the ACL has increased over the past decade. The indications for surgery include the type of recreational or occupational activities of the patient and whether the patient is able to modify these activities. The number of women playing competitive athletics has increased dramatically. This population has a disproportionate number of ACL injuries. The number of athletically active baby boomers and seniors has increased. Several recent papers have documented success in ACL reconstruction in patients over the age of 50 (10,11).

The success of current technique for ACL-reconstructed knees is well documented. The senior author has performed over 3500 of these operations over his 18-year career. Over the last 15 years, there has been continual interest in finding the "ideal" graft. The advantages of using autogenous tissue grafts such as bone-patella tendon-bone, hamstring, and quadriceps tendon autografts include the strength of the grafts and the elimination of rejection and disease transmission risks. The disadvantages include graft site morbidity, more postoperative pain, and a larger incision. Allograft tissues that are used in ACL reconstruction include Archilles tendon, bone-patella tendon-bone (BPB), and anterior tibialis tendon grafts. The disadvantages of allograft tissue include a decrease in tensile strength, a prolonged healing time, disease transmission risks, and, occasionally, difficulty obtaining tissue. The search for the ideal replacement for a torn ACL has led to continued exploration into biological enhancement and tissue engineering.

The two most commonly used autograft tissues are bone-patella tendon-bone and semitendinous-gracilis (ST-G) hamstring grafts. The BPB graft is taken from the central third of the tendon and has bone plugs on both ends. The healing process is bone-to-bone healing in the femoral and tibial tunnels. The ST-G graft heals in a tendon-to-bone fashion. The graft undergoes a ligamentazation process over 12 weeks but takes up to several years to complete (12).

III. REQUIREMENTS FOR TISSUE-ENGINEERED ACL

Tissue engineering strategies to reconstruct the ACL involve many factors. First, the factors that affect the healing of the graft at its fixation points within the tunnel must be considered. Next, which growth factors contribute to the "ligamentazation" process? Third, what is the sequence for growth factor delivery and function and what is their effective life span? Fourth, what ways are used to transport these factors to the graft site? Fifth, what regulatory process exists to keep these factors optimally functioning and yet not causing other harmful side effects?

The use of ligament and tendon grafts in orthopedic surgical procedures depends on the healing of the grafts to the native bone. This is independent of the fixation device that is used. The replication of either a direct or indirect attachment to bone must occur in the reconstructed tissues. Direct attachments contain four distinct layers from bone to tendon. They are the tendon, a fibrocartilage insertion, cartilaginous insertion, and then bone. The indirect insertions are fibers that extend from tendon to bone, i.e., Sharpey's fibers. Ligament grafts usually contain a bone block on at least one end of the graft. Examples of this include rotator cuff surgery, medial collateral elbow reconstruction, and ACL reconstruction. ACL reconstruction will be used as an example.

The causation of early failure after ACL surgery is failure at the ends of fixation (5). The type of fixation is dependent upon what type of tissue is present within the osseous tunnel. Many graft choices are available to use when performing ACL reconstruction. These include BPB autograft and allograft, ST-G hamstring autografts, quadriceps tendon autograft, and tibialis anterior (TA) allograft. The BPB graft choice contains bone plugs at both ends and will heal with bone-to-bone healing within the osseous reconstruction tunnels. The ST-G and TA grafts contain tendon ends, so there is tendon-to-bone healing within the osseous tunnels. The quadriceps graft has a tendon end and a bone plug end, so it has implications in both types of healing. Bone-to-bone healing displays rigid bony fixation upon healing. The BPB and the ST-G are the most commonly used grafts and will be representative of the two types of osseous healing.

Soft-tissue grafts that depend on a bone-to-tunnel-tissue junction may have advantages. Clinically, there is a reported reduction in anterior knee pain and postoperative morbidity (5). However, there is fibrous tissue growth into bone at 6 weeks postimplantation that does not restore the direct insertion that is normally found in the native ACL (25). Controversy exists over the long-term healing and stability of ACL reconstruction using BPB and ST-G grafts since late failure of ACL-reconstructed knees occurs within the intra-articular portion of the ACL (5). Therefore, the importance of graft-to-tunnel healing appears to be limited to the time it takes to complete.

The tendon-bone interface heals with collagen fibers that resemble indirect insertion, i.e., Sharpey's fibers, by 12 weeks (26,27). Perpendicular collagen fibers have been found within a sheep model at 8 weeks. These fibers were circumferential around the graft by 12 weeks. The bone tunnel was well defined by 24 weeks. When the grafts were biomechanically tested, they failed at pullout from the bone tunnel up to 12 weeks after reconstruction. When the 24–52-week specimens were tested, they all ruptured through the intra-articular portion of the graft. This serves as further evidence that the grafts had incorporated within the tunnels (28). The incorporation of the bone plug has been shown to be completed at 12 weeks after reconstruction. The tendon insertion was shown to have four distinct zones, histologically similar to the native ACL (29).

Others studied bone-bone versus bone-tendon healing in a rabbit patella tendon model (30). The lateral 4 mm of the tibial side of the patella tendon was removed with either a tendon edge or a bone block edge. This was then inserted into a bony tunnel. The bone-bone group showed stronger biomechanical properties with regard to maximum stiffness and tensile load at 4 and 8 weeks. However, at 12 weeks the two groups were equal. This difference also was seen in clinical and anatomical analysis of biopsies taken from ACL insertion sites during revision ligament reconstruction (31).The hamstring grafts had three distinct zones in healing to the bone. These were the graft, a woven bone zone that entered the bone at oblique angles, and the lamellar bone of the tibia. The patella tendon graft had four characteristic zones. These were the graft, a zone of unmineralized fibrocartilage, a zone of mineralized fibrocartilage, and the bone. This had the appearance of the normal chondral enthesis found in the native ACL (31). Ohtera et al. demonstrated increased tendon-bone healing in tendon that was wrapped with periosteum prior to insertion into the bone tunnel. A fibrocartilaginous insertion with increased mechanical strength versus control was demonstrated (32).

Efforts to improve tendon-bone healing have led to studies of growth factors that can influence this process. Aspenberg and Forsund found that there was an increase in tendon callus size and strength at an earlier time when treated with cartilage-derived morphogenetic protein 1 and 2. Bone morphogenetic protein (BMP), specifically osteogenic protein 1 (OP-1), induced bone formation in the tendon. However, this was at the expense of mechanical strength of the tendon itself (33).

This previous study has been taken further with tissue-engineered ACL tendon grafts. Martinek et al. evaluated the effect of BMP-2 on tendon bone healing in a rabbit model. An adenoviral gene vector was used. The BMP-2 gene transfer to ACL hamstring grafts resulted in enhanced biomechanical and biological effects on tendon-bone healing. There was a single application of the growth factor and it was shown to have prolonged fibroblastic effect within the bone tunnel. This provides some data to support the sustained effect of gene transfer. The bone tunnel healing differed between the control group, which demonstrated indirect tendon-bone healing with Sharpey's fibers, and the BMP-2-treated group, which displayed healing with qualities similar to the bone-bone tunnel direct healing. This latter group had osteoblastic activity, neo-ossification of the tendon, and chondral-appearing tissue at the interface (34).

Biomechanical testing of the two groups showed that the tissue-engineered ACL group was almost twice as stiff as the control group. The ultimate load was greater than twice that of the control group. The most interesting point was that the control group failed at the insertion site whereas the tissue-engineered group failed midsubstance. This has application to the clinical concerns regarding early graft failure at tendon-bone insertion sites (34).

The use of biological fixation devices is now limited to biodegradable screws. Recently, screws made of allograft bone have become available. The incorporation of these screws may be enhanced with applications of the previously discussed studies using growth factors. One study compared type I collagen bone anchors to metal anchors. It was shown in a sheep model that collagen integration occurred by 6 weeks. The devices showed no difference in strength (35).

Growth factors that have elicited a positive effect on ACL fibroblast metabolism include PDGF-AB, EGF, and bFGF (13). Therefore, there is evidence that these factors in the right environment may improve ACL graft healing. Gene therapy provides the ability to provide growth factors to the healing graft site and is one potential approach to tissue engineering an effective ACL. The goal is to provide the transfer of the defined genes for these factors to the target site. The successful application of gene therapy would allow therapeutic levels of growth factor proteins at the site of injury or inflammation in the reconstruction of a deficient ACL (14).

DNA for each desired growth factor must be held in a vector that will transport the genetic information into the host cell. Once the DNA is within the nucleus of the host cell it either integrates itself into the host cell's chromosomes or it will remain extrachromosomal or episomal. If the DNA is integrated into the host genetic information it will continue to propagate with cell division. Episomal DNA will be lost when the cell divides. The inserted gene is transcribed into messenger RNA (mRNA). This mRNA is transported to the cell cytoplasm and is the template for ribosomes to produce each specific, therapeutic growth factor protein. The effect of the vector is described as either transduction, which is defined as stable genetic alteration (seen with viral vectors), or transfection, which is transient genetic alteration (seen with naked DNA).

Two main categories of vectors exist—nonviral and viral vectors. Nonviral vectors include liposomes, DNA-ligand complexes, and DNA-gene gun. The nonviral vectors transmit DNA that remains episomal. They are less immunogenic and less expensive than the viral vectors. The liposome vector has the weakness of having a low efficiency of gene delivery. The liposome vector has the weakness of having a low efficiency of gene delivery. The DNA-ligand complexes seek out cells with a marker and have so-called "target delivery." These vectors can be incorporated with an adenoviral protein, which may show beneficial effects of both vector categories. DNA-gene gun vectors are 1–7-μm particles of gold coated with DNA and accelerated into the tissue at high velocity. This is a highly effective way to transfect cells.

Viral vectors include adenovirus, retrovirus, adeno-associated virus, and herpes simplex virus. The viral vectors now available are more efficient in gene transfer than nonviral vectors (15). The use of viral vectors requires that all genes for viral replication are removed and the desired gene for specific growth factors replaces the native pathogenic protein. Viral vectors have the ability to infect the desired tissue target by attaching to the cell via receptor and transporting the DNA of the desired growth factor protein to the nucleus of the target cells. Each of the previously mentioned viral vectors has individual characteristics. There is continued work in finding viral vectors that are less cytotoxic and immunogenic (14).

Gene delivery to cells can occur through either systemic or local gene delivery. Systemic delivery involves injecting the gene vector into the bloodstream. The vector is responsible for finding the target tissue. The vector is disseminated throughout the body. This is a favorable technique if the target organ is difficult to approach. Markers on some cells will be able to signal for the attachment of the gene vector. The difficulties with systemic gene delivery are that there is a low specificity of gene expression and a low quantity of the gene vectors at the target site, which may result in a subtherapeutic concentration of the growth-factor-specific gene. The systemic delivery system is unable to provide large amounts of gene vectors to tissues with poor blood supplies such as the meniscus or articular cartilage (14,15).

The local gene delivery system is able to deliver the gene vectors specifically to the target site. Gene vectors can be injected into the host tissue, the in vivo technique, or the cells can be removed from the target tissue and genetically altered in vitro and reinjected to their original site within the body, the ex vivo technique. The in vivo technique is easier to do because it requires only injection to the site of interest. The ex vivo technique requires several steps and is therefore more invasive. However, the cells are genetically altered outside the body in a controlled in vitro environment. Viral particles and DNA are not injected directly into the body and this may be a safer method. Ex vivo cells can be tested for safety prior to reinjection. The ex vivo technique allows the cells that express high levels of the growth factor to be chosen to be reinjected (15).

The techniques described above have been used to study the effect, timing, and concentration of these factors on ligament healing. Growth factors, including fibroblast growth factor, platelet-derived growth factor, and TGF-β1, have been shown to express themselves within ACL grafts. The initial work was to evaluate the effects of these growth factors on ligaments. PDGF-PB was shown to increase stiffness, ultimate load, and increase the cross-sectional area of the MCL when applied with a fibrin sealant (16). The cells themselves vary in their response to these factors. Age of the animal and location of the cell have both been shown to influence the effect of PDGF, bFGF, and EGF on fibroblasts (8,17). Fibroblast cell outgrowths explanted from the MCL show more outgrowth than those from the ACL (18). These differences may help to account for some of the differences in the healing capacities.

The healing process after ACL reconstruction shows that the concentration and timing of growth factors varies. Kuroda and associates evaluated the expression of multiple growth factors within an ACL graft (41). The growth factors were noted to increase during the early postoperative period, peaking at 3 weeks and reaching preoperative levels by 12 weeks. This increase correlates with ACL graft revascularization. Growth factors display a synergy with each other. Part of this is based on their concentrations and feedback mechanisms. The combination, concentration, and timing of the interaction between these proteins affects ligament healing. Dog ACL fibroblasts display increased activity with TGF-β1. This has been shown to be dose-dependent. TGF-β1 has a synergistic effect on PDGF-AB at certain doses. However, at increased concentrations TGF-β1 will decrease the activity of PDGF (19).

The strength of scar tissue is dependent on collagen. The protein decorin has been shown to limit the necessary increase in collagen size. Nakamura et al. were successful in down-regulating decorin (20). This led to increased collagen fibrillogenesis and an increase in collagen size and scar strength. Nakamura et al. then took this a step further by utilizing the nonviral gene vector HVJ-liposome in suspension using a local, in vivo technique to deliver PDGF-B to rat patella ligaments. The ligament was directly injected with the suspension. PDGF displayed an increase in expression for up to 4 weeks after transfection. There was an increase in both angiogenesis and collagen deposition. This group has shown similar results with a rabbit ligament scar model (21).

Cell therapy provides a conduit for the transfer of genes. Various cells have been shown to be capable of multipotential differentiation including cells derived from bone marrow, bone, and periosteum (2). Our center has emphasized the advantages of muscle-based tissue engineering. Muscle tissue provides satellite cells, which are mononucleated precursor cells. They are capable of persistent gene expression once triggered. Mesenchymal stem cells are also found in muscle. Cells within muscle tissue are capable of differentiating into different tissue lineages and, therefore, may be capable of regenerating different types of tissues. The use of muscle-cell-mediated ex vivo gene therapy may have the ability to achieve persistent local gene expression and growth factory delivery to ligaments (22).

Stem cell research has gained a great deal of attention owing to the political and legal issues involved. However, the in vitro transfection of these cells that are capable of participating in the healing process has been extensively studied. Gerich et al. transplanted fibroblasts into the patella tendons of rabbits (23). The fibroblasts were transduced with a retroviral vector and these cells could be observed for 6 weeks after transduction. The transplanted cells integrated themselves within the crimp of the tendon. Menetrey et al. used muscle-cell-mediated ex vivo genetic transfer to deliver epidermal growth factor, platelet-derived growth factor, and TGF-β to rabbit ligament through an adenovirus carrier. These proteins at the site of the ACL influenced fibroblasts and myoblasts. This has two significant ramifications. First, the delivery of proteins, which are capable to facilitate ligament healing and graft maturation, may enhance healing rates. Second, the myoblasts response may accelerate vasularization of the graft (24).

IV. LIGAMENTIZATION OF GRAFTS

The ST-G graft has been shown to undergo a similar ligamentazation process as the patellar tendon graft. Improving the strength, quality of tissue, and time to heal of the ligamentazation process is an important goal. It has direct ramifications within the athletic population since it may dictate the timing of return to play. Animal studies show that the graft begins a transition from random fiber orientation to longitudinal orientation over the first 12 weeks after surgery. The graft maturation pattern correlated with histological evidence of the sinusoidal crimp pattern. In one study, this process was seen up to the 52-week point of observation (36). The remodeling of the graft has been described as continuing for several years. The expression of growth factors during ligament healing is also dependent upon mechanical stress. The regulation of tenascin-C matrix protein has been shown to be regulated by mechanical strain in vivo. Tenacin-C is a matrix protein found in highest quantity during hyperplastic processes within tissues, which is important in ligament graft maturation. Stress is a major regulator of this expression in fibroblasts and chondrocytes (37).

One concern when taking a graft for knee ligament reconstruction is the resultant effect on the knee. This occurs due to graft site morbidity as well as the loss of that tissue whether ST-G, BPB, or quadriceps tendon on function. Recently, there has been radiographic evidence that hamstring tendons will regenerate. The application of tissue engineering principles to facilitate this regeneration and ensure quality regenerative tissue would enable surgeons to eliminate these concerns. CDMP-2 has been shown to enhance healing of tendons under mechanical load (38).

V. OTHER TISSUE ENGINEERING STRATEGIES

The use of tissue engineering in developing scaffolds or other graft sources would help eliminate the risks involved in the use of allograft tissue or the perioperative and postoperative complications previously mentioned with autografts. The ability to use both cell and gene therapy to deliver cells and growth factors to the bone tunnel and intra-articular portions of grafts could potentially lead to a readily usable graft option. The use of porcine, intestinal submucosa as an ACL scaffold is being evaluated (39). Murray et al. have shown that fibroblasts from the ACL migrate into a collagen-glycosaminoglycan scaffold (40). The ideal graft would reproduce the biomechanical functions of the native ACL and reproduce the insertion sites of the native ligament. The knee would regain the neuromuscular feedback that it receives from the native ligament. Currently, this graft does not exist.

Knowledge of the growth factors involved in the ligamentazation process of the ACL graft and the timing of their function allows for the potential to modulate these biological responses. The half-life of growth factors is limited to a few days. This necessitated the novel approach to keep concentrations of growth factors elevated for longer time periods that led to investigations of gene therapy. Gene therapy allows for the incorporation of genes specific for growth factors to stimulate and regulate healing over a longer period of time (2). Healing is a multistep process and different cytokines need to peak at various times to get the best results (15). The application of these findings makes tendon and ligament tissue engineering one of the most exciting research areas within orthopedics today.

VI. FUNCTIONAL TISSUE ENGINEERING

One area of interest within tissue engineering is functional tissue engineering (42). This discipline of tissue engineering addresses the biomechanical factors seen in repair tissues. There are several issues within tissue engineering within an in vivo environment. These include the baseline mechanical factors required by the native tissues, the parameters required for the engineered tissue, the effects of physical factors on cellular activities, and whether there could be a benefit in stimulating the tissue prior to implantation (43).

VII. SUMMARY

The healing of ligaments and tendons is regulated by a highly orchestrated sequence of events. Understanding this sequence of events, the delivery of growth factors and cells to the site of healing tissue, is crucial to future developments directed toward enhancing clinical outcomes. Tissue engineering of ligaments and tendons incorporates cell therapy, gene therapy, and biological scaffolding.

Tissue engineering of ligament grafts involves biologically influencing the healing of grafts to the native bone. Efforts to improve tendon-to-bone healing have led to investigations of growth factors. The final analysis of the success of enhancing healing will involve the biomechanical evaluation of the resulting graft. The important issues will be the increase in strength, graft fixation, and healing potential.

There are different strategies for tissue engineering. These include local and systemic delivery systems, the development of scaffolds, and functional tissue engineering. The development of advanced biological techniques for ligament and tendon healing may utilize some or all of these techniques.

REFERENCES

1. Frank CB, Bray RC, Hart DA, et al. Soft tissue healing. In: Fu FH, Harner CD, Vince KG, eds. Knee Surgery. 1st ed. Baltimore, MD: Williams & Wilkins, 1994; 189–229.
2. Woo SL, Hildebrand K, Watanabe N, et al. Tissue engineering of ligament and tendon healing. Clin Orthop 1999 Oct, (367 Suppl):S312–323.
3. Murphy PG, Grank CB, Hart DA. The cell biology of ligaments and ligament healing. In: Jackson DW, ed. The ACL: Current and Future Concepts. New York: Raven Press, 1993; 165–177.
4. Woo SL. Ligaments. Orthopaedic Basic Science. Rosemond, IL: AAOS1994.
5. Fu FH, Bennett CH, Lattermann C, et al. Current trends in ACL reconstruction. Am J Sports Med 2000; 27:821–829.
6. Lyon, RM, Akeson WH, Amiel D, et al. Ultrastructural differences between the cells of the medial collateral and the anterior cruciate ligaments. Clin Orthop 1991; 272:279–286.
7. Nagineni CN, Amiel D, Green MH, et al. Characterization of the intrinsic properties of the anterior cruciate and medial collateral ligament cells: an in vitro cell culture study. J Orthop Res 1992; 10:465–475.
8. Scherping SC Jr., Schmidt CC, Georgescu III, Kwoh CK, Evans CH, Woo SL. Effect of growth factors on the proliferation of ligament fibroblasts from skeletally mature rabbits. Connect Tissue Res 1997; 36(1):1–8.
9. Cao M, Stefanovic-Racic M, Georgescu HI, et al. Does nitric oxide help explain the differential healing capacity of the ACL, PCL and MCL? Am J Sports Med 2000; 28:176–182.
10. Miller M, Sullivan R. Anterior cruciate ligament reconstruction in an 84-year-old man. Arthroscopy 2001; 17(1):70–72.
11. Heier KA, Mack DR, Moseley JB, et al. An analysis of ACL reconstruction in middle-aged patients. Am J Sports Med 1997; 25:527–532.
12. Arnoczky SP, Rarvin GB, Marshall JL. Anterior cruciate ligament replacement using patellar tendon. J Bone Joint Surg Am 1982; 64:217–224.
13. Scherpling SC Jr, Schmidt CC, Georgescu HI, et al. Effect of growth factors on the proliferation of ligament fibroblasts from skeletally mature rabbits. Connect Tissue Res 1997; 36:1–8.

14. Martinek V, Fu FH, Huard J. Gene therapy and tissue engineering in sports medicine. Phys Sportsmed 2000; 28:35–51.

15. Evans CH, Robbins PD. Possible orthopaedic applications of gene therapy. J Bone Joint Surg 1995; 77:1105–1114.

16. Hildebrand KA, Woo SL, Smith DW, et al. The effects of platelet derived growth factor-BB on healing of the rabbit medial collateral ligament: an in vivo study. Am J Sports Med. 1998; 26:549–554.

17. Schmidt CC, Georgescu HI, Kwoh CK, et al. Effect of growth factors on the proliferation of fibroblasts from the medial collateral and anterior cruciate ligaments. J Orthop Res 1995; 13:184–190.

18. Hannafin JA, Attia E, Warren RF, et al. The effect of cytokines on the chemotactic migration of canine knee ligament fibroblasts. Tran Orthop Res Soc 1997; 22:50.

19. DesRosiers EA, Yahia L, Rivard C-H. Proliferative and matrix synthesis response of canine anterior cruciate ligament fibroblasts submitted to combined growth factors. J Orthop Rres ; 14:200–208.

20. Nakamura N, Hart DA, Boorman RS, et al. Decorin antisense gene therapy improves functional healing of early rabbit ligament scar with enhanced collagen fibrillogenesis in vivo. J Orthop Res 2000, 18:517–523.

21. Nakamura N, Shino K, Natsuume T, et al. Early biological effect of in vivo gene transfer of platelet-derived growth factor (PDGF)-B into healing patellar ligament. Gene Ther 1998; 5(9):1165–1170.

22. Musgrave DS, Huard J. Muscle-based tissue engineering for the musculoskeletal system. Gene Ther Mol Biol 1999; 3:207–221.

23. Gerich TG, Kang R, Fu FH, et al. Gene transfer to ligaments and menisci. Gene Ther 3:1089–1093.

24. Menetrey J, Kasemkijwattana C, Day CS, et al. The potential of growth factors to improve muscle regeneration following injury. J Bone Joint Surg Am 1998.

25. Rodeo SA, Arnoczky SP, Torzilli PA, et al. Tendon-healing in a bone tunnel: a biomechanical and histological study in the dog. J Bone Joint Surg Am 1993; 75:795–803.

26. Tomita F, Yasuda K, Mikani S. Comparisons of introsseous graft healing between the double flexor tendon graft and the bone patella tendon bone graft in ACL reconstruction. Arthroscopy 2001; 17(5):461–476.

27. Shaieb MD, Singer DI, Grimes J, et al. Evaluation of tendon bone reattachment: a rabbit model. Am J Orthop 2000; 29(7):537–542.

28. Goradia VK, Rochat MC, Grana WA, et al. Tendon bone healing of a semitendonosus tendon autograft used for ACL reconstruction in a sheep model. Am J Knee Surg. 2000; 13(3):143–151.

29. Yoshiya S, Nagaro M, Kurosaka M, et al. Graft healing in the bone tunnel in ACL reconstruction. Clin Orthop 2000; 376:278–286.

30. Park, MJ, Lee, MC, Seong SC. A comparative study of the healing of tendon autograft and tendon-bone autograft using patellar tendon in rabbits. Inter Orthop Mar 2001; 25:35–39.

31. Peterson W, Laprell H. Insertion of autologous tendon grafts to the bone: a histological and immunohistochemical study of hamstring and patellar tendon grafts. Knee Surg Sports Traum Arthrosc 2000; 8(1):26–31.
32. Ohtera K, Yamada Y, Aoki M, et al. Effects of periosteum wrapped around tendon in a bone tunnel: a biomechanical and histological study in rabbits. Crit Rev Biomed Eng 2000; 28(1–2):115–118.
33. Aspenberg P, Forsund C. Bone morphogenetic proteins and tendon repair. Scand J Med Sci Sports 2000; 10(6):372–275.
34. Martinek V, Lattermann C, Usas Arvydas, et al. Enhancement of the tendon-bone integration of ACL tendon grafts with BMP-2 gene transfer: a hisological and biomechanical study. J Bone Joint Surg. In revision.
35. Harrison JA, Wallace D, Van Sickle, et al. A novel suture anchor of high-density collagen compared with a metallic anchor. results of a 12-week study in sheep. Am J Sports Med 2000; 28(6):883–887.
36. Goradia VK, Rochat MC, Kida M, et al. Natural history of a hamstring tendon autograft used for anterior cruciate ligament reconstruction in a sheep model, Am J Sports Med 2000; 28(1):40–46.
37. Jarvinen TA, Jozsa L, Kannus P, et al. Mechanical loading regulates tenascin-C expression in the osteotendinous junction. J Cell Sci 1999; 18:3157–3166.
38. Forslund C, Aspenberg P. Tendon healing stimulated by injected CDMP-2. Med Sci Sports Exerc 2001; 33(5):685–687.
39. Badylak S, Arnoczky S, Plouhar P, et al. Naturally occurring extracellular matrix as a scaffold for musculoskeletal repair. Clin Orthop 1999; 367(Suppl): 333–343.
40. Murray MM, Martin SD, Spector M. Migration of cells from human ACL explants into collagen-glycosaminoglycan scaffolds. J Orthop Res 2000; 8:557–564.
41. Kuroda R, Kurosaka M, Yoshiya S, et al. Localization of growth factors in the reconstructed anterior cruciate ligament: immunohistological study in dogs. Knee Surg Sports Trauma 2000; 8(2):120–126.
42. Guilak F, Butler DL, Goldstein SA. Functional tissue engineering: the role of biomechanics in articular cartilage repair. Clin Orthop 2001:S295–305.
43. Butler DL, Goldstein SA, Guilak F. Functional tissue engineering: the role of biomechanics. J Biomech Eng 2000; 122(6):570–575.

16

Functional Engineered Skeletal Muscle

Robert G. Dennis

Harvard-MIT Division of Health Sciences and Technology, and
MIT Artificial Intelligence Laboratory, University of Michigan,
Ann Arbor, Michigan, U.S.A.

I. INTRODUCTION

Skeletal muscle constitutes over 45% of the body mass of the typical adult human. Muscle is both an excitable tissue (like nerve), and a tissue capable of generating active force, work, and mechanical power. The function most commonly associated with muscle tissue is the generation of force, but muscle tissue performs many other functions critical to the survival of higher animals. Muscle plays an important role in thermogenesis and the thermal management associated with homeostasis in warm-blooded animals. Adult phenotype skeletal muscle is both highly metabolically active and postmitotic, and has recently been proposed for use as an implantable protein factory (1–7). As a structural element, muscle can act as a *motor* (to actively generate positive mechanical displacement, force, work, and power), as a *brake* (to dissipate mechanical energy), as a *spring* (to elastically store mechanical energy for later recovery), and as a *strut* (to transmit mechanical loads from one location to another within as animal) (8). Skeletal muscle is a "smart material," with integrated sensors for force (Golgi tendon organs in the tendons of muscles), strain, and strain rate (muscle spindles). Muscle allows an animal to adapt to the changing mechanical demands of the environment over a wide range of time scales. As a result of increased mechanical demands from the environment, skeletal muscle can undergo functional adaptation, such as hypertrophy (an increase in muscle fiber diameter) or hyperplasia (an increase in the total number of muscle fibers). Functional adaptation is a relatively slow process, generally requiring weeks to months. Skeletal muscle also reacts rapidly to changing mechanical demands by modulating its viscoelastic properties directly, through neuromotor activation. The viscoelastic properties of muscle can change in a matter of tens of milliseconds as a result of muscle activation, either by reflex or by volitional neuromotor commands.

II. APPLICATIONS FOR ENGINEERED SKELETAL MUSCLE

The tacit assumption is that engineered tissues are ultimately intended to provide suitable replacement materials for the surgical correction of tissue trauma, disease, or congenital deformity. The surgical applications are one important application of engineered tissues, but there are many others. For striated muscles, these applications include: (1) an in vitro model for basic scientific research of tissue development, aging, injury, disease, and gene therapy; (2) an in vitro model for commercial applications, such as drug screening and testing; (3) cell and tissue-based micro actuators to power BioMEMS devices; (4) macroscopic living actuators for biomimetic robots and hybrid (tissue + synthetic) prosthetic devices; (5) replacement tissues for the correction of congenital deformity or tissue damage due to trauma (the most commonly recognized application); and (6) food. Although the final application for engineered muscle (as food) is perhaps furthest from realization given our current technology, several factors may ultimately drive the technology in this direction, including the need to harvest animal tissues under aseptic conditions (relevant in light of recent concerns about prion disease), the need to generate animal proteins as food during prolonged space flight, and the growing social consciousness of and distaste for the need to slaughter animals for food.

III. MUSCLE AS A MECHANICAL ACTUATOR

The use of engineered muscle as a mechanical actuator should not be too lightly discounted. Based upon well-established figures of merit (FoM) (9,10), muscle compares very favorably with every available synthetic actuator technology, and in many respects is vastly superior (9). In particular, in terms of quantitative FoM muscle has an extraordinarily high power per unit mass ($\sim$50–250 W/kg), greater than any synthetic actuator when the total required actuator mechanism is considered. Muscle also has a very high mechanical efficiency, especially in light of the fact that the chemomechanical energy transduction in muscle takes place at nearly equilibrium temperature conditions, unlike, for example, a diesel engine combustion reaction. In addition to these direct functional comparisons, living muscles have many advantages that far exceed the most hopeful technological potential envisioned for synthetic actuator technologies. Muscle operates almost silently, can functionally adapt to changing environment demands, is self-organizing, self-repairing, and self-regulating, has built-in sensors, and is scalable from tens of microns to tens of meters in dimension (consider blue whales) simply by adding contractile proteins and cells either in parallel or in series. Muscle also has an astonishing capacity for architectural plasticity; striated muscles can form rods, cones, plates, fans, hollow tubes, and spheres.

IV. MUSCLE TISSUE DEVELOPMENT AND REGENERATION

There are many approaches to engineering skeletal muscle tissue, but each requires an understanding of muscle tissue development and regeneration in vivo, and the relationship between structure and function. It was originally thought that muscle tissue regeneration following trauma recapitulated the events during initial tissue development, though it is becoming increasingly clear that the events surrounding tissue regeneration may be more complex than those involved in initial tissue genesis (11). Nonetheless, the processes bear some important similarities, and can be summarized as follows. In the embryo, skeletal muscles develop from three separate cell lineages, one giving rise to the muscles of the head, one giving rise to the muscles of the back, and one giving rise to the muscles of the abdomen, intercostals, and limbs (11). Adult muscle fibers are polynucleated, forming from the fusion of many myogenic precursor cells. During embryonic tissue genesis and tissue regeneration after trauma, skeletal muscle cells occur in a range of developmental states (12). *Myogenic precursor (muscle progenitor)* cells are embryonic cells that, in a permissive environment, will normally develop into muscle tissue. Specific molecular markers for cells at this level of development are yet to be fully defined. *Myoblasts* are thought to be fully determined, mitotically active (proliferating), mononucleated muscle cells, of several different types, that express a subset of the four identified myogenic determination factor genes (MyoD, myf-5, myogenin, and MRF4). *Satellite cells* are quiescent myoblasts that are in close physical proximity to a single muscle fiber in vivo (11,12). Satellite cells lie within small depressions on the periphery of adult myofibers, and are enclosed by the same basal lamina. Satellite cells generally remain quiescent until activated in response to growth, muscle injury, or remodeling. When activated, satellite cells swell away from the surface of the myofiber with which they are associated (11,13). *Myocytes* are terminally differentiated, mononuclear (not yet fused) muscle cells. Myocytes are postmitotic, so they are unable to proliferate, but they are able to fuse with other myocytes or with myotubes, and they express several muscle specific proteins. *Myotubes* are multinucleated, forming from the fusion of two or more myocytes. Myotubes have centrally located nuclei, and are also postmitotic. *Muscle fibers (myofibers)* are mature myotubes, generally exhibiting peripherally located nuclei and a predominance of cross striations resulting from the arrangement of contractile proteins organized into regular arrays of myofibrils. Myofibers also surround themselves with a basal lamina.

Because a muscle fiber is not a single cell by a strict definition of the term, having up to several hundred nuclei within a single plasma membrane, somewhat confusing terminology has been developed: sarcolemma (instead of plasma membrane), sarcoplasm (cytoplasm), sarcosome (mitochondrion), and sarcoplasmic (as opposed to endoplasmic) reticulum. Nonetheless, the fusion of many cells to form a single "cell" has several interesting and potentially useful consequences. Individual myonuclei within the myotube/myofiber do not have to contain identical genetic material, and it can be readily shown that each nucleus has a "nuclear domain" along the length of the myotube/myofiber, for example, by promoting the fusion of a genetically engineered myocyte that will express a reporter gene (such as β-gal)(G. Salvatori, personal communication). Thus, in principle, a single myofiber could be engineered to exhibit a variable genotype (and subsequent phenotype) as a function of position along the length of the myofiber, which may confer a desirable engineering property, such as differential expression of contractile proteins, mitochondrial density, integrins, or other cytoskeletal or transmembrane structures at desired locations along individual myofibers. The extent to which this can be utilized for engineered muscle tissue remains largely unexplored.

FIGURE 1 Cell culture of primary skeletal muscle cells from adult mammals: (A) dissociated porcine skeletal muscle precursor cells (myoblasts and fibroblasts), excised from the lower superfacial abdominal muscles of a freshly slaughtered pig, (B) bovine (Jersey cow) myogenic precursor cells at confluence in culture, immediately before the onset of myocyte fusion, (C) myotubes resulting from the fusion of rat myocytes after the reduction of the serum concentration in the cell culture media. The 100-division reticule in each photograph indicates a total dimension of 1.0 mm, with 10-μm spacing between the smallest divisions.

A

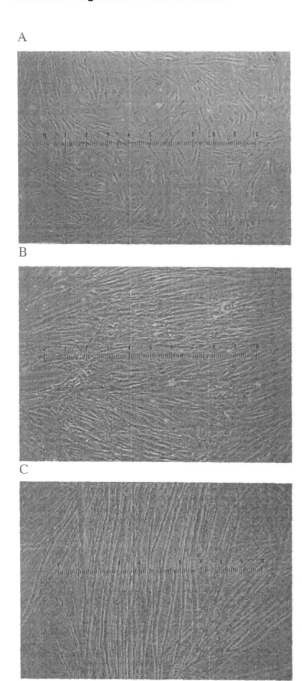

B

C

V. MUSCLE TISSUE STRUCTURE

For a detailed treatment of the subcellular structure, arrangement of the contractile proteins, generation of action potentials, and excitation-contraction coupling in skeletal and cardiac muscles, the reader is referred to any recent textbook of physiology (14). Although muscle contractility arises from action of subcellular structures, it is at the level of *tissues*, the integrated architecture of the extracellular matrix (ECM) and arrays of cells controlled and acting in concert, that the tissue engineer much invariably distinguish his work from that of the cell biologist. We will therefore focus the remainder of this chapter on a discussion of muscle tissue resolved to the structural level of individual myofibers.

Adult skeletal muscle if comprised principally of long polynucleated myofibers, ranging from 40 to 100 μm in diameter, the diameter depending on many factors, including the age and species of the animal. Myofibers can be many centimeters in length in the large limb muscles of humans. Locally, myofibers tend to be aligned in parallel, that is, it is unusual for skeletal myofibers to criss-cross when viewed on the scale of a few myofibers. On the global scale of entire muscle organs, however, the fiber orientations can be quite complex.

Muscle architecture is often described in terms of a global description of the fiber orientation within the muscle. A whole muscle organ may be predominantly comprised of long parallel bundles of myofibers, each myofiber spanning the entire length of the muscle from tendon to tendon. This is conceptually the simplest muscle architecture, but it rarely occurs in natural whole muscle. In a typical muscle, the individual myofibers do not span the entire length of the whole muscle organ, nor are they precisely aligned in parallel with the force-generating axis of the muscle. More frequently, the individual myofibers are, on average, some fraction of the length of the whole muscle organ, giving rise to the ratio L_f/L_o and L_f/L_m, where L_f is the mean myofiber length, L_m is defined as the distance from the origin of the most proximal myofibers to the insertion of the most distant fibers, where the muscle is fixed at the neutral physiological length (15), and L_o is the overall muscle organ length, when the muscle is at its optimal length for force generation. Thus, L_m is a measure based upon musculoskeletal anatomy, whereas L_o is a measure based upon whole muscle physiology. Both measures are approximate, and in practice there are often approximately equivalent. Measures of L_f are most frequently made by nitric acid digestion or microdissection of formalin-fixed whole muscle organs (16,17) maintained at L_m in the case of cadaveric studies, or L_o in the case of whole excised muscle organs for physiological experiments. Typical values for L_f/L_o in the limb musculature of mammals range from ~0.4 to 0.8.

The pennation angle (θ) is defined as the angle between the force-generating axis of a muscle organ and an individual myofiber. In mammalian muscle at rest, θ varies from ~0 to $30°$ (15), and can increase to as high as $60°$ when a muscle is fully activated (18). Thus, while contracting the pennation angle in muscle can change significantly, which means that during contraction, the myofibers can both shorten and rotate with respect to the axis of force generation of the whole muscle organ. For whole muscle organs the architecture is roughly classified on the basis of the pennation angle: *longitudinal*, in which the myofibers all run approximately parallel to the force-generating axis; *unipennate*, in which the myofibers run at a single fixed angle to the force-generating axis; and *multipennate*, in which the myofibers run at several distinct angles to the force-generating axis (15). Most mammalian muscles fall into the *multipennate* category. Even within whole muscles with multipennate architectures, locally the myofibers run in approximately parallel arrays, the fiber arrangement appearing like a bundle of straws rather than a mesh of crossing or skewed fibers.

The myofiber diameter does not vary a great deal within a single muscle, so the *contractility* of whole muscle organs is dominated by the architectural arrangement of the myofibers. Contractility is essentially the *active* mechanical function of whole muscle organs, and is described in terms of the peak force-generating capacity (P_o) of the muscle (15).

The fiber architecture is quantitatively related to the force-generating capacity of whole muscle organs by calculation of the physiological cross-sectional area (PCSA). PCSA has been defined in two separate ways:

$$PCSA = [m \cos(\theta)]/(\rho L_f) \tag{1}$$

$$PCSA = m/(\rho L_f) \tag{2}$$

where m is the total muscle mass, θ represents the pennation angle measured at the surface of the whole muscle, ρ is the muscle density (~1060 kg/m^3 for mammalian muscle), and L_f is the fiber length. The units of each parameter should be selected such that the resulting cross-sectional area is in units of square meters (m^2) so that force generation can be readily normalized to units of kN/m^2 (or kPa). The assumptions in these equations are that the measured tissue mass is contributed by functional myofibers (not extracellular matrix, tendon, or adipose tissue), that the pennation angle remains constant (though we know it generally does not), that the muscle is normally hydrated, and that all fibers within the muscle are the same length, which we also know to be generally incorrect. In addition, in Eq. (2), the pennation angle θ is assumed to be "small" (less than $\sim 10°$), for which $\cos(\theta)\sim 1 (19–21)$. These approximations are widely used by muscle physiologists to allow the normalization of contractile properties. Force is normalized by dividing by the appropriate area (in this case, PCSA) to allow the direct comparison of contractility of muscles of vastly differing mass and fiber architecture, as well as muscles from differing species (e.g., ants, frogs, chickens, and humans). The errors in the estimate of the PCSA have serious implications for the accurate prediction of force, fiber-shortening velocity, and length-tension behavior in whole muscle organs, when basing the calculations upon the physiology of isolated myofibers. Thus, an accurate estimate of the PCSA is essential for the quantitative evaluation of muscle contractility.

VI. MEASUREMENT OF MUSCLE FUNCTION

Classical muscle physiology provides an excellent starting point for the assessment of the function of engineered muscle. The methods of assessment of the contractility of both normal and diseased muscle tissue have been recently reviewed (22). The primary functional assessments of engineered muscle must include both the tissue contractility (the ability to generate mechanical force, work, and power) and *excitability* (the stimulus required to elicit a contraction, in terms of stimulus pulse amplitude and duration) (23–28). In the normal course of muscle physiological research, the quantitative assessment of excitability had faded from common use until it was necessitated by the emergence of functional engineered muscle tissues that were electrically excitable (25) and the availability of implantable electrical stimulator technology capable of maintaining the mass and contractility of denervated whole muscles in vivo (29–33).

The classic definition of tissue excitability is illustrated in Figure 2, by the strength-duration curve (14). Nominally developed to describe the excitability of single nerve axons, the strength-duration curve illustrates that a stimulus pulse must be both of sufficient amplitude (voltage or current) and duration to elicit an action potential. Because an action potential in both muscle and nerve is an all-or-nothing response (14), the curve on the chart in Figure 2 is the clear demarcation between the two possible outcomes: the generation or failure to generate an action potential. For nerve axon depolarization, two terms have been employed to quantify the excitability of tissues: *rheobase* and *chronaxie.*

Classically defined, excitability is measured as follows: the tissue is stimulated using a "wide" pulse, and the pulse amplitude (either current or voltage) is adjusted until the threshold for stimulation is determined. The resulting amplitude is defined as the *rheobase.* The stimulus amplitude is then fixed at twice the rheobase, and the pulse width is then adjusted until the

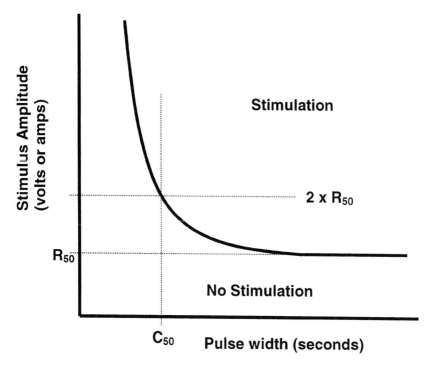

FIGURE 2 A modification of the classical strength-duration curve for excitable tissues to assess the excitability of functional engineered tissues. Rheobase (R_{50}) and chronaxie (C_{50}) are defined by the tissue twitch response to electrical stimulation.

stimulus threshold is again identified. The resulting pulse width is defined as the *chronaxie*. In practical tissue preparations, the rheobase will be dependent on the geometry of the electrodes and the tissue specimen, so rheobase must be determined using parallel electrodes of known surface area, to allow normalization as either V/m (voltage field strength between electrodes separated by a known distance, in m), or amps/m^2 (current flow per unit area, between parallel plate electrodes). The chronaxie is known to be less sensitive to differences between experimental setups, and is therefore considered to be a reliable metric for the comparison of tissue excitability for different preparations (14). This classic definition of excitability is suitable for nerve tissue and individual myofibers, but modifications are required before it can be employed for engineered muscle tissue (23–28). The response of contractile tissues to stimulus pulses is graded, in contrast to the all-or-nothing response of isolated nerve axons. At the tissue level, the response is sigmoidal with respect to pulse amplitude, and curvilinear with a plateau in response to increasing pulse duration (25). As a result, when stimulated by a single electrical pulse, a muscle will respond with a twitch force ranging between zero and maximal twitch force (P_t). By defining the threshold value for the response at 50% of P_t, the excitability of muscle can be quantified in terms of rheobase (R_{50}) and chronaxie (C_{50}) using the classic procedure (25), as illustrated in Figure 2. One important point to consider is that higher values for R_{50} and C_{50} indicate reduced excitability. The relative excitability of rodent skeletal muscle tissues [adult, juvenile, denervated, and engineered from satellite cells in culture (23)] is illustrated in Figure 3, where the highest excitability occurs at the lower left corner of the plot.

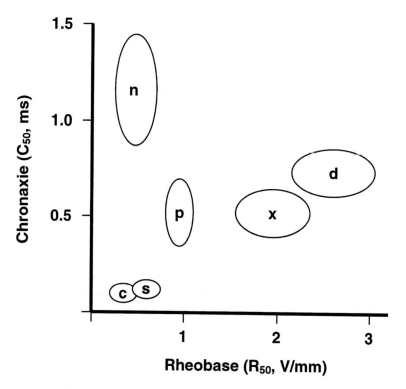

FIGURE 3 Excitability of muscle, native and engineered. Greatest excitability is in the lower left corner of the plot; (c) control muscle from adult rats; (d) chronically denervated rat muscle; (s) denervated-stimulated rat muscle; (n) neonatal and juvenile rat muscles; (p) self-organized muscle engineered in culture from primary myogenic cells; (x) self-organized muscle engineered in culture from immortalized myogenic cells.

The quantitative assessment of muscle contractility requires "supramaximal" electrical stimulation to assure the generation of peak force. The excitability of the muscle tissue must therefore be established to assure that supramaximal stimulation is applied. The excitability of control skeletal muscle from mammals and amphibians is extremely consistent, so much so that it is rarely or never verified before contractility measures are made. As a result of some muscle pathologies, such as chronic denervation, the excitability can fall dramatically, depending upon the species and duration of denervation. The arrested developmental state of many forms of engineered skeletal muscle absolutely necessitates the determination of tissue excitability prior to the measurement of tissue contractility (25). Once the excitability of pathological or engineered muscle tissue has been established, the contractility can be reliably measured.

Specific instrumentation and protocols for the measurement of the contractility of engineered muscle have been described in detail (22,26). Briefly, the muscle specimens are placed between parallel electrodes and are mechanically affixed to a force transducer at one end. A means for adjusting the muscle length must also be provided, allowing the isometric measurements of peak twitch force (P_t), peak isometric tetanic force (P_o), specific force (sP_o), baseline force (P_b), force-frequency, and length-tension to be made. Optionally, a servo motor is provided to allow the measurement of dynamic contractile properties, such as maximum velocity of contraction, work, and power.

VII. APPROACHES TO MUSCLE TISSUE ENGINEERING

The broadest definition of muscle tissue engineering might be: the application of externally controlled signals to muscle tissue or myogenic cells to guide the formation and architecture of muscle tissue toward a specific desired outcome. By this definition, many classes of muscle tissue engineering can be considered. In general, these classes can be categorized on the basis of the general area of application, such as clinical, basic research, or industrial applications, or on the bases of the techniques actually employed in the engineering process. A systematic organization of all forms of muscle tissue engineering is yet to be fully described. For simplicity, the strategy taken in this chapter will be to categorize the approaches on the basis of the materials that are employed (tissues, cells, and synthetic materials), beginning with native tissues altered in vivo, progressing to muscle tissues that are engineered entirely in culture from isolated cells.

A. Resistance Training

Resistance training is the least invasive form of skeletal muscle tissue engineering. It is commonly employed by athletes and physical therapists to promote significant changes in the architecture of whole-muscle groups, typically involving noticeable changes in the force-generating capacity and mass of the muscles of the limb and trunk. Such tissue engineering frequently results in significant enhancements in athletic performance and mobility. This is a well-developed approach with an extensive literature. The relevance of this form of tissue engineering of skeletal muscle should not be discounted too lightly, in part due to the clinical significance of resistance training in rehabilitation medicine, and in part because it will become increasingly necessary to translate the science of exercise into mechanical stimulation protocols to guide the development of muscle tissues in vitro, as more successful culture systems of functional engineered muscle tissue are developed. Current strategies for the use of resistance training to guide muscular development in vivo have been treated in detail by Fleck and Kraemer (34).

B. Surgical Tissue Engineering of Skeletal Muscle

The use of skeletal muscle tissue to replace the function of lost or injured tissues is a well-established surgical practice (35). Muscle and musculotaneous "flaps" are used to cover exposed vital structures, prosthetic appliances, and grafts. This surgical form of skeletal muscle tissue engineering is commonly employed by general, orthopedic, cardiothoracic, vascular, neurosurgeons, and gynecological surgeons. Muscle and musculotaneous flaps are one means by which surgeons are able to achieve large tissue transpositions, which are often more effective than skin flaps in terms of subsequent wound healing and the minimization of external contour defects (Fig. 4). Applications include breast reconstruction and the correction of massive injury to the extremities. The use of muscle flaps also allows restoration of some specialized muscular functions, such as facial reanimation after paralysis (35).

FIGURE 4 Example of surgical skeletal muscle tissue engineering: use of a muscle flap to cover an open wound. (A) Open wound in lower limb, (B) surgical elevation of soleus muscle flap, (C) completed muscle flap. (Photographs courtesy of William Kuzon M.D., Ph.D., University of Michigan, Department of Surgery, Section of Plastic and Reconstructive Surgery).

A

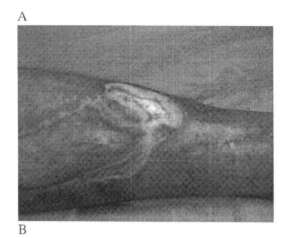

B

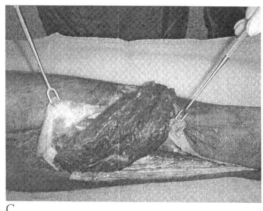

C

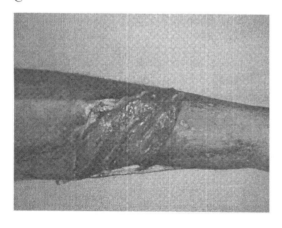

VIII. FIBER-TYPE TRANSFORMATION

One particularly useful tool in the engineering of skeletal muscle is the induction of fiber-type transformation (35–43). Each adult phenotype muscle fiber can be characterized as either fast or slow twitch, on the basis of myosin ATPase. Fiber type is not inherent to individual muscle fibers; rather it is known to be defined by the motor nerve activity. Thus, every motor unit contains a homogeneous population of fiber types, either fast or slow, but not both. Although there is evidence to suggest that fast-twitch muscle generates higher specific force (sP_o) than slow-twitch muscle, the difference is probably less than 10%, and often does not achieve statistical significance in measurements of muscle contractility. The functional significance of fiber type relates to both the peak power output capacity and the fatigability of the muscle. Fast-twitch muscle can generate 225–250 W/kg of mechanical power, approximately 3 times more powerful than slow-twitch muscle at 75–100 W/kg (44,44a). However, the oxidative metabolism of slow-twitch muscles allows the generation of power over much longer periods of time than is possible for fast-twitch muscle, permitting predominantly slow-twitch muscles to work continuously to perform such functions as the maintenance of posture and musculoskeletal tonus.

There are several approaches to induction of fiber-type transformation in skeletal muscles. The first is to cross-innervate, that is, to transect motor nerves and coapt the fast nerve to the nerve stump on a slow muscle, and vice versa (43). For example, the soleus muscle in rodents is almost entirely slow twitch, whereas the extensor digitorum longus (EDL) muscle is almost entirely fast twitch. The motor nerves supplying each can be transected and "switched," such that the slow soleus muscle is now innervated by a fast motor nerve, and the fast EDL is innervated by a slow motor nerve. Within a matter of weeks, the fiber types within each muscle will have transformed. Many experiments in this area have demonstrated that slow motor nerves can cause almost complete transformation of a fast-twitch muscle to the slow-twitch phenotype, whereas the converse, the conversion of slow-twitch to fast-twitch phenotype under the influence of a fast motor nerve, is significantly less complete (42). It is also of clinical significance that the transformative plasticity of regenerating fibers is greater than that of nonregenerating fibers (44,44a). The use of cross-innervation to induce fiber type transformation has clinical significance for the treatment of irreversible facial palsy (41).

An alternative to cross-innervation is to induce fiber-type transformation by electrical stimulation of the motor nerve using an implantable stimulator device. Electrical stimulation in vivo is applied to muscles for three basic purposes: (1) stimulation of normally innervated muscle to induce fiber-type transformation, (2) stimulation of muscle masses that have been denervated to restore function, also known as functional electrical stimulation (FES), and (3) electrical stimulation of denervated muscle simply to retain mass and contractility, with the ultimate goal of re-establishing innervation and normal function. For the purposes of inducing fiber-type transformations in muscle, the implantable stimulator is programmed to deliver stimulus pulses commensurate with the desired muscle fiber type: fast or slow. One major advantage of the use of electrical stimulation to induce fiber-type transformation is that it is not necessary to transsect the motor nerves, thus minimizing collateral tissue damage. The stimulator is used to directly stimulate an intact motor nerve, typically via cuff electrodes placed around the nerve at some distance from the target muscle, or bracketing the neuromuscular junction on the surface of the target muscle. All motor axons within the nerve are depolarized with the imposed stimulus pattern from the implanted stimulator, and the resulting action potentials are transmitted to the target muscle, thereby controlling the pattern of contractile activity of the muscle and inducing fiber-type transformation. This approach has several technical limitations, since many nerves are "mixed" nerves, containing both efferent (motor) and afferent (sensory) nerves, so the application of electrical stimulation can cause severe discomfort. Also, the placement of nerve cuff electrodes often causes a focal pressure gradient along the nerve axons, which is known to disrupt longitudinal flow of cytoplasmic material along nerve axons, often resulting in nerve damage. Typically, to cause conversion of a fast muscle to the slow phenotype, the stimulator would supply a low-frequency ($\sim$10 Hz) stimulus pattern, either continuously, or for long periods of time with brief intervals of rest. To promote slow-to-fast fiber-type transition, the stimulator would be programmed to provide brief high-frequency pulse trains (100–150 Hz), with long intervals of inactivity. For practical reasons, fast-to-slow transformations are more frequently employed. As an example, during electrical stimulation to induce a slow-to-fast fiber-type transformation there would be low-level tonic activity in the intact slow motor nerve between the brief high-frequency bursts from the electrical stimulator, thus in part defeating the imposed "fast" stimulus pattern. Most human muscles are mixed, that is, they contain both slow and fast motor units, so the fiber-type transformations will shift the relative proportions of fiber types within a muscle to a more desirable distribution for the application at hand. For most clinical surgical purposes, a fast-to-slow fiber-type transformation is desirable, because the objective is the restoration of function involving contractility and fatigue resistance commensurate with slow, not fast, twitch muscle function, as in the case of graciloplasty and cardiomyoplasty.

The technical issues surrounding the electrical stimulation of denervated skeletal muscle are different and more challenging than the stimulation of innervated skeletal muscle. Denervation of skeletal muscle typically results in a loss of excitability. So it is often necessary to provide electrical stimulation pulses that are much greater in both amplitude and pulse duration to elicit a muscle contraction. Often, the energy requirement for the stimulation of chronically denervated muscle is 100–1000 times that required to stimulate normally innervated skeletal muscle at an equivalent level of contraction (23,31–33). For this reason, the stimulation of denervated muscle has usually been done with externally powered stimulator systems (29,30). Recent developments have allowed the use of fully implantable stimulators (23,31). The stimulus pattern can be chosen either to maintain the original fiber types in the muscle or it may be used to transform the fibers within the denervated muscle. Because fiber-type transformation can be induced in totally denervated muscles, it is believed that the activity pattern, rather than other nerve-derived (chemical or trophic) factors, defines the fiber type within muscles (46,47).

IX. ENGINEERING SKELETAL MUSCLE FOR RESTORATION OF FUNCTION: GRACILOPLASTY AND CARDIAC ASSIST

Transposition of the gracilis muscle followed by chronic electrical stimulation, a technique referred to as "dynamic graciloplasty," allows restoration of function of the anal sphincter to treat both congenital atresia and acquired incontinence following excision of the anal sphincter due to a malignancy (47). In dynamic graciloplasty, the fast-twitch gracilis muscle is re-engineered in two important ways: (1) the muscle shape and position are surgically altered to allow it to function as a neosphincter, and (2) chronic, low-frequency electrical stimulation is applied via an implantable pulse generator, causing a muscle-fiber-type transformation from fast (type II) to slow (type I). The function of the anal sphincter requires continuous, tonic contractions, which are only possible with type I fibers. A remote control device then allows the patient to control defecation voluntarily (47). With this method, continence can often be re-established within 2 months.

The use of skeletal muscle to assist the pumping action of the heart in the case of end-stage cardiovascular disease has become increasingly common (36,48–56). Like mechanical artificial hearts, skeletal-muscle-based cardiac assist technologies are primarily employed as a bridge until a suitable transplant organ becomes available, though it is ultimately envisioned that a permanent cardiac assistance can be provided by engineered skeletal muscle (36). The use of surgically modified skeletal muscle, transposed from a nearby site within the patient, has great potential and many significant advantages over fully synthetic cardiac assist devices. Most notably, skeletal muscle draws energy from the available sources within the body, so the external energy requirement of a skeletal-muscle-based pump is very low, requiring only that a micropower implantable muscle stimulator, similar to a cardiac pacemaker, be provided. The energy for mechanically pumping the blood is derived from the normal intake of food and oxygen. Issues of rejection and biocompatibility are mitigated as well. Several approaches have been proposed and are currently undergoing detailed clinical testing in humans and animals. The most conservative approach is to fashion a left ventricular assist device (LVAD) from a transposed muscle, which is subsequently wrapped around one or both of the heart ventricles. This approach is termed *cardiomyoplasty*, and skeletal muscle pumps constructed for this purpose have also been termed *biological left ventricular assist devices* (BLVAD). The most frequently used muscle for this purpose is the latissimus dorsi (LD) muscle, though others have also been employed, such as the diaphragm, rectus abdominis, pectoralis major, and serratus anterior (36). Early attempts to utilize skeletal musclegenerally involved the use of the diaphragm (54–56), but these early attempts were generally not successful owing to fatigue of the transposed muscle (36). It is possible to induce fiber-type transformations in the LD muscle to yield both slow-twitch and fast-twitch, oxidative-type fibers, by applying the correct protocol of electrical stimulation to the muscle (36,37,39,40). A similar surgical approach, termed *aortomyoplasty*, is also under development. In aortomyoplasty the skeletal muscle is wrapped around either the ascending or descending aorta. Both cardiomyoplasty and aortomyoplasty are considered to be "conservative" surgical approaches because they do not present new endothelial surfaces to the circulating blood, but the mechanical pumping is less efficient owing to the geometrical limitations of the existing organs, and the fact that the skeletal muscle power is used both to deform the existing tissue (ventricle or aortic wall) and to pump blood. Skeletal muscle can also be formed into a separate auxiliary pump, termed a *skeletal muscle ventricle* (SMV), allowing freedom of design in terms of chamber size, the primary constraint being the geometry and fiber orientation of the original skeletal muscle tissue (36–48). To synchronize stimulation and contraction of the assisting skeletal muscle structures, the R wave of the patient's ECG is often used as a trigger. Depending on the cardiac demand, it is not necessary for the skeletal muscle to contract with each heartbeat. Rather, a *synchronization ratio* is employed, in which the skeletal muscle is stimulated for only for one out of every 2–16 beats. This reduced workload results in good long-term performance while reducing the problems associated with skeletal muscle fatigue (36). In the case of an SMV, stimulation can be timed to provide effective counterpulsation.

A. Explanted Whole-Muscle Organs

Explanted whole muscles generally do not retain their contractility for longer than a few hours. The muscles are maintained for a short period of time in an oxygenated bath of a physiological saline solution. The primary reason for employing explanted whole muscles is to evaluate the contractility of the tissue after an intervention of scientific interest, such as aging, contraction-induced injury, dietary supplementation, etc. This approach is generally restricted to whole muscles from small animals for research purposes. Currently, whole-muscle explants are used in basic research, as well as in drug testing and screening. Explants of large bundles of muscle fibers are also used in the diagnosis of congenital disease of muscle, such as malignant hyperthermia.

B. Acellularized/Recellularized Muscle

Within a whole-muscle organ, each individual myofiber is surrounded by a thin sheath of fibrous extracellular matrix (ECM). It is possible to remove the cellular components of skeletal muscle tissue by exposing the tissue to a series of surfactants, thereby producing a natural scaffold that retains many of the architectural details of the original muscle tissue, such as the size, length, and orientation of each myofiber. Very small muscle masses (less than $\sim$40 mg) can be removed whole and soaked directly in the acellularization solutions. Larger tissue masses can be cannulated and perfused with the acellularization solutions, a process that rapidly yields very satisfactory results for well-vascularized tissues of almost any mass. For at least some protocols, the acellularized ECM is nonantigenic, so it is possible to utilize the resulting ECM as a scaffold for implantation into a different individual. The two general approaches currently under development include (1) the explicit reintroduction of cells into the acellularized matrix in culture, and (2) the implantation of the ECM scaffold into a tissue recipient, with the intent of promoting cellular infiltration into the scaffold. The potential advantages of this approach are that the scaffold architecture can provide a template for the formation of architecturally complex muscle tissues, such as those of the facial musculature, that the scaffold retains important architectural features of the critical tissue interfaces (neuromuscular junction, vascular bed, and the myotendinous junction), and that the natural scaffold can, in principle, be modified prior to implantation to incorporate desired growth factors and antithrombogenic agents.

C. Engineered-Scaffold Approaches

A process such as casting or molding defines the size and shape of engineered scaffolds. Scaffolds can be engineered from materials of both synthetic and natural origin. An excellent series of articles on the commonly employed natural and synthetic polymer scaffold materials and the processes that are used for manipulating them for tissue engineering has been published by Atala and Lanza (58). Scaffold materials comprised chiefly of naturally derived substances that have been used for skeletal muscle often include Matrigel, fibrin gels, and collagen (60–67).

Engineered scaffolds are designed to advantageously provide an initial template for tissue genesis in terms of overall size and shape, to incorporate adhesion molecules and growth factors to promote cell differentiation and tissue formation, and in many cases to use resorbable matrix materials, allowing the cells in the formed tissue to break down the engineered matrix by degrees as the cells take over the demands of producing a natural ECM to bear the mechanical loads (57–59).

The use of engineered scaffolds has proven to be effective for certain types of tissues, such as bone, skin, and articular cartilage, but not for functional skeletal muscle. Skeletal muscle tissue regularly undergoes large mechanical strains (> 10%) as a result of normal activity. Although some scaffold materials can, in principle, tolerate such high strains (such as alginate), a suitable synthetic scaffold material for skeletal muscle has not been identified. Additionally, many scaffold materials currently available inhibit the cell-cell interactions and cell fusion that is required for the formation of long, multinucleated myofibers. This limitation poses a significant challenge when engineering skeletal muscle, but is less limiting for cardiac or smooth muscle constructs because the latter two tissue types do not involve cell fusion into myotubes during development and differentiation.

D. Self-organized Muscle Tissue

When cultured for an adequate period of time, a confluent monolayer of spontaneously contracting myotubes will form in culture, as first demonstrated by Lewis in 1915 (68,69). Since that time, many two-dimensional skeletal muscle cell culture systems have been used to study the cell biology of myotubes. The ability of primary myogenic cells to self-organize into three-dimensional muscle organs in vitro was first demonstrated in 1990 by Strohman et al. (70). In this experiment, primary cells were cultured on Saran film pinned to a SYLGARD (PDMS, polydimethylsiloxane) substrate. The cell monolayer partially detached from the Saran while remaining attached to each of the seven pins, arranged in a circle, resulting in the formation of a starfish-shaped, three-dimensional skeletal muscle organ in culture. Although the tissue mass was not tested for contractile function, it was a large, stable, three-dimensional structure, several hundred microns thick and spanning approximately 3 cm. On the basis of this important demonstration, it became evident that myogenic precursor cells could self-organize into three-dimensional structures in an appropriate environment.

To promote self-organization of myogenic precursors into three-dimensional structures it is necessary to: culture a cohesive monolayer of confluent myogenic cells, predominantly composed of myocytes or myotubes; control the level of adhesion of the cell monolayer to the substrate material, to allow gradual detachment of the cell monolayer at a defined time point in culture, a process called "delamination"; provide anchor materials to which the cell monolayer will remain attached during the delamination process, to define the axis of the forming muscle organ and to provide points against which the self-organizing tissue can mechanically

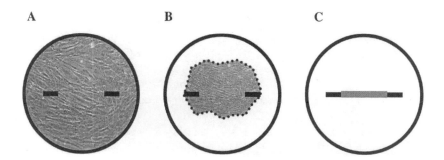

FIGURE 5 Self-organization of muscle cells into a functional, three-dimensional structure in culture (24,25,28). (A) Myogenic precursor cells, including myoblasts and fibroblasts, are plated onto an engineered substrate material (laminin-coated PDMS). The substrate has two anchor materials pinned into place to serve as artificial tendon. (B) The cells grow to eventually form a confluent monolayer, followed by fusion of the myocytes into long, poly-nucleated myotubes. The myotubes begin to spontaneously contract as a syncytium, leading to detachment of the cell monolayer, process called *delamination*, progressing radially inward from the periphery. (C) Delamination progresses for several days, driven by contracting cells within the monolayer, while the monolayer remains attached at the two anchor points. When the cell monolayer has completely detached from the substrate it remains under tension between the anchor points, and remodels into a cylindrical, self-organized muscle organ, with myotubes aligned along the axis defined by the location of the two anchor points. By this process, cylindrical muscle organs can be engineered in culture without the need for an artificial scaffold to define the size and shape of the contractile tissue.

react; and provide chemical cues to promote differentiation of the cells at the appropriate time point in culture. The process of cell monolayer delamination is summarized in Fig. 5. By carefully controlling the culture conditions it is possible to induce simultaneous formation of many skeletal muscle constructs in culture (Fig. 6).

A great deal of important work has been done using both two-dimensional and three-dimensional skeletal muscle cell culture models (3–7,23–28,65–67,71–99). The two-dimensional models have categorically demonstrated that many cellular processes, including metabolism, protein production, and cellular differentiation, are mediated by the mechanical environment external to the cell (100). The three-dimensional skeletal

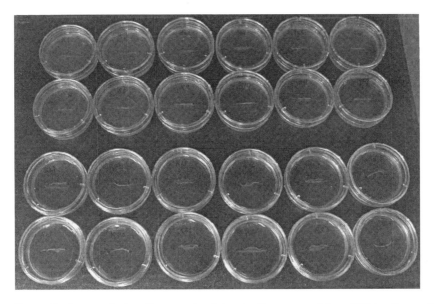

Figure 6 Array of simultaneously delaminating myooids, ~520 h after cell plating. Each plate is 35 mm in diameter, and has been coated with PDMS and laminin. In each culture plate the delamination of the cohesive monolayer of myotubes and fibroblasts is mediated by mechanical events related to both the passive stress generated in the cell monolayer (~5 kPa), due primarily to the action of fibroblasts, and the active stress arising from spontaneous contractions of the myotubes. By employing careful process control during the preparation of the culture substrate and cell harvesting and seeding, the process of cell monolayer delamination and tissue self-organization becomes a predictable and controllable process, with minimal variation in terms of both the resulting tissue morphology and contractility.

muscle tissue models have allowed the quantitative study of the contractility of muscle tissue in culture. The three-dimensional skeletal muscle constructs have been variously termed "organoids," "bioartificial muscles (BAMs)," and "myooids." The tissue constructs can be subjected to externally applied mechanical and electrical fields to induce myocyte and myotube alignment and differentiation toward an adult phenotype (101–104).

Several methods have been developed to measure the isometric contractility of three-dimensional skeletal muscle engineered in vitro (Fig. 7). In the first reported values for the contractility of skeletal muscle constructs, Vandenburgh et al.(94) were able to elicit a contractile response from four organoids, engineered from avian muscle cells, by elevation of the extracellular potassium to 75 mM, resulting in a 91% increase in force

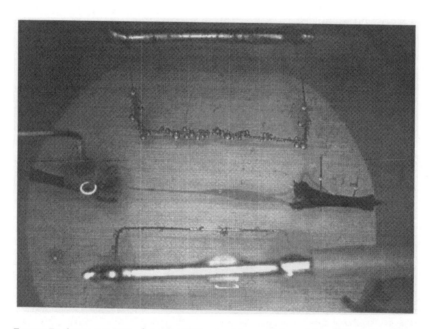

Figure 7 Assessment of excitability and isometric contractility of self-organized muscle tissue in vitro. A self-organized muscle organ (myooid), 12 mm in length, is suspended in culture between two anchors (laminin-coated braided silk suture). Each anchor is held in place by two insect pins, affixed through the anchor and into the PDMS substrate below (visible on the anchor at right). The suture anchor at left has been detached from the PDMS substrate by removal of the insect pins, and has been affixed to the arm of a force transducer. Parallel wire electrodes (36 AWG platinum) have been placed on either side of the myoid to provide electrical stimulation for the quantitative assessment of tissue excitability and contractility.

above resting tension. More recently, electrical stimulus pulses are used to elicit contractions in tens of milliseconds (24–28). The forces generated by three-dimensional muscle contracts in culture are typically only on the order of tens or hundreds of micronewtons, and as a result the vast majority of reports on engineered muscle to date do not include quantitative measures of contractility, the data being limited to biochemical or histological assessments. Measurements of isomeric contractility include the physiological cross-sectional area (CSA), rheobase (R_{50}, pulse *amplitude* required to elicit a twitch), chronaxie (C_{50}, pulse *duration* required to elicit a twitch), resting baseline force (P_b), twitch force (P_t), time to peak tension (TPT), half relaxation time [$\frac{1}{2}$RT], and peak isometric force (P_o). Specific force (sP_o) is calculated by dividing P_o by the cross-sectional area (CSA) of the tissue construct. The sP_o generated by the myoids from a range of primary and immortal mammalian myogenic cells was 1–8% of that generated by control adult skeletal muscles ($\sim$285 kPa). The current hypothesis for the low level of contractility of engineered muscle is that the tissue is arrested at an early developmental phenotype. This results from the culture conditions: the myoids or organoids are cultured without innervation, vascularization, or perfusion, and often under isomeric conditions.

Current research with in vitro-engineered skeletal muscle involves the use of bioreactors to apply controlled electrochemical and chemical interventions in an attempt to guide cellular development and tissue architecture. Myotubes in culture require the application of mechanical strain for the myotubes to fully develop (3,74,78,83,94–96). In addition, myotube orientation is strongly influenced by the application of mechanical strain (94–99). Myotubes will align in parallel with the principle axis of strain when the substrate is subjected to uniaxial, monotonic tension. Since 1841 it has been known that active contractions of skeletal muscle are critical for the maintenance of mass and contractility of skeletal muscle (101). Chronic electrical stimulation promotes the physical alignment of myocytes (102) and expression of adult myosin isoforms in cultured rat and avian skeletal muscle (103,104), and can maintain mass and contractility of denervated muscle indefinitely in vivo (23,31–33). Thus, it is currently hypothesized that active contractile activity, and not necessarily innervation, is essential for the maintenance of adult muscle phenotype, provided that an appropriate electrical stimulation protocol is applied (31,32,45,46).

ACKNOWLEDGMENTS

The author is thankful to the following individuals for their assistance during the preparation of materials for use in this chapter. William Kuzon, M.D., Ph.D.; Krystyna Pasyk, M.D., Ph.D.; Paul Kosnik, Ph.D.

REFERENCES

1. Jiao S, Schultz E, Wolff JA. Intracerebral transplants of primary muscle cells: a potential 'platform' for transgene expression in the brain. Brain Res 1992; 575(1):143–147.
2. Miller RR, Rao JS, Burton WV, Festoff BW. Proteoglycan synthesis by clonal skeletal muscle cells during in vitro myogenesis: differences detected in the types and patterns from primary cultures. Int J Dev Neurosci 1991; 9: 259–267.
3. Perrone CE, Fenwick-Smith D, Vandenburgh HH. Collagen and stretch modulate autocrine secretion of insulin-like growth factor-1 and insulin-like growth factor binding proteins from differentiated skeletal muscle cells. J Biol Chem 1995; 270(5):2099–2106.
4. Powell C, Shansky J, Del Tatto M, Forman DE, Hennessey J, Sullivan K, Zielinski BA, Vandenburgh HH. Tissue–engineered human bioartificial muscles expressing a foreign recombinant protein for gene therapy. Hum Gene Ther 1999; 10:565–577.
5. Vandenburgh HH, Hatfaludy S, Sohar I, Shansky J. Stretch-induced prostaglandins and protein turnover in cultured skeletal muscle. Am J Physiol 1990; 259(2 Pt 1):C232–240.
6. Vandenburgh H, Del Tatto M, Shansky J, Lemaire J, Chang A, Payumo F, Lee P, Goodyear A, Raven L. Tissue-engineered skeletal muscle organoids for reversible gene therapy. Hum Gene Ther 1996; 7(17):2195–2200.
7. Vandenburgh H, Del Tatto M, Shansky J, Goldstein L, Russel K, Genes N, Chromiak J, Yamada S. Attenuation of skeletal muscle wasting with recombinant human growth hormone secreted from a tissue–engineered bioartificial muscle. Hum Gene Ther 1998; 9:2555–2564.
8. Dickinson MH, Farley CT, Full RJ, Koehl MAR, Kram R, Lehman S. How animals move: an integrative view. Science 2000; 288:100–106.
9. Hollerbach JM, Hunter IW, Ballantyne J. A comparative analysis of actuator technologies for robotics. Robotics Review 2. Cambridge, MA: MIT Press 1991:299–342.
10. Full RJ, Meijer K. Metrics of natural muscle. In: Bar-Cohen, Y, ed. Electro Active Polymers (EAP) as Artificial Muscles, Reality Potential and Challenges. Bellingham, WA: SPIE & William Andrew/Noyes Publications, 2001:67–83.
11. Hawke TJ, Garry DJ. Myogenic satellite cells: physiology and molecular biology. J Appl Physiol 2001; 91:534–551.
12. Engel AG, Franzini-Armstrong C. Myology. Vol. I. Basic and Clinical. New York: McGraw-Hill, Inc.1994.
13. Rosenblatt JD, Lunt AI, Parry DJ, Partridge TA. Culturing satellite cells from living single muscle fiber explants. In Vitro Cell Dev Biol Anim 1995; 31(10):773–779.
14. Berne RM, Levy MN. Physiology. 2d ed. St. Louis: Mosby, 1988.
15. Lieber RL, Friden J. Functional and clinical significance of skeletal muscle architecture. Muscle Nerve 2000; 23:1647–1666.

16. Gans C, Bock, WJ. The functional significance of muscle architecture: a theoretical analysis. Adv Anat Embryol Cell Biol 1965; 38:115–142.
17. Gans C, De Vries F. Functional basis of fiber length and angulation in muscle. J Morph 1987; 192:63–85.
18. Zuurbier CJ, Huijing PA. Changes in geometry of actively shortening unipennate rat gastrocnemius muscle. J Morphol 1993; 218:167–180.
19. Close RI. Dynamic properties of mammalian skeletal muscles. Physiol Rev. 1972; 52:129–197.
20. Close R, Hoh JFY. Force:velocity properties of kitten muscles. J Physiol 1967; 192:815–822.
21. Close R. Dynamic properties of fast and slow skeletal muscles of the rat during development. J Physiol 1964; 173:74–95.
22. Faulkner JA, Brooks SV, Dennis RG. Measurement of recovery of function following whole muscle transfer, myoblast transfer, and gene therapy. In: Morgan JR, Yarmush ML, eds. Methods in Tissue Engineering. Tissue Engineering Methods and Protocols. Totowa, NJ: Humana Press Inc.,1997:18: 155–172.
23. Dennis RG, Dow DE, Hsueh A, Faulkner JA. Excitability of engineered muscle constructs, denervated and stimulated-denervated muscles of rats, and control skeletal muscles in neonatal, young, adult and old mice and rats. Biophys Abstr Feb 2002; 82(1):364A.
24. Dennis RG, Kosnik PE, Gilbert ME, Faulkner JA. Excitability and contractility of skeletal muscle engineered from primary cultures and cell lines. Am J Physiol Cell Physiol 2001; 280:C288–C295.
25. Dennis RG, Kosnik PE. Excitability and isometric contractile properties of mammalian skeletal muscle contracts engineered in vitro. In Vitro Cell Dev Biol Anim 2000; 36:327–335.
26. Dennis RG, Kosnik PE. Mesenchymal cell culture: instrumentation and methods for evaluating engineered muscle. In: Atala A, Lanza R, eds. Methods of Tissue Engineering. San Diego: Academic Press, 2001:307–315.
27. Kosnik PE, Dennis RG. Mesenchymal cell culture: functional mammalian skeletal muscle constructs. In: Atala A, Lanza R, eds. Methods of Tissue Engineering. San Diego: Academic Press, 2001:299–305.
28. Kosnik PE, Faulkner JA, Dennis RG. Functional development of engineered skeletal muscle from adult and neonatal rats. Tissue Eng. 2001; 7:573–584.
29. Eken T, Gundersen K. Electrical stimulation resembling normal motor-unit activity: effects on denervated fast and slow rat muscles. J Physiol 1988; 402:651–669.
30. Gundersen K, Eken T. The importance of frequency and amount of electrical stimulation for contractile properties of denervated rat muscles. Acta Physiol Scand 1992; 145:49–57.
31. Dennis RG. Bipolar implantable stimulation for long-term denervated-muscle experiments. Med Biol Eng Comput 1998; 36:225–228.
32. Dow DE, Dennis RG, Hassett CA, Faulkner JA. Electrical stimulation protocol to maintain mass and contractile force in denervated muscles. BMES-

EMBS 1st Joint Conference, Session 6.1.2 Functional Neuromuscular Stimulation, Paper # 573, 1999.

33. Dow DE, Dennis RG, Hassett CA, Faulkner JA. Electrical stimulation to maintain functional properties of denervated EDL muscles of rats. 31st Annual Neural Prosthesis Workshop, National Institutes of Health, Lister Hill Center, Oct. 25–27, 2000.

34. Fleck SJ, Kraemer WJ. Designing Resistance Training Programs. 2d ed. Champaign, IL: Human Kinetics, 1997.

35. Chang, CN, Mathes SJ. Muscle and musculocutaneous flaps. In: Georgiade SG, Riefkohl R, Levin LS, eds. Plastic, Maxillofacial and Reconstructive Surgery. Baltimore: Williams & Wilkins, 1997:29–33.

36. Salmons S. Permanent cardiac assistance from skeletal muscle: a prospect for the new millennium. Art Organs 1999; 23(5):380–387.

37. Salmons S. Exercise, stimulation and type transformation of skeletal muscle. Int J Sports Med 1994; 15:136–141.

38. Pette D, Vrbova G. Adaptation of mammalian skeletal muscle fibers to chronic electrical stimulation. Rev Physiol Biochem Pharmacol 1992; 120:116–202.

39. Jarvis JC, Sutherland H, Mayne CN, Gilroy SJ, Salmon S. Induction of a fast oxidative phenotype by chronic muscle stimulation: mechanical and biochemical studies. Am J Physiol 1996; 270:C306–312.

40. Mayne CN, Sutherland H, Jarvis JC, Gilroy SJ, Craven AJ, Salmons S. Induction of a fast-oxidative phenotype by chronic muscle stimulation: histochemical and metabolic studies. Am J Physiol 1996; 270:C313–320.

41. Nehrer-Tairych GV, Rab M, Kamolz L, Deutinger M, Stohr HG, Frey M. The influence of the donor nerve on the function and morphology of a mimic muscle after cross innervation: an experimental study in rabbits. Br J Plast Surg 2000; 53(8):669–675.

42. Chammas M, Coulet B, Micallef JP, Prefaut C, Allieu Y. Influence of the delay of denervation on slow striated muscle resistance to slow-to-fast conversion following cross-innervation. Microsurgery 1995; 16(12):779–785.

43. Romanul FC, Van der Meulen JP. Reversal of the enzyme profiles of muscle fibers in fast and slow muscles by cross-innervation. Nature 1966; 212(68):1369–1370.

44. Brooks SV, Faulkner JA, McCubbrey DA. Power outputs of slow and fast skeletal muscles of mice. J Appl Physiol 1990; 68(3):1282–1285.

44a. Donovan CM, Faulkner JA. Plasticity of skeletal muscle: regenerating fibers adapt more rapidly than surviving fibers. J Appl Physiol 1987; 62(6):2507–2511.

45. Adams L, Carlson BM, Henderson L, Goldman D. Adaptation of nicotinic acetylcholine receptor, myogenin, and MRF4 gene expression to long-term muscle denervation. J Cell Biol 1995; 131(5):1341–1349.

46. Goldman D, Brenner HR, Heinemann S. Acetylcholine receptor α, β, γ, and δ-subunit mRNA levels are regulated by muscle activity. Neuron 1988: 329–333.

47. Rosen HR, Novi G, Zoech G, Feil W, Urbarz C, Schiessel R. Restoration of anal sphincter function by single-stage dynamic graciloplasty with a modified (split sling) technique. Am J Surg 1998; 175:187–193.

48. Acker MA, Hammond RL, Mannion JD, Salmons S, Stephenson LW. Skeletal muscle as the potential power source for a cardiovascular pump: assessment in vivo. Science 1987; 236:324–327.

49. Cararro U, Barbiero M, Docali G, Cotogni A, Rigatelli G, Casarotto D, Muneretto C. Demand dynamic cardiomyoplasty: mechanograms prove incomplete transformation of the rested latissimus dorsi. Ann Thorac Surg 2000; 70:67–73.

50. Guldner NW, Klapproth P, Großherr M, Brugge A, Sheikhzadeh A, Tolg R, Rumpel E, Noel R, Sievers HH. Biochemical hearts: muscular blood pumps, performed in a 1-step operation, and trained under support of clenbuterol. Circulation 2001; 104:717–722.

51. El Oakley RM, Jarvis JC. Effects of a new cardiomyoplasty technique on cardiac function. Cardiovasc Surg 2001; 9:50–57.

52. Park SE, Cmolik BL, Lazzara RR, Trumble DR, Magovern JA. Right latissimus dorsi cardiomyoplasty augments left ventricular systolic performance. Ann Thorac Surg 2001; 71:2077–2078.

53. Carraro U, Docali G, Barbiero M, Brunazzi C, Gealow K, Casarotto D, Muneretto C. Demand dynamic cardiomyoplasty: Improved clinical benefits by non-invasive monitoring of LD flap and long-term tuning of its dynamic contractile characteristics by activity-rest regime. Basic Appl Myol 1998; 8:11–15.

54. Kantrowitz A, McKinnon W. The experimental use of the diaphragm as an auxiliary myocardium. Surg Forum 1959; 9:266–268.

55. Kantrowitz A. Functioning autogenous muscle used experimentally as an auxiliary ventricle. Trans Am Soc Artif Intern Organs 1960; 6:305–310.

56. Nakamura K, Glenn WL. Grafts of diaphragm as a functioning substitute for the myocardium. J Surg Res. 1964; 4:435–439.

57. Lanza RP, Langer R, Chick WL. Principles of Tissue Engineering. Austin: R.G. Landes Company, Academic Press1997.

58. Atala A, Lanza RP. Methods of Tissue Engineering. San Diego: Academic Press, 2002.

59. Putnam AJ, Mooney DJ. Tissue engineering using synthetic extracellular matrices. Nature Med 1996; 2(7):824–826.

60. Okano T, Matsuda T. Tissue engineered skeletal muscle: preparation of highly dense, highly oriented hybrid muscular tissues. Cell Transplant 1998; 7:71–82.

61. Okano T, Matsuda T. Muscular tissue engineering: capillary-incorporated hybrid muscular tissues in vivo tissue culture. Cell Transplant 1998; 7(5):435–442.

62. Okano T, Satoh S, Oka T, Matsuda T. Tissue engineering of skeletal muscle: Highly dense, highly oriented hybrid muscular tissues biomimicking native tissues. ASAIO J 1997; 43:M749–M753.

63. van Wachem PB, Brouwer LA, van Luyn MJ. Absence of muscle regeneration after implantation of a collagen matrix seeded with myoblasts. Biomaterials 1999; 20:419–426.

64. van Wachem PB, van Luyn MJ, da Costa ML. Myoblast seeding in a collagen matrix evaluated in vitro. J. Biomed Mater Res 1996; 30:353–360.
65. Swasdison S, Mayne R. In vitro attachment of skeletal muscle fibers to a collagen gel duplicates the structure of the myotendinous junction. Exp Cell Res 1991; 193:227–231.
66. Swasdison S, Mayne R. Formation of highly organized skeletal muscle fibers in vitro: comparison with muscle development in vivo. J Cell Sci 1992; 102:643–652.
67. Mayne R, Swasdison S, Sanderson RD, Irwin MH. Extracellular Matrix, Fibroblasts and the Development of Skeletal Muscle. Cellular and Molecular Biology of Muscle Development. New York: Alan R. Liss, Inc.1989:107–116.
68. Lewis MR. Rhythmical contraction of the skeletal muscle tissue observed in tissue cultures. Am J Physiol 1915; 38:153–161.
69. Lewis WH, Lewis MR. Behavior of cross striated muscle in tissue cultures. Am J Anat. 1917; 22:169.
70. Strohman RC, Bayne E, Spector D, Obinata T, Micou-Eastwood J, Maniotis A. Myogenesis and histogenesis of skeletal muscle on flexible membranes in vitro. In Vitro Cell Dev Biol 1990; 26:201–208.
71. Chromiak JA, Shansky J, Perrone C, Vandenburgh HH. Bioreactor perfusion system for the long-term maintenance of tissue-engineered skeletal muscle organoids. In Vitro Cell Dev Biol Anim 1998; 34:694–703.
72. Chromiak JA, Vandenburgh HH. Glucocorticoid-induced skeletal muscle atrophy in vitro is attenuated by mechanical stimulation. Am J Physiol 1992; 262(6 Pt 1):C1471–1477.
73. Chromiak JA, Vandenburgh HH. Mechanical stimulation of skeletal muscle cells mitigates glucocorticoid-induced decreases in prostaglandin production and prostaglandin synthase activity. J Cell Physiol 1994; 159(3):407–414.
74. Hatfaludy S, Shansky J, Vandenburgh HH. Metabolic alterations induced in cultured skeletal muscle by stretch-relaxation activity. Am J Physiol 1989; 256(1 Pt 1):C175–181.
75. Samuel JL, Vandenburgh HH. Mechanically induced orientation of adult rat cardiac myocytes in vitro. In Vitro Cell Dev Biol 1990; 26(9):905–914.
76. Shansky J, Chromiak J, Del Tatto M, Vandenburgh HH. A simplified method for tissue engineering skeletal muscle organoids in vitro. In Vitro Cell Dev Biol Anim 1997; 33:659–661.
77. Vandenburgh H, Chromiak J, Shansky J, Del Tatto M, LeMaire J. Space travel directly induces skeletal muscle atrophy. FASEB J 1999; 13:1031–1038.
78. Vandenburgh H, Kaufman S. In vitro model for stretch-induced hypertrophy of skeletal muscle. Science 1979; 203(4377):265–268.
79. Vandenburgh H, Kaufman S. Protein degradation in embryonic skeletal muscle. Effect of medium, cell type, inhibitors, and passive stretch. J Biol Chem 1980; 255(12):5826–5833.
80. Vandenburgh HH, Hatfaludy S, Karlisch P, Shansky J. Mechanically induced alterations in cultured skeletal muscle growth. J Biomech 1991; 24(suppl 1): 91–99.

81. Vandenburgh HH, Hatfaludy S, Karlisch P, Shansky J. Skeletal muscle growth is stimulated by intermittent stretch-relaxation in tissue culture. Am J Physiol 1989; 256(3 Pt 1):C674–682.

82. Kosnik PE. Contractile Properties of Engineered Skeletal Muscle [Doctoral Thesis]. University of Michigan, Ann Arbor, Michigan. 2000.

83. Vandenburgh HH, Karlisch P, Farr L. Maintenance of highly contractile tissue-cultured avian skeletal myotubes in collagen gel. In Vitro Cell Dev Biol 1988; 24(3):166–174.

84. Vandenburgh HH, Karlisch P, Shansky J, Feldstein R. Insulin and IGF-I induced pronounced hypertrophy of skeletal myofibers in tissue culture. Am J Physiol 1991; 260(3 Pt 1):C475–484.

85. Vandenburgh HH, Karlisch P. Longitudinal growth of skeletal myotubes in vitro in a new horizontal mechanical cell stimulator. In Vitro Cell Dev Biol 1989; 25(7):607–16.

86. Vandenburgh HH, Kaufman S. Coupling of voltage-sensitive sodium channel activity to stretch-induced amino acid transport in skeletal muscle in vitro. J Biol Chem 1982; 257(22):13448–13454.

87. Vandenburgh HH, Kaufman S. Stretch-induced growth of skeletal myotubes correlates with activation of the sodium pump. J Cell Physiol. 1981; 109(2):205–214.

88. Vandenburgh HH, Lent CM. Relationship of muscle growth in vitro to sodium pump activity and transmembrane potential. J Cell Physiol 1984; 119(3):283–295.

89. Vandenburgh HH, Shansky J, Karlisch P, Solerssi RL. Mechanical stimulation of skeletal muscle generates lipid-related second messengers by phospholipase activation. J Cell Physiol 1993; 155(1):63–71.

90. Vandenburgh HH, Shansky J, Solerssi R, Chromiak J. Mechanical stimulation of skeletal muscle increases prostaglandin F2 alpha production, cyclooxygenase activity, and cell growth by a pertussis toxin sensitive mechanism. J Cell Physiol 1995; 163(2):285–294.

91. Vandenburgh HH, Sheff MF, Zacks SI. Soluble age-related factors from skeletal muscle which influence muscle development. Exp Cell Res 1984; 153(2):389–401.

92. Vandenburgh HH, Solerssi R, Shansky J, Adams JW, Henderson SA, Lemaire J. Response of neonatal rat cardiomyocytes to repetitive mechanical stimulation in vitro. Ann NY Acad Sci 1995; 752:19–29.

93. Vandenburgh HH, Solerssi R, Shansky J, Adams JW, Henderson SA. Mechanical stimulation of organogenic cardiomyocyte growth in vitro. Am J Physiol 1996; 270(5 Pt 1):C1284–1292.

94. Vandenburgh HH, Swasdison S, Karlisch P. Computer-aided mechanogenesis of skeletal muscle organs from single cells in vitro. FASEB J 1991; 5(13):2860–2867.

95. Vandenburgh HH. A computerized mechanical cell stimulator for tissue culture: effects on skeletal muscle organogenesis. In Vitro Cell Dev Biol 1988; 24(7):609–619.

96. Vandenburgh HH. Cell shape and growth regulation in skeletal muscle: exogenous versus endogenous factors. J Cell Physiol 1983; 116(3):363–371.
97. Vandenburgh HH. Dynamic mechanical orientation of skeletal myofibers in vitro. Dev Biol 1982; 93(2):438–443.
98. Vandenburgh HH. Mechanical forces and their second messengers in stimulating cell growth in vitro. Am J Physiol 1992; 262(3 Pt 2):R350–355.
99. Vandenburgh HH. Motion into mass: how does tension stimulate muscle growth?. Med Sci Sports Exercise 1987; 19(5 Suppl):S142–149.
100. Harris AK. Physical forces and pattern formation in limb development. In: Hinchliffe JR, Hurle JM, Summerbell D, eds. Developmental Patterning of the Vertebrate Limb. New York: Plenum Press, 1991:203–210.
101. Reid J. On the Relation between muscular contractility and the nervous sytem. London Edinburgh Monthly J M 1841; 1:320–329.
102. Hinkle L, McCaig CD, Robinson KR. The direction of growth of differentiating neurones and myoblasts from frog embryos in an applied electric field. J Physiol 1981; 314:121–135.
103. Naumann K, Pette D. Effects of chronic stimulation with different impulse patterns on the expression of myosin isoforms in rat myotube cultures. Differentiation 1994; 55:203–211.
104. Wehrle U, Dusterhoft S, Pette D. Effects of chronic electrical stimulation on myosin heavy chain expression in satellite cell cultures derived from rat muscles of different fiber-type composition. Differentiation 1994; 58(1):37–46.

17

Gene Therapy to Enhance Bone and Cartilage Repair

Jay R. Lieberman
David Geffen School of Medicine at UCLA,
Los Angeles, California, U.S.A.

I. INTRODUCTION

Gene therapy involves the transfer of genetic information to cells. When a gene is properly transferred to a target cell, the cell synthesizes the protein encoded by the gene. Therefore, with gene therapy the genetic message is delivered to a particular cell, which then synthesizes the protein (1–3). In general, the duration of protein synthesis after gene transfer depends on the techniques used to deliver the gene to the cell. Both short-term and long-term expression are possible. Although gene therapy was originally conceived as a treatment modality to treat genetic diseases or life-threatening disorders such as cancer, it is now quite evident that it is a potentially novel form of therapy that is particularly applicable for the treatment of musculoskeletal problems. There are a number of potential clinical applications for gene therapy including treatment of nonunions, cartilage defects, and arthritic diseases, enhancement of ligament, tendon, and fracture healing, fusion of the spine, and regeneration of injured discs, nerves, and tendons. In addition, the management of diseases that affect the development of the skeleton, including osteogenesis imperfecta, Gaucher's disease, achondroplasia, multiple epiphyseal dysplasia, and spondyloepiphyseal dysplasia, may also be amendable to treatment with gene therapy (4,5). In this review we will restrict ourselves to potential uses of gene therapy to problems related to bone and cartilage repair.

II. GENE THERAPY STRATEGIES

The duration of protein production required and the anatomical location where the protein must be delivered clearly influence the type of gene therapy that will be employed. Several different gene therapy options are available. First, gene therapy can be either systemic or regional. Second, the gene can be introduced directly to a specific anatomical site (in vivo technique) or specific cells can be harvested from the patient, genetically manipulated, and then reimplanted (ex vivo technique). The specific cell targeted for gene delivery can also be specified when using an ex vivo gene transfer strategy. Third, the vehicle or vector for gene delivery can be either viral or nonviral (4,6,7).

A. Regional vs. Systemic Gene Therapy

Gene therapy can be used to either treat a disorder resulting from a single gene mutation or enhance the production of a specific protein. Osteogenesis imperfecta and Gaucher's disease are two examples of genetic diseases that are potentially amendable to gene therapy but would likely require a systemic approach because every host cell has a defective gene. Osteoporosis is another condition that may require a systemic approach since multiple anatomical sites have deficient mineralization. In contrast, regional therapy may be a better choice to heal fracture nonunions, fuse a spine, or treat cartilage defects or an inflammatory joint (4,5,7).

B. Ex Vivo vs. In Vivo Approach

In vivo gene transfer involves the introduction of a specific gene directly into the body. The expectation is that this gene will reach the target cell. This approach is attractive because it is technically simple and requires only one surgical procedure. The disadvantage of the direct in vivo approach lies in the less efficient transduction of specific target cells. Direct injection of viral particles carries the potential risk of systemic spread and a systemic inflammatory response. Direct or in vivo gene therapy approaches must rely on vectors, which have been made less immunogenic and have a high affinity for a surface molecule on a target cell or that have a tissue specific promoter (7).

In ex vivo gene transfer, cells are harvested from the patient and the DNA is subsequently transferred to the cells. In most strategies, the cells are expanded in tissue culture and then the cells are genetically manipulated and subsequently administered to the patient. However, strategies are now being developed in which cells could be harvested from the patient, genetically manipulated, and then delivered to the patient during the same operative procedure (8). An advantage of the ex vivo approach is that one can select a specific cell type that is to be genetically manipulated. For example, when trying to enhance bone repair, one can deliver an osteoinductive gene such as bone morphogenic protein (BMP) to a specific anatomical site and also select the cellular delivery vehicle. Bone marrow cells are attractive as a delivery vehicle for bone repair since there is a potential benefit of obtaining both an autocrine and a paracrine response. The bone marrow cells can respond to the BMP that they are overexpressing. Another potential advantage of the ex vivo approach is the ability to ensure more consistent results by implanting only cells that express the protein of interest at high levels. The disadvantage of the ex vivo approach is that it is complicated and potentially time consuming, and it may not be cost-effective (4,5).

III. VECTORS

Vectors are agents that enhance the entry and expression of DNA into a target cell. Vectors may be of viral or nonviral origin. Viruses are efficient vectors because the delivery and expression of DNA is a critical aspect of their normal life cycle. When a virus is used as a vector, essential portions of its genome must be deleted to render it replication-deficient and create a space in its genome for the insertion of the therapeutic DNA. Insertion of therapeutic DNA in exchange for a portion of the viral genome, which would otherwise confer upon the virus the ability to replicate, is accomplished by a process known as *homologous recombination* (5,7,9,19). The process that involves the transfer of functional genetic information from the recombinant vector (virus) into the target cell is known as transduction. The virus that contains the therapeutic DNA binds to the cell, usually via a receptor-mediated process, and then enters that cell. The DNA then enters the nucleus of the cell where it may become integrated into the host genome or it may remain extrachromosomal or episomal. It is then possible for the transduced cell to produce and secrete the growth factor encoded by the DNA (7).

A major concern with the use of viral vectors is the subsequent recombination of the defective virus with viruses in the host cell resulting in the generation of replication-competent viruses with the ability to multiply in the patient. In addition, cells infected with certain viruses (e.g., adenoviruses) produce not only the transgene product but also other viral proteins. These viral proteins may elicit an immune response in the host, which can limit the duration of protein expression by the transduced cells. Specific therapeutic needs associated with different clinical conditions require that viruses with a variety of properties be investigated as potential vectors for clinical use. These vectors include: retroviruses, adenoviruses, adeno-associated viruses, and herpes simplex viruses. A critical issue with viral vectors is whether the genetic information transferred will integrate into the host cell's chromosome or remain episomal because this is the critical factor in determining the duration of protein production (7,9).

Retroviruses are enveloped single-stranded RNA viruses that transfer their genetic information into the genome of the target cell resulting in the potential for long-term expression. Retroviruses have minimal antigenicity and immunogenicity. Disadvantages of retroviral vectors include the potential for toxicity associated with chronic overexpression of the protein and the ability of retroviral vectors to integrate randomly in the host cell genome, which can potentially cause insertional mutagenesis or activate a proto-oncogene. These vectors are generally used in ex vivo gene transfer strategies to facilitate the testing of cells after infection and because retroviruses can only infect dividing cells (7,9).

Adenoviral vectors are currently under study for both in vivo and ex vivo applications. These vectors are attractive because they can be produced in high titers and can infect both replicating and nonreplicating cells. However, the episomal position of the inserted DNA and the nonspecific inflammatory response induced by the adenoviral proteins may limit gene expression. This is clearly a problem when chronic protein production is necessary to treat a disease associated with a single gene defect. However, the treatment of many bone and cartilage repair problems may require only short-term gene production. Therefore, the limited transgene expression associated with adenoviral gene therapy may be advantageous in this clinical setting (5,10). Investigators are at present attempting to develop third-generation adenoviral vectors in which a majority of viral sequences are deleted in the hope that these vectors will be less immunogenic (11).

Adeno-associated viruses also have substantial potential for bone repair applications. Adeno-associated viruses are human parvoviruses that demonstrate preferential integration into a particular region of the host genome (short arm of chromosome 19). The advantages of this vector include: (1) the ability to transduce nondividing cells, (2) production of high titers, (3) site-specific integration into the host genome, and (4) long-term transgene expression (12). This type of vector could be potentially used in cases where intermediate or long-term protein production is required such as osteoporosis, or the treatment of large segmental defects associated with revision total joint arthroplasty, or tumor resection. Major disadvantages of adeno-associated viruses include the fact that the genome is relatively small and the maximum cDNA that can be incorporated is 4–8 kb. Large quantities of the virus are difficult to produce because efficient packaging cells have not been developed and there are potential problems with contamination by the adenovirus used to help to produce the vector. If the adenoassociated virus is not purified of adenovirus there is potential for production of adenoviral proteins along with the transgene product resulting in the induction of an immune response (12–14).

Herpes simplex virus is a large, enveloped, double-stranded DNA virus that has the ability to incorporate approximately 30 kb. These viruses can also infect both dividing and nondividing cells. A major limitation of this vector is the associated cytotoxicity, which can reduce its overall efficacy (15).

To avoid some of the problems of viral vectors, nonviral vectors are being developed as gene delivery vehicles. Nonviral vectors are usually easier to produce, have greater chemical stability than their viral counterparts, and are easier to manufacture for large-scale use. In addition, there are fewer safety concerns with nonviral vectors because they are typically less immunogenic than viral vectors. The major disadvantage of nonviral vectors is that they are generally less efficient in delivering genetic material to cells. Examples of nonviral vectors include naked DNA, liposomes, and DNA-ligand complexes. Strategies need to be developed to increase the transfection rate of these nonviral vectors to enhance their clinical potential (4,16,17).

IV. FRACTURE HEALING AND NONUNION

Approximately 5–10% of fractures heal slowly (delayed union) or do not heal at all (nonunion) (18). Problems with bone healing are associated with a number of risk factors including the degree of soft-tissue injury, location of the fracture, amount of bone lost, and presence of infection. Physiology of bone formation and repair is influenced by growth factors and cytokines that can regulate critical cellular functions including cell proliferation, differentiation, and matrix synthesis (19). A number of growth factors that can enhance bone repair have been identified. In particular, the bone morphogenic proteins (BMPs) have been shown to induce bone formation in both human clinical trials and preclinical animal models (20–24). Although these proteins are clearly osteoinductive, there are concerns that a single dose of exogenous protein may not induce an adequate osteoinductive response. In many clinical situations, the healing potential of bone may be compromised by poor blood supply, limited bone stock, and abundant fibrous tissue formation. In addition, bone repair may be inhibited in diabetic, elderly, or nicotine-addicted patients (3,4,25). In two clinical trials in humans, large doses of BMP were required to induce adequate bone repair (20,21). This suggests that the mode of BMP delivery still requires further optimization. Gene therapy has the potential to provide more sustained protein release and to deliver proteins to a specific anatomical site in a more physiological manner than recombinant proteins (3,4,19,25).

A. In Vivo Gene Therapy

Both in vivo and ex vivo gene transfer strategies have been used in preclinical animal models to enhance bone repair. In vivo strategies using either viral or nonviral delivery methods have been used successfully to induce bone formation. Baltzer et al. used a first-generation adenoviral vector containing the cDNA for BMP-2 to heal critical-size femoral defects in New Zealand white rabbits (Fig. 1). The healing of bone defects was noted in all animals 12 weeks after direct injection of the BMP-2-containing adenovirus into the bone defect (26). Although this direct injection of the adenovirus induced sufficient bone formation to heal a critical-size defect, there are concerns about the immune response to production of adenoviral proteins in humans. Okubo et al. noted bone formation after injection of the BMP-2-containing adenovirus only when Wistar rats were immunosuppressed with cyclophosphamide. No osteoinduction occurred without cyclophosphamide treatment (27). A reduction in the immunogenic response to adenoviral proteins is necessary before direct adenoviral injection into an anatomical site will be approved for human use.

Nonviral delivery strategies are also being developed to avoid the potential problems associated with various viral vectors. Nonviral vectors include liposomes, DNA ligand complexes, and naked DNA. Naked DNA placed in a gene-activated matrix (GAM) is an example of a nonviral delivery method that has been successfully used to promote bone repair in a rat femoral defect model. In this strategy, the DNA for PTH 1–34 or BMP-4 was incorporated into a collagen matrix and then implanted into a bone defect. The goal of this strategy is to turn local fibroblasts into bioreactors for the synthesis of PTH or BMP-4 protein, which will then induce bone formation (16,17). This strategy was used successfully to heal 5-mm defects in rats (16). Recently, Bonadio et al. noted in vivo protein production of PTH 1–34 for 6 weeks after a GAM was implanted into a canine tibial defect. Unfortunately, insufficient bone was produced to heal a critical-size tibial defect in this canine model (17). The results of this study suggest that either the local transfection efficiency is low or perhaps a more osteoinductive

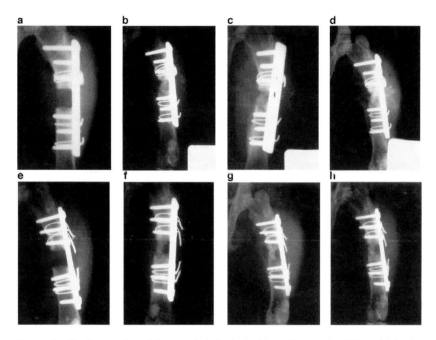

FIGURE 1 Radiographs of femoral defects in New Zealand white rabbits treated with either an adenoviris containing the BMP-2 or luciferase gene. Representative radiographs of defects treated with the BMP-2 gene at the time of
operation (a) and 5 weeks (b), 7 weeks (c), and 12 weeks (d) after the operation. Representative radiographs of defects receiving the luciferase gene at
the time of operation (e) and 5 weeks (f), 7 weeks (g), and 12 weeks (h) after
the operation. None of the defects treated with the luciferase gene healed.
(Adapted from Ref. 26.)

protein than PTH 1–34 must be used to enhance bone repair using this strategy. Overall, the use of a GAM is an attractive gene transfer strategy, but
further study is necessary to determine the appropriate cDNA to use with
the GAM.

B. Ex Vivo Gene Therapy

Ex vivo gene transfer strategies are also being investigated in animal models because not only can an osteoinductive gene be implanted in an appropriate anatomical site, but this strategy allows the surgeon to select
specific cells for genetic manipulation. The use of bone marrow cells,
muscle cells, or stem cells may enhance the bone repair process because
both an autocrine and paracrine response can be elicited with secretion

of the desired gene. Ex vivo methods are also attractive when working
with an adenovirus because no viral particles or DNA complexes are
directly injected into the body and this may reduce the immunogenic reaction normally associated with direct adenoviral injection. The selection
of specific cells to use in an ex vivo gene strategy may play a critical role
in determining the success of these techniques when employed in humans.
Bone marrow cells are an obvious candidate to use with this type of strategy because they are osteogenic themselves and bone marrow harvests
are a well-established technique (3,4,5,7). In addition, methods have been
developed to produce a pure population of mesenchymal cells. These purified mesenchymal cells can be expanded in tissue culture and they have
demonstrated the ability to induce sufficient bone formation to heal critical-size defects in both and rats and canine animal models (28,29).
However, bone marrow cells alone probably do not have sufficient
osteoinductive potential to heal bone defects in humans and therefore
genetic manipulation of these cells to produce an osteoinductive protein
would further enhance the bone repair response.

Lieberman et al. used an ex vivo gene transfer strategy to heal critical-
size femoral defects in a rat model (10). Autologous rat bone marrow cells
were transduced with a BMP-2-containing adenovirus and these BMP-producing bone marrow cells were then successfully used to heal femoral
defects (Fig. 2). Histomorphometric analysis revealed a more robust pattern of bone formation in femoral defects treated with the BMP-2 protein.
It was hypothesized that the more robust bone formed by transduced
BMP-2-producing cells was a result of a more physiological release of
BMP-2 protein compared to the kinetics of BMP release from a collagen
sponge. In addition, the more vigorous osteogenic activity may have been
noted because both the paracrine and autocrine response were induced by
the BMP-producing bone marrow cells (10).

A variety of the cell types have also been used to induce bone formation. BMP-7-transfected rat skin fibroblasts were used to heal critical-sized
calvarial defects in Lewis rats (30). Fibroblasts are attractive cellular delivery vehicles because they are easy to harvest and readily available in all
patients. There is some concern about using skin fibroblasts to enhance
bone repair because fibrous tissue can actually inhibit bone formation and
is present in fracture nonunion sites.

Muscle-derived stem cells may contain osteogenic precursor cells.
Lee et al. demonstrated that muscle cells transduced with a BMP-2-con-
taining adenovirus could successfully heal calvarial defects in SCID mice.
A small percentage of muscle-derived cells implanted in calvarial defects
actually differentiated into osteoblasts in vivo. Both the muscle cells and
bone marrow cells have a similar advantage in ex vivo transfer strategies in

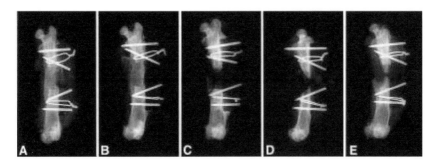

FIGURE 2 Radiographs of the specimens made 2 months after the operation. Twenty milligrams of guanidine hydrochloride-extracted demineralized bone matrix was used as a substrate in all defects. (A) Group I—BMP-2-producing bone-marrow cells [5 x 10⁶]. Dense, coarse trabecular bone, which was remodeling to form a new cortex, was present in these defects. (B) Group II—rhBMP-2 (20 μg). The healed defect is filled with lace-like trabecular bone. (C, D, E) Group III—β-galactosidase-producing rat-bone-marrow cells, Group IV—uninfected rat-bone-marrow cells, and Group V—demineralized bone matrix alone. Minimum bone formation was noted in these three groups. (Adapted from Ref. 10.)

that they not only deliver an osteoinductive signal but they contain osteogenic precursor cells (31).

Recently, fat has been identified as another source of mesenchymal stem cells. Human adipose tissue obtained by liposuction yields a fibroblast-like population of cells that have the potential to be used in different types of tissue engineering strategies (32). When grown in the appropriate media, these adipose-derived stem cells have been shown to differentiate into either bone, cartilage, fat, or muscle. The full osteogenic potential of these cells has not been characterized in vivo. However, when these adipose-derived stem cells are transduced with a BMP-2-containing adenovirus and implanted into a muscle pouch in SCID mice, bone formation is induced (33). Further work with these cells is now being performed in our laboratory.

V. SPINE FUSION

Over 980,000 spinal fusions are performed in the United States each year and approximately one third of these procedures require a bone graft (34). In general, autogenous bone graft is a successful technique for inducing a spine fusion but nonunion rates still range from 5 to 35% (35). The ability to obtain a successful spine fusion is generally influenced by a variety of factors, including: mechanical instability of the spine, stability of fixation, quality of bone, vascularity of the surrounding soft tissue, type of bone graft used, and the concurrent use of medications and drugs such as nicotine. Recently, the Food and Drug Administration has approved the use of the combination of a recombinant BMP-2 in a collagen sponge and a tapered titanium cage to enhance fusion of the spine. As previously discussed, large doses of BMP-2 were required to induce spinal fusion and therefore other protein delivery methods still require investigation to improve the efficiency of this process.

LIM mineralization protein-1 (LMP-1) is a transcription factor that promotes endogenous expression of bone morphogenic proteins. Bone marrow cells transduced with a cDNA for LMP-1 were assessed in a single intertransverse process lumbar spine fusion model in rats. Successful spine fusion was obtained in all 11 sites treated with the LMP-1-transduced bone marrow cells. Spine fusion was not obtained in animals treated with a reverse copy of the cDNA that does not express LMP-1 or with control bone marrow cells alone (36). The same investigators have used buffy coat cells that have been transduced with an adenovirus containing the cDNA for LMP-1 (Fig. 3). Rabbits treated with these transduced peripheral blood-derived cells developed solid spine fusions (8). These peripheral blood cells are attractive as cellular delivery vehicles because they are easier to harvest in bone marrow cells. However, a potential disadvantage of these cells is that they do not possess the same autocrine effects that are seen with transduced bone marrow cells. The results of LMP-1 in these preclinical models are quite impressive and could be adapted to treat other bone repair problems such as fracture nonunions. However, there is minimal information regarding the biology of LMP-1 particularly related to the potential side effects associated with overexpression of this transcription factor (7).

Recombinant adenovirus containing the BMP-2 cDNA has been used successfully to induce an intertransverse lumbar spinal fusion in rats. Bone marrow cells were harvested from Lewis rats, expanded in tissue culture, and then infected with the BMP-2-containing adenovirus. These transduced cells were then either loaded onto a collagen sponge or guanidine-extracted demineralized bone matrix and implanted into the appropriate fusion site. These BMP-2-producing bone marrow cells induced a fusion in all 15 spines that were treated. Bone marrow cells that were not transduced did not induce fusion of the spine (37).

The ability to deliver growth factors via gene therapy may lead to the development of less invasive operative techniques such as laparoscopic spine fusion. These minimally invasive surgical techniques have the potential to reduce operative morbidity and soft-tissue injury and decrease costs (38). Although gene therapy will not be necessary to treat all patients, it

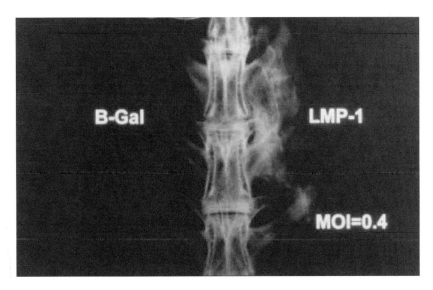

FIGURE 3 Radiograph made 5 weeks after arthrodesis performed with bone-marrow-derived buffy coat infected with AdLMP-1 (right) or AdBgal (adeno-virus containing the cDNA for β-galactosidase, negative control (left) (MOI = 0.4 pfu/cell) for 10 min and implanted on a rabbit devitalized bone matrix carrier (rDVBM) (guanidine hydrochloride-extracted demineralized bone matrix). A continuous spinal fusion mass formed on the side treated with cells infected with AdLMP-1, while minimal bone formed on the side treated with cells infected with AdBgal. (Adapted from Ref. 8.)

does have the potential to enable orthopedic surgeons to treat difficult bone repair problems that cannot be handled successfully with out present technology.

VI. ARTICULAR CARTILAGE REPAIR

Chondrocytes do not possess the inherent ability to regenerate themselves. Therefore, the repair of cartilage defects results in the formation of fibrocartilage repair tissue rather than normal cartilage (5). The prevention of the development of end-stage arthritis after cartilage injury is a significant clinical problem. At present, potential treatment options for cartilage defects include: autologous chondrocyte transplantation (39), marrow-stimulating procedures such as abrasion, arthroplasty (40), or the micro-fracture technique (41), and osteochondral allografts (42). However, none of these techniques have been consistently successful in producing normal cartilage. The repair of a cartilage defect requires the re-establishment of the microarchitecture of the extracellular matrix that is synthesized by normal chondorcytes, and union of the new cartilage that is formed to the host cartilage. In addition, the new cartilage that is formed must unite to the underlying subchondral bone. The repair tissue that is produced with the aforementioned surgical techniques does not meet these requirements and, therefore, deteriorates over time with weight bearing (7,43).

Recently, attention has been focused on using growth factors to enhance cartilage repair. Such growth factors as transforming growth factor beta (TGF-β), insulin growth factor (IGF), and bone morphogenic proteins (BMP) have been used to enhance cartilage repair (44–47). However, using exogenous growth factors to treat cartilage defects also has potential problems. It is not clear that a single exposure to an exogenous growth factor will induce an adequate healing response because it is difficult to deliver these growth factors intra-articularly. In addition, there are concerns that the carriers used to deliver the growth factor may inhibit cartilage repair as they degrade. If biological degradation of the carriers is associated with an inflammatory response in the joint, healing of the cartilage defect could be inhibited.

Several potential gene therapy strategies could be used to heal cartilage defects. First, one can use an in vivo technique in which the gene of interest is injected into the surrounding synovium (48–50). Another in vivo option is the development of light-activated adeno-associated viruses, which could potentially be used to trigger cartilage healing (51). Finally, an ex vivo strategy in which autologous chondrocytes or chondroprogenitor cells are harvested from the patient, genetically manipulated, and then reimplanted has clinical potential.

It has already been demonstrated that synovium can be readily transduced by a wide variety of different vectors and it has also served as a site of gene transfer in a clinical study related to treatment of arthritis in gene therapy (48). The cDNAs for various growth factors are easily delivered to the synovium and then the synovium can serve as intra-articular source of diffusible transgene products. The concept for this strategy has been demonstrated in rabbit knee joints (49). Administration of either IGF-1 or BMP-2 cDNA via adenoviral gene transfer to the synovium increases articular cartilage matrix systhesis in the knee joint by approximately 50% (50–52). One of the major limitations of gene transfer to synovium alone is that when trying to heal cartilage defects, one also needs to provide a matrix. This may not be done via an in vivo gene transfer strategy unless a technique similar to a gene-activated matrix used for bone repair would be employed.

Autologous chondrocyte transplantation is already a commonly used clinical technique (39). In this strategy chondrocytes are harvested from a patient, expanded in tissue culture, and then reimplanted into the articular cartilage defect. Therefore, it is not unreasonable to consider genetically manipulating these chondrocytes or chondroprogenitor cells to help enhance the repair process. Chondrocytes have been demonstrated to be easily transduced by viral and nonviral vectors (53,54).

Adenoviral gene transfer using the cDNAs encoding IGF-1 and BMP-7 have been used in in vivo animal models (52,55,56). These studies have demonstrated increases in matrix production and the presence of the growth factor in the joint. However, long-term production of durable, bio-mechanically stable articular cartilage has not been demonstrated at this point. Another option for ex vivo gene transfer strategies, instead of articular chondrocytes, is to use chondroprogenitor cells such as mesenchymal stem cells or adipose-derived stem cells. It has been demonstrated that, under the appropriate in vitro tissue culture conditions, these cells can differentiate into chondrocytes. Wakitani et al. have demonstrated in a rabbit model that mesenchymal stem cells can be used to heal articular cartilage defects (57). Another potential option is to use a modification of the present mosaicplasty technique. Autologous cartilage can be harvested from the patient and treated with an adeno-associated virus containing a cDNA such as IGF-1 or BMP-7 (58). The transduced cartilage that has been transplanted into the defect is then activated with a laser and the cartilage repair would be enhanced by expression of the growth factor. Some in vitro work has demonstrated the potential of this technique and further studies using this strategy are worthwhile.

The major difficulty in developing cartilage repair strategies is not only the type of vector to use but also selecting an appropriate scaffolding to deliver the cells. As stated previously, one of the major problems in developing cartilage repair strategies is producing cartilage that is durable enough to sustain weight bearing over long periods of time. Scaffolding that could deliver transduced cells or proteins that would be released over time and then could be incorporated into the cartilage matrix could provide a significant advantage for this type of strategy. A successful implementation of a gene therapy program for cartilage repair will require a more comprehensive understanding of the biology of chondrocyte matrix synthesis and cartilage repair.

VII. CONCLUSION

It is clear that to solve difficult clinical problems, innovative treatment strategies need to be developed. Gene therapy is a potentially novel approach to deliver particular proteins to a specific anatomical site. Clearly, gene therapy will not be appropriate for every patient. However, the development of gene therapy as a clinical tool is an evolutionary process. Preclinical studies discussed in the chapter have demonstrated the potential clinical application of gene therapy in a number of different models of both bone repair and cartilage repair. It is clear that clinical trials to enhance bone repair will be appropriate within the decade. The development of gene therapy for cartilage repair is more difficult because this is a much more complex biological process. However, it is clearly worth the effort to try to develop cartilage repair strategies using gene therapy because we may be able to develop new treatment modalities and also learn more about the biology of cartilage itself.

REFERENCES

1. Evans CH, Robbins PD. Possible orthopaedic applications of gene therapy. J Bone Joint Surg Am 1995; 77:1103–1114.
2. Evans CH, Ghivizzani SC, Smith P, Shuler FD, Mi Z, Robbins PD. Using gene therapy to protect and restore cartilage. Clin Orthop 2000; 379(suppl): S214–219.
3. Oakes DA, Lieberman JR. Osteoinductive applications of regional gene therapy: ex vivo gene transfer. Clin Orthop 2000; 379(suppl):S101–112.
4. Scaduto AA, Lieberman JR. Gene therapy for osteoinduction. Orthop Clin North Am 1999; 30:625–633.
5. Lieberman JR, Ghivizzani SC, Evans CE. Gene transfer approaches to the healing of bone and cartilage. Mol Ther 2002. In press.
6. Crystal RG. Transfer of genes to humans: early lessons and obstacles to success. Science 1995; 270:404–410.
7. Hannallah D, Peterson B, Lieberman JR, Fu F, Huard J. Gene therapy in orthopaedic surgery. J Bone Joint Surg Am 2002; 84:1046–1061.
8. Viggeswarapu M, Boden SD, Liu Y, Hair GA, Louis-Ugbo, Murakami H, Kim HS, Mayr MT, Hutton WC, Titus L. Adenoviral delivery of LIM mineralization protein-1 induces new-bone formation in vitro and in vivo. J Bone Joint Surg Am 2001; 83:364–376.
9. Anderson WF. Human gene therapy. Nature 1998; 392(suppl):25–30.
10. Lieberman JR, Daluiski A, Stevenson S, Wu L, McAllister P, Lee YP, Kabo JM, Finerman GAM, Berk AJ, Witle ON. The effect of regional gene therapy with bone morphogenetic protein-2 producing bone-marrow cells on the repair of segmental femoral defects in rats. J Bone Joint Surg Am 1999; 81:905–917.
11. Sato M, Suzuki S, Kubo S, Mitani K. Replication and packaging of helper-dependent adenoviral vectors. Gene Ther 2002; 9:472–476.

12. Schwartz EM. The adeno-associated virus vector for orthopaedic gene therapy. Clin Orthop 2000; 379(suppl):S31–39.
13. Berns KI, Bohenzky RA. Adeno-associated viruses: an update. Adv Virus Res 1987; 32:243–306.
14. Goater J, Muller R, Kollias G, Firestein GS, Sanz I, O'Keefe RJ, Schwarz EM. Empirical advantages of adeno associated viral vectors in vivo gene therapy for arthritis. J Rheumatol 2000; 27:983–989.
15. Oligino T, Ghivizzani S, Wolfe D, Lechman E, Krisky D, Mi Z, Evans C, Robbins P, Glorioso J. Intra-articular delivery of a herpes simplex virus IL-1Ra gene vector reduces inflammation in a rabbit model of arthritis. Gene Ther 1999; 6:1713 1720.
16. Fang J, Zhu YY, Smiley E, Bonadio J, Rouleau JP, Goldstein SA, McCauley LK, Davidson BL, Roessler BJ. Simulation of new bone formation by direct transfer of osteogenic plasmid genes. Proc Natl Acad Sci USA 1996; 93: 5753–5758.
17. Bonadio J, Smiley E, Patil P, Goldstein S. Localized, direct plasmid gene delivery in vivo: prolonged therapy results in reproducible tissue regeneration. Nat Med 1999; 5:753–759.
18. Praemer M, Furnes S, Rice D. Musculoskeletal Conditions in the United States. Park Ridge, IL: American Academy of Orthopaedic Surgeons 1992.
19. Lieberman JR, Daluiski A, Einhorn T. The role of growth factors in the repair of bone. J Bone Joint Surg Am 2002; 84:1032–1045.
20. Boden SD, Zdeblick TA, Sandhu HS, Heim SE. The use of rhBMP-2 in interbody fusion cages: definitive evidence of osteoinduction in humans: a preliminary report. Spine 2000; 25:376–381.
21. Friedlaender GE, Perry CR, Cole JD, Cook SD, Cierny G, Muschier GF, Zych GA, Calhoun JH, LaForte AJ, Yin S. Osteogenic protein-1 (bone morphogenetic protein-7) in the treatment of tibial nonunions. J Bone Joint Surg Am 2001; 83(suppl 1(Pt 2)):S151–158.
22. Yasko AW, Lane JM, Fellinger EJ, Rosen V, Wozney JM, Wang EA. The healing of segmental bone defects, induced by recombinant human bone morphogenetic protein (rhBMP-2): a radiographic, histological, and biomechanical study in rats. J Bone Joint Surg Am 1992; 74:659–670.
23. Bostrom M, Lane JM, Tomin E, Browne M, Berberian W, Turek T, Smith J, Wozney J, Schildhauer T. Use of bone morphogenetic protein-2 in the rabbit ulnar nonunion model. Clin Orthop 1996; 327:272–282.
24. Cook SD, Salkeld SL, Brinker MR, Wolfe MW, Rueger DC. Use of an osteoinductive biomaterial (rhOP-1) in healing large segmental bone defects. J Orthop Trauma 1998; 12:407–412.
25. Lieberman JR. Fracture healing and other nongenetic problems of bone. Clin Orthop 2000; 379S:S156–158.
26. Baltzer AW, Lattermann C, Whalen JD, Wooley P, Weiss K, Grimm M, Ghivizzani SC, Robbins PD, Evans CH. Genetic enhancement of fracture repair: healing of an experimental segmental defect by adenoviral transfer of the BMP-2 gene. Gene Ther 2000; 7:734–739.

27. Okubo Y. Bessho K, Fujimara K, Iizuka T, Miyatahe SI. Osteoinduction by bone morphogenetic protein-2 via adenoviral vector under transient immunosuppression. Biochem Biophys Res Communm 2000; 7:382–387.
28. Bruder SP, Kurth AA, Shea M, Hayes WC, Jaiswal N, Kadiyala S. Bone regeneration by implantation of purified, culture-expanded human mesenchymal stem cells. J Orthop Res 1998; 16:155–162.
29. Bruder SP, Kraus KH, Goldberg VM, Kadiyala S. The effect of implants loaded with autologous mesenchymal stem cells on the healing of canine segmental bone defects. J Bone Joint Surg Am 1998; 80:985–996.
30. Krebsbach PH, Gu K, Franceschi RT, Rutherford RB. Gene therapy-directed osteogenesis: BMP-7 transduced human fibroblasts form bone in vivo. Hum Gene Ther 2000; 11:1201–1210.
31. Lee JY, Musgrave D, Pelinkovic D, Fukushima K, Cummins J, Usas A, Robbins P, Fu FH, Huard J. Effect of bone morphogenetic protein-2-expressing muscle-derived cells on healing of critical-sized bone defects in mice. J Bone Joint Surg Am 2001; 83:1032–1039.
32. Zuk PA, Zhu M, Mizuno H, Huang J, Futrell JW, Katz AJ, Benhaim P, Lorenz HP, Hedrick MH. Multilineage cells from human adipose tissue: implications for cell-based therapies. Tissue Eng 2001; 7:211–228.
33. Bruder SP, Jaiswal N, Haynesworth SE. Growth kinetics, self-renewal, and the osteogenic potential of purified human mesenchymal stem cells during extensive subcultivation and following cryopreservation. J Cell Biochem 1997; 64:278–294.
34. Deutsche Banc AB. Estimates and Company Information. 2001.
35. Boden SD. Biology of lumber spine fusion and use of bone graft substitutes: present, future and next generation. Tissue Eng 2000; 6:383–399.
36. Boden SD, Titus L, Hair G, Viggeswarapu M, Nanes MJ, Barahowski C. Lumber spine fusion by local gene therapy with a cDNA encoding a novel osteoinductive protein (LMP-1). Spine 1998; 22:2486–2492.
37. Wang J, Kanim L, Yoo S, Campbell P, Berk A, Dawson E, Lieberman JR. Gene therapy for spinal fusion: transformation of marrow cells with an adenoviral vector to procduce BMP-2. J Bone Joint Surg Am 2003; 85:905–911.
38. Boden SD, Martin GJ, Horton WC, Truss TL, Sandhu HS. Laparoscopic anterior spinal arthrodesis with rhBMP-2 in a titanium interbody threaded cage. J Spinal Disord 1998; 11:95–101.
39. Brittberg M, Lindahl A, Nilsson A, Ohlsson C, Isaksson O, Peterson L. Treatment of deep cartilage defects in the knee with autologous chondrocyte transplantation. N Engl J Med 1994; 331:889–895.
40. Johnson LL. Arthroscopic abrasion arthroplasty: a review. Clin Orthop 2001; 391(Suppl):S306–317.
41. Steadman JR, Rodkey WG, Rodrigo JJ. Microfracture: surgical technique and rehabilitation to treat chondral defects. Clin Orthop 2001; 391(suppl):S362–369.
42. Meyers MH, Akeson W, Convery FR. Resurfacing of the knee with fresh osteochondral allograft. J Bone Joint Surg Am 1989; 71:704–713.

43. Buckwalter JA, Mankin HJ. Articular cartilage repair and transplantation. Arthritis Rheum 1998; 41:1331–1342.

44. Shuler FD, Georgescu HI, Niyibizi C, Studer RK, Mi Z, Johnstone B, Robbins RD, Evans CH. Increased matrix synthesis following adenoviral transfer of a transforming growth factor betal gene into articular chondrocytes. J Orthop Res 2000; 18:585–592.

45. Hunziker EB, Driesang IM, Morris EA. Chondrogenesis in cartilage repair is induced by members of the transforming growth factor-beta superfamily. Clin Orthop 2001; 391(suppl):S171–181.

46. Sellers RS, Peluso D, Morris EA. The effect of recombinant human bone morphogenetic protein-2 (rhBMP-2) on the healing of full-thickness defects of articular cartilage. J Bone Joint Surg Am 1997; 79:1452–1463.

47. Sellers RS, Zhang R, Glasson SS, Kim HD, Peluso D, D'Augusta DA, Beckwith K, Morris EA. Repair of articular cartilage defects one year after treatment with recombinant human bone morphogenetic protein-2 (rhBMP-2). J Bone Joint Surg Am 2000; 82:151–160.

48. Evans CH, Robbis PD, Ghivizzani SC, Herndon JH, Kang R, Bahnso AB, Barranger JA, Elders EM, Gay S, Tomaino MM, Wasko MC, Wa SC, Whiteside TL, Glorioso JC, Lotze MT, Wright TM. Clinical trial to assess the safety, feasibility, and efficacy of transferring a potentially anti-arthritic cytokine gene to human joints with rheumatoid arthritis. Hum Gene Ther 1996; 7:1261–1280.

49. Mi Z, Ghivizzani SC, Lechman ER, Jaffurs D, Glorioso JC, Evans CH, Robbins PD. Adenovirus-mediated gene transfer of insulin-like growth factor 1 stimulates proteoglycan synthesis in rabbit joints. Arthritis Rheum 2000; 43:2563–2570.

50. Brittberg M, Tallheden T, Sjorgren-Jansson B, Lindahl A, Peterson L. Autologous chondrocytes used for articular cartilage repair: an update. Clin Orthop 2001; 391(suppl):S337–S348.

51. Smith P, Shuler FD, Georgesci HI, Ghivizzani SC, Johnstone B, Niyibizi C, Robbins PD, Evans CH. Genetic enhancement of matrix synthesis by articular chondrocytes: comparison of different growth factor genes in the presence and absence of interleukin-1. Arthritis Rheum 2000; 43:1156–1164.

52. Nixon AJ. Insulinlike growth factor-I gene therapy applications for cartilage repair. Clin Orthop 2000; 379(suppl):S201–213.

53. Kang R, Marui T, Ghivizzani SC, Nita IM, Georgescu HI, Suh JK, Robbins PD, Evans CH. Ex vivo gene transfer to chondrocytes in full-thickness articular cartilage defects: a feasibility study. Osteoarthritis Cartilage 1997; 5:139–143.

54. Madry H, Trippel SB. Efficient lipid-mediated gene transfer to articular chondrocytes. Gene Ther 2000; 7:286–291.

55. Mason JM, Grande DA, Barcia M, Grant R, Pergolizzi RG, Breitbart AS. Expression of human bone morphogenic protein 7 in primary rabbit periosteal cells: potential utility in gene therapy for osteochondral repair. Gene Ther 1998; 5:1098–1104.

56. Hidaka C, Quitoriano M, Warren RF, Crystal RG. Enhanced matrix synthesis and in vitro formation of cartilage-like tissue by genetically modified chondrocytes expressing BMP-7. J Orthop Res 2001; 19:751–758.

57. Wakitani S, Goto T, Pineda SJ, Young RG, Mansour JM, Caplan AI, Goldberg VM. Mesenchymal cell-based repair of large, full-thickness defects of articular cartilage. J Bone Joint Surg Am 1994; 76:579–592.

58. Urlich-Vinter M, Maloney M, Goates J, Soballe K, Goldring MB, O'Keefe RJ, Schwartz EM. Light activated gene transduction (LAGT) enhances adeno-associated virus vector-mediated gene expression in human articular chondrocytes. Arthritis Rheum. In press.

Index

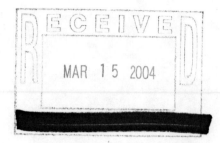